Praise for *God's Hotel*

"Transcendent . . . Readable chapters go down like restorative sips of cool water, and its hard-core subversion cheers like a shot of gin. . . . *God's Hotel* [is] a tour de force. . . . Others have written about the relationship between time and medical care with similar eloquence and urgency, but the centuries of perspective that Dr. Sweet brings infuse the point with unforgettable clarity."   —*The New York Times*

"A radical and inspiring alternative vision of caring for the sick."
—*Vanity Fair*

"Engaging . . . You might not expect a book about San Francisco's most downtrodden patients to be a page-turner, but it is. With its colorful cast of characters battling the tide of history, *God's Hotel* is a remarkable journey into the essence of medicine."   —*San Francisco Chronicle*

"A beautifully written and illuminating book . . . [Sweet's] metaphors are poetic and hint at the mystical, but then she pulls back with the educated eye of a scientist . . . For both the agnostic and the believer, Sweet pinpoints the element of medicine that makes it a calling rather than a job: the unique and sustaining love that is sparked between a doctor and patient."   —*The New York Review of Books*

"Sweet writes fluidly and well. . . . She weaves a fascinating account of the historical forces that transformed our view of the body. . . . It's high time that someone gets medieval on modern medicine's morass, and Victoria Sweet is just the woman to do it."   —*The Cleveland Plain Dealer*

"Captivating . . . With this humane and thoughtful work, Sweet joins physician-authors such as Oliver Sacks, Jerome Groopman, and Abraham Verghese."   —*The Dallas Morning News*

"Sweet's tone in *God's Hotel* nicely matches her subject. Her writing has a lovely, antique quality. . . . This hospital, with its chronically ill patients, crumbling buildings, and never-ending budget woes, was 'a gift.' In this beautiful and unique book, she shares that gift with us generously."
—*The Boston Globe*

O9-ABE-907

"Intelligent and moving . . . In this often lyrical book, Dr. Sweet reveals a deep spirituality and unsentimental compassion."

—*Minneapolis Star Tribune*

"Sweet paints a dynamic portrait . . . [which] is at its core testimonial to the body's remarkable ability to heal when it is provided with the simple ingredients of time and care."

—*Utne Reader*

"Visionary . . . thoroughly subversive in all the best ways . . . Sweet proposes ways that we might reimagine our way forward by looking into the distant past . . . This book's lessons and conclusions should challenge doctors, nurses, hospital administrators, and policy makers to stop and rethink their core beliefs."

—*Journal of Health Affairs*

"Contains no medical jargon . . . Nothing too gory or gut-wrenching; just descriptive stories of patients, unusual treatments, a hospital in transition, and a doctor on a journey, learning to practice 'a beautiful art.' "

—*East Bay Express*

"[Our] health care system might function a lot better if every single American citizen, health care professional, politician, and legislator would read Victoria Sweet's insightful, beautifully written, and moving book."

—*BookPage*

"Victoria Sweet writes beautifully about the enormous richness of life at Laguna Honda, the chronic care hospital where she has spent the last twenty years, and the intense sense of place and community that binds patients and staff there. Such community in the medical world is vanishingly rare now, and Laguna Honda may be the last of its kind. *God's Hotel* is a most important book, which raises fundamental questions about the nature of medicine in our time. It should be required reading for anyone interested in the 'business' of health care—and especially those interested in the *humanity* of health care."

—Oliver Sacks, MD, author of
The Man Who Mistook His Wife for a Hat and *Hallucinations*

"[A] watershed book . . . Vital, exquisitely written, and spectacularly multi-dimensional, Sweet's clinically exacting, psychologically discerning, practical, spiritual, and tenderly funny anecdotal chronicle steers the politicized debate over health care back to medicine and compassion."

—*Booklist* (starred review)

"This is a unique book about a healer and those in need of her healing. Charting her journey in *God's Hotel*, Victoria Sweet shows us that medicine is still fundamentally a sacred calling. By illuminating this truth, [Sweet] provides comfort and inspiration."

—Jerome Groopman, MD, Recanati Professor, Harvard Medical School, author of *How Doctors Think* and coauthor of *Your Medical Mind*

"A remarkable, poignant portrait of a committed physician on a quest to understand the heart, as well as the art, of medicine . . . A marvelous, arresting read."

—*Library Journal* (starred review)

"Victoria Sweet is a master storyteller and a consummate physician. Her beautifully written stories from the frontline of health care document the struggle of all modern-day healers to hold fast to the immortal soul of medicine despite the pressures of economics, the self-interest of politics, and the reductionism of science. *God's Hotel* reminds us of the fundamental truth that medicine is and has always been an act of love and brotherhood . . . and of the vulnerabilities we share and the compassion we aspire to."

—Rachel Naomi Remen, MD, author of *Kitchen Table Wisdom* and *My Grandfather's Blessings*

"Remarkably honest . . . Sweet's warm, anecdotal style shines . . . [Her] compelling argument for Laguna Honda's philosophy of 'slow medicine' will make readers contemplate if perhaps the body should be viewed more as a garden to be tended rather than a machine to be fixed."

—*Kirkus Reviews*

"A profoundly moving account of a remarkable hospital and the people who inhabit it, *God's Hotel* reveals intimate knowledge of the shift in modern medicine, from personal tending to industrialized 'health care.' Victoria Sweet embodies the traits of a persevering and compassionate doctor, while conveying the wisdom of a philosopher, and the instincts of a born storyteller."

—Julie Salamon, author of *Hospital* and *Wendy and the Lost Boys*

"Sweet's tales of her hospital, patients, colleagues, and herself offer a fresh linking of medicine past and present." —*Publishers Weekly*

"It almost always annoys me when someone who isn't a professional writer produces a great book, but Victoria Sweet has written the best nonfiction book I've read this year." —Jesse Kornbluth, HeadButler.com

GOD'S HOTEL

A Doctor, a Hospital, and a Pilgrimage
to the Heart of Medicine

VICTORIA SWEET

RIVERHEAD BOOKS
New York

RIVERHEAD BOOKS
Published by the Penguin Group
Penguin Group (USA) Inc.
375 Hudson Street, New York, New York 10014, USA

USA / Canada / UK / Ireland / Australia / New Zealand / India / South Africa / China

Penguin Books Ltd., Registered Offices: 80 Strand, London WC2R 0RL, England
For more information about the Penguin Group, visit penguin.com.

All of the names and identifying characteristics of the patients have been changed.

The Library of Congress has catalogued the Riverhead hardcover edition as follows:

Sweet, Victoria.
God's hotel : a doctor, a hospital, and a pilgrimage to the heart of
medicine / Victoria Sweet.
p.   cm.
ISBN 978-1-59448-843-6 (hardback)
1. Sweet, Victoria.   2. Physicians—United States—Biography.
3. Laguna Honda Hospital (San Francisco, Calif.)—History.
4. Hospital care—California—San Francisco—Anecdotes.   I. Title.
R154.S925A3   2012   2011049340
610.92—dc23
[B]

First Riverhead hardcover edition: April 2012
First Riverhead trade paperback edition: April 2013
Riverhead trade paperback ISBN: 978-1-59448-654-8

PRINTED IN THE UNITED STATES OF AMERICA

10   9   8

Cover design by Kristen Haff
Cover art by Sabina Hahn
Book design by Amanda Dewey

While the author has made every effort to provide accurate telephone numbers and Internet
addresses at the time of publication, neither the author nor the publisher is responsible
for errors, or for changes that occur after publication. Further, the publisher does not have
any control over and does not assume any responsibility for author or third-party
websites or their content.

*Penguin is committed to publishing works of quality and integrity.
In that spirit, we are proud to offer this book to our readers;
however, the story, the experiences, and the words
are the author's alone.*

FOR MY PARENTS

and

FOR THE PATIENTS OF LAGUNA HONDA HOSPITAL
IN SAN FRANCISCO, CALIFORNIA

Contents

GOD'S HOTEL

Introduction

HOW I CAME TO GOD'S HOTEL

I T WAS MY FIRST AUTOPSY, my first day in the clinical clerkship of medical school called pathology.

Of course, I had seen and even taken apart dead bodies before, in the first months of medical school, but those had been bodies that were clearly ex-bodies. They smelled like the formaldehyde no longer running in their veins, and my hands and fingers were wrinkled from touching them. Except for that smell, they might as well have been made out of plastic.

But when the covers were lifted from *this* body's face, I was stunned. It was Mr. Baker! One of my first-ever real patients! A short, stocky, cigarette-smoking "blue bloater," whose emphysema had destroyed his lungs and given him his barrel chest; thick, short neck; and gravelly voice. Whose arteries and veins had been so difficult to get blood from, and who had been so understanding, so cheerful, so lively. I was sure he'd done well, been discharged, gone home. But apparently not.

emphysema

As I looked at this body, however, I began to have doubts. I knew that it was Mr. Baker, but, really, it didn't look like him. Or rather it resembled Mr. Baker the way the figures in a wax museum look like Clark Gable or Winston Churchill—like them, but not them.

I watched as the pathologist set to work with his electric saw. He opened the chest wall and removed the soggy, honeycombed lungs. He weighed them each separately, first the right lung, then the left. Then he took out the large and heavy heart, with its right side hypertrophied from lung disease, and documented its weight in grams. Next he opened the abdomen and ditto the liver, the spleen, the pancreas, the kidneys. Each organ was removed and weighed, and its weight in grams tallied. The blood vessels, large and small, were inspected and commented upon. Then the saw attacked the head. Sure enough, there it was—the brain—looking just like it did in the books, gray, spongy, with a texture kind of like pâté—homogeneous, boring. Then Mr. Baker was done. We were done. Finished. That was it. Nothing more inside.

I found myself strangely disappointed. There was nothing else to see. No hidden place, unexplored and unexplorable, no unopenable, small black box, hidden in all those wiggly intestines. It was undeniable— Mr. Baker had completely disappeared. Autopsied, his body was nothing more than a suit of clothes lying disregarded in the corner.

Something was missing. But what? Mr. Baker's breathing? His movement? His warmth? What I had expected, I later came to realize, was some sort of *thing,* some unopenable last nubbin, like what you find at the center of a baseball when you unroll it. I had expected some thing that was, well, ineradicably Mr. Baker, something the pathologist's saw could not open and destroy. But there was no such thing; I could see for myself.

Much later I learned that medicine had once had a name for this, this something present in the living body but missing from the corpse. 下化 Two names, actually. There was *spiritus*, from which we get the English *spirit*, although the Latin *spiritus* was not as insubstantial as "spirit." *Spiritus* was the breath, the regular, rhythmic breathing of the live body that is so shockingly absent from the dead. *Spiritus* is what is exhaled in the last breath.

And there was *anima*. Usually translated as *soul*, the Latin is better for conveying the second striking distinction between Mr. Baker's dead body and Mr. Baker—its lack of movement. Because *anima* is not really the abstraction, "soul." *Anima* is the invisible force that *animates* the body, that moves it, not only willfully but also unconsciously—all those little movements that the living body makes all the time. The slight tremor of the fingers, the pounding of the heart that shakes the living frame once a second, the gentle rise and fall of the chest. Those movements by which we perceive that someone is alive. *Anima*, ancient medicine had observed, is just as absent from the dead body as *spiritus*.

By the time medicine got to me, however, words like *spiritus* and *anima* had been banished from the medical vocabulary. I had no concepts for describing what I'd seen. Perhaps it had been autopsy—from the Greek *auto-opsia*: seeing for oneself—that brought about the disappearance of those words from the Western vocabulary. Perhaps it was the absence of that little black box.

I formed no hypothesis, at the time, about the absence of Mr. Baker's *spiritus* or *anima* at the autopsy of his body. I didn't even know that such concepts had once existed. But I did tuck away in the back of my mind the image of his dead body as a crumpled suit of clothes, abandoned in the corner of a sterile white room.

❖

When my family learned I was going to medical school, they were shocked. No one in the family—and our family history goes way back—had ever been a doctor, medicine being too physical a profession for our businessmen and intellectuals. Medicine was too physical for me also, but it intrigued me with its possibility of engaging with what Catholics call the last things: death, resurrection, heaven, hell, and purgatory. Also, I liked that medicine would require me to meet with everyone on a kind of equal basis. Anyhow, I reassured them, I was going into medicine through a side door that was not physical at all—the door of psychiatry. The work of Carl Jung fascinated me, and I hoped to imitate his life—seeing brilliant, well-paying patients in the morning in my stone house on Lake Zurich, writing and lecturing in the afternoon.

After the first two years of medical school, which teach the basics of medicine—anatomy, physiology, biochemistry, and pharmacology— there are the two clinical years, when the student gets to apply this learning to real patients. I hadn't expected to like this part, but I did. There was a lot of psychology to it. I discovered that I loved taking the "history"—the story that the patient tells, within which is hidden the real meaning of his condition. I loved the physical examination of the patient, on whose body was written, if I could only read it, the real diagnosis. And I loved analyzing the facts and reaching a conclusion, which is the diagnosis, the treatment, and the plan.

After medical school I started my psychiatric training. But psychiatry, I soon realized, had changed since Jung. Madness was now located in the brain and caused by a chemical imbalance; its treatment was not analysis but medication, which often worked remarkably well. So instead of becoming a psychiatrist, I went out and practiced medicine in a county clinic, and then in a rural private practice. Eventually I went back for more training and finished the three years of a medical residency. After that I practiced in a community clinic and became its medical director.

During all those years I was ever more impressed by the power of modern medicine—by its logic, its method for arriving at a diagnosis and a treatment. Yet every now and again I had other experiences like that with Mr. Baker—experiences that left me wondering. The moment of birth. The moment of death. A mysterious knowing of just when a patient was about to get ill. All evidence of some subtle but shared world, where beings popped up and disappeared, of invisible connections with visible effects.

Naturally, I assumed that modern medicine had investigated such phenomena, and I began to research what it had learned about them. They had acquired very boring names, I immediately discovered: the "doctor-patient relationship"; the "placebo effect"; "psychosomatism"; the "effect of prayer." Also, they had been assigned to the realm of psychology, where they had been psychologized—separated, that is, from the body where I'd seen and felt them.

Next, I looked at alternative medicine for answers. Chinese and Indian medicine did give me some insights, since the body they described was a body of flows and blockages, balances and imbalances, a body that might explain the borderless energy I'd felt in my patients. But the languages and cultures of Chinese and Indian medicine were just too different; they stood in the way of my integrating their point of view into my own.

It was at this discouraging moment that I stumbled across a book that surprised me. It was the record of a German nun's medical practice from the Middle Ages, translated from the Latin. Hildegard of Bingen, I learned in its introduction, had been a twelfth-century

German mystic, theologian, and, amazingly, medical practitioner, and she had written a book about her medicine. And, although *Hildegard of Bingen's Medicine* was not a great book, it was thrilling. Because the world underlying *its* medicine was just the kind of world in which the observations I had tucked away for so many years had been known and used—in the West.

So I began to study Hildegard's medicine. I began to realize that our medicine, modern medicine, had not been the first Western system for explaining the body, but the second. Before the reductive modern medicine I'd learned in medical school, there had been a different medical system in the West. This "premodern medicine" had originated with Hippocrates in the fifth century BC, and it had once been how everyone understood the body. Its approach, I realized as I studied Hildegard's medicine, was not mechanistic: The body was not imagined as a machine nor disease as a mechanical breakdown.

But if the body was not imagined as a machine, I wondered, then how had it been imagined in the 2,500 years that preceded my medical education? Could it be that the West did have explanations for the difference between the dead body and the living, and for the other experiences I'd had in my medical life? And that these explanations had been thrown out with the triumphs of modern medicine? Did premodern medicine and modern medicine perhaps make up a unit— one thing seen from two perspectives, like those drawings that show two different images at the same time?

I didn't know. But I was intrigued, and I resolved to find out.

To do so, I needed time, however, and time was another concept left out of modern medicine. In the premodern world, medicine had not been a full-time profession but a craft, transmitted through families and learned as an apprentice. Most practitioners, therefore, were not only doctors, but doctors and something else. The elite were doctors and professors; the majority were doctors and farmers, doctors and herbalists, doctors and barbers. This had some advantages. For the patient, it meant that doctors had more than one point of reference; for the doctor, he or she had time to think about other things in other ways.

In the modern world, though, medical training was arduous and costly; physicians were obliged, both professionally and financially, to be available to their patients at every hour of the day and night. Personal time was scarce, and part-time positions unheard of. Today this is no longer the case. Medicine has completed its metamorphosis from craft to profession to commodity, and health-care providers now sell their wares—that is, their time—by the piece on the open marketplace. Back then, however, I spent several months looking for a position that would allow me to practice medicine and also pursue a doctorate in the history of medicine. Without success.

Until I contacted Dr. Major, the medical director of Laguna Honda Hospital in San Francisco. On the telephone, Dr. Major assured me that she could accommodate my requirement for a part-time position; many of the doctors she'd hired did other things with their lives. She had doctor-musicians, doctor-sculptors, doctor-physicists, and doctor-mothers. She knew that time was the special perk she had to offer.

So I drove over, somewhat skeptically, for my interview.

When I saw Laguna Honda for the first time, I was taken aback. During my medical training I'd occasionally had a patient admitted to it, but, like most physicians in the city, I'd never visited. If asked, I would have said that I imagined it as a concrete parking structure where patients were stacked one on top of another, floor by floor, in some dusty, industrial part of the city. Instead, what I saw as I drove in the front gate and past the gatekeeper's abandoned cottage was an elegant, though somber, riff on a twelfth-century Romanesque monastery. High on a hill, its peach-colored, red-roofed buildings overlooked the ocean. Each of the six wings of the hospital was lined with rows of windows, and at the end of each wing was a turret, with swallows flying in and out of its open arches.

I met Dr. Major in her office and, after our interview, she took me out for the tour. Laguna Honda was an almshouse, she explained as we started, or, as the French called it, an Hôtel-Dieu—God's Hotel—a kind of hospital from the Middle Ages that evolved as a way of taking care of those who couldn't take care of themselves. At one time, almost every county in the United States had an almshouse, she told me, as well as a county hospital. They had functioned together. The county hospital took care of the acutely ill, and the almshouse took care of the chronically disabled. In theory. In practice, the almshouse had been a catchall for everyone who didn't fit someplace else—it was a shelter, a farm for the unemployed, a halfway house, and a rehabilitation center, as well as a hospital. Over the last forty years, though, just about all the almshouses in the United States had closed, except for Laguna Honda. Laguna Honda, Dr. Major said, was probably the last almshouse in America, and with its 1,178 patients, it was as large as a village.

We walked under a delicate, wooden statue of Saint Francis, the patron saint of our city, and then into a wide central hall with floor-to-ceiling windows. There were vending machines and small round tables, and the hall was filled with patients, smoking, drinking coffee, playing poker. Then we turned and walked through heavy doors into a ward. We passed a small working kitchen, a dining room, a doctor's office, and the nurses' station, and then we entered the long, open ward.

It was lined with beds, fifteen to a side, and each bed was set next to an open window. By each bed was a bureau for the patient's belongings, a chair for visitors, and a small table. At the end of the ward was a round room, windowed and sunny, the solarium, designed so that each patient could have access to sunlight and fresh air without leaving the ward. (So that was the purpose of the turrets!) There were thirty-eight wards in the hospital, Dr. Major explained, and they were more or less identical. They'd been designed before the antibiotic era so that, in case of infection, every ward could be quarantined from the rest of the hospital and still function as a separate minihospital.

Then we strolled back through the hall with its vending machines and patients. We passed a 1950s-era beauty salon with steel-helmet hair dryers and Naugahyde swivel chairs, and we peeked in at the barbershop, which had a miniature barber's pole inside. We went upstairs to see the operating room, with celadon tile and glass cabinets, and the laboratory, with black benches, a microscope, and a centrifuge. Dr. Major showed me the little store that sold candy, batteries, and shaving cream, and a book-lined library with oak tables and newspapers on wooden racks.

We went down more stairs and came to the theater. Its cement floors were painted and polished; there were red velvet curtains drawn across a stage and carved box seats behind us. In the old days, Dr. Major said, the theater had been used for silent movies, handcranked by the superintendent's son; now it was mainly used for the Christmas show and the Valentine's Day dance. Next to the theater was the chapel. It was not the neutral "Quiet Room" of a modern hospital. No. The chapel of Laguna Honda was more like a small church. Its stained-glass windows were large and real; its pews were made of polished wood; and the Stations of the Cross lined its walls.

Then Dr. Major took me outside.

Laguna Honda covered sixty-two acres, she told me, and this was because it originally had been as much a farm as a hospital. Patients had been expected to work if they could. They grew most of the hospital's vegetables; they took care of the dairy; they raised pigs, cows, and sheep; ran the laundry; and sewed, mended, and cooked. If they could do nothing else, they gardened. And, as we walked, I could see the remains of old orchards and flower beds now run wild. There were apple trees and quince, olive trees and fig. Scattered among the trees were medicinal herbs: digitalis, rosemary, nasturtium, lavender, geranium, and valerian. Finally, we came to the end of the tour—the greenhouse, the aviary, and the barnyard.

The greenhouse smelled of humus and plants. On Saturdays, Dr. Major explained, the therapists brought patients out to sit at the wooden benches and pot their own plants. Next to the greenhouse was the aviary, with doves, parakeets, pigeons, chickens, and incubators. Later I would discover that the AIDS ward had even had its own incubator and its own chicken, which had hatched on the ward. It roamed the ward and pecked around the patients' beds until the state found out and had her taken away to a fate unknown but guessed.

Last we looked in at the barnyard. There were wooden coops for the rabbits on the right, for the chickens on the left, and, free to root in the green lawn in the middle, two miniature black pigs. Behind a short fence at the back was a pond for ducks and geese, and hillocks for a turkey and two goats. On certain holidays, Dr. Major told me, the therapists would put the animals in little carts to visit the bedbound patients. They would dress the animals in appropriate holiday attire—the goats with little Pilgrim hats for Thanksgiving, the turkey in dark glasses and a tie for the Fourth of July.

Then we walked back to her office and sat down. It was a plain office—one large desk, bookcases with reports and manuals, a window that gave out onto a parking lot, where ambulances were coming and going.

Dr. Major offered me the position.

I wasn't sure. Laguna Honda was like no hospital I'd ever seen or even imagined. But it was the only situation where my criterion of time was satisfied. So I accepted, but only temporarily. Two months, I told her. I could make only a two-month commitment. It was a way of hedging my bets. I didn't think she would accept; two months wasn't much for the amount of paperwork my employment would entail.

But Dr. Major knew something I didn't know: Laguna Honda cast a kind of spell. Most everyone came for just a few months, maybe a year or two, and most everyone stayed for decades—thirty, forty, even fifty years. She herself had come to the hospital for only four weeks of consulting, two and a half years before.

Dr. Major was pretty sure I would fall under that spell.

She was right. I would fall under it.

I would stay at Laguna Honda not for two months but for more than twenty years. I would finish a PhD in Hildegard's medicine; I would go off on a medieval pilgrimage and come back; and I would be present as the old almshouse was transformed, for better and for worse, into a modern health-care facility. Above all, I would take care of 1,686 of its patients, and what they taught me would change me and how I practiced medicine in ways I would never have imagined.

To my surprise, Dr. Major accepted my offer of two months.

I would be assigned to the admitting ward, she told me, where I would be replacing Dr. Judd, who was moving to a different ward. I would start in three weeks. On my first day, I should stop off in personnel to sign the papers, then pick up a white coat in the laundry and meet Dr. Judd on the admitting ward. He would show me around and turn his patients over to me.

One

FIRST YEARS

T WAS EARLY MORNING ON MY FIRST DAY, and Dr. Judd was waiting for me.

As Dr. Major had instructed, I stopped first at personnel and then at the laundry, where I picked up a white coat—highly starched, neatly pressed, slightly frayed. Then I went up the stairs, down the hallway, through the double doors of the admitting ward, and into the doctors' office. The doctors' office was small and narrow, no larger than a single patient's room. But it was familiar, with the same bareness, plainness, down-to-earthness that I was used to in the kind of medicine I practiced—businesslike, if your business was taking care of the sick poor.

I was taking over the patients of Dr. Judd, who was transferring to another ward. Somber, even a little withdrawn, he handed me his index cards. These were the cards on which he, like all of us at the time, wrote down the basic information about his patients: name and medical number, date of admission, list of diagnoses and medications.

He was anxious to be on his way. Nevertheless, we left the doctors' office together to go on rounds, so that he could introduce his
patients to me and summarize their medical problems. There's an art
to it—in a few sentences to tell the essence of a patient, past, present,
and future—and Dr. Judd was good at it.

First on our rounds was Mr. Tarn, who had Parkinson's disease.
He had consequently fallen and broken his hip, and needed daily
manipulation of his many medications. Mr. Benturi had been hit by a
car and was recovering from head trauma and multiple orthopedic
injuries. Mr. Davis also had a fracture and the additional problems of
alcoholism and diabetes. There was Fred S., disabled from a brain
tumor and on dialysis; Mrs. Lorenz with Alzheimer's; and Mrs.
Roche, rehabilitating after a stroke. We were treating Betty Wilson
for fractures of both arms, both legs, and pelvis, and Ms. Devlin for
the rare and inexorable disease of spinocerebellar degeneration. Mr.
Demmings was at Laguna Honda with terminal alcoholic cirrhosis—
bleeding, confusion, and jaundice—although he was improving.

Dr. Judd's patients were familiar to me, not specifically but in
general; they were just like the patients I'd managed throughout my
medical training. Complex, fragile, and unstable, in need of close
monitoring of medications and laboratory tests, the only thing surprising about my new patients was that they were at Laguna Honda
and not in an acute hospital. Although, as we walked around the ward
and I thought about the last few years in medicine, having the patients
at Laguna Honda and not at an acute hospital did make sense, in a
way. What with the changes in medical financing of health maintenance organizations (HMOs) and diagnosis-related groups (DRGs),
doctors and hospitals were now paid for "maintaining health," not for
treating disease. Often, to encourage health-care efficiency, doctors
simply received a fixed amount per patient per month, and hospitals a

fixed amount per disease, regardless of how sick a patient was. Doctors, therefore, tried to retain only their healthy patients, and hospitals tried to ensure the shortest possible stays and the speediest possible workups. But patients like Mr. Tarn, Ms. Devlin, and Mr. Demmings had no health to maintain. They were very ill, and the only way for the acute hospital to be efficient and not lose money taking care of them was to discharge them as soon as possible. Which they did, if they could find a chronic hospital willing to admit such patients. In San Francisco that hospital was Laguna Honda. So while I was surprised by how sick my new patients were for a chronic care hospital, I wasn't astonished.

Until we came to Mr. Hickman.

Mr. Hickman was thirty-nine years old, Dr. Judd told me, and he was odd. He lived, no one knew quite how, on the streets. He rarely spoke. He'd been sent to Laguna Honda because he'd failed the usual treatment for his disease, which was tuberculosis. He hadn't taken the four daily medications necessary to kill the tuberculous bacteria, which, consequently, had multiplied in his lungs, forming pockets of pus that were inaccessible to medication. He'd been taken to surgery, therefore, and his infected lung was removed, along with much of his chest wall—ribs, sternum, and skin—so that he could heal from the inside out. It was an old-fashioned treatment, Dr. Judd explained to me, an "Eloesser flap," developed before there'd been medications for tuberculosis. Our job was to dress the open wound twice a day, and make sure Mr. Hickman took his medicines.

With this, Dr. Judd introduced me to Mr. Hickman, who was skinny and taciturn, and lying in bed, staring up at the ceiling. He did not shake my hand or turn his head to look at me. I went over to the left side of the bed and Dr. Judd went over to the right, and he turned back the covers. Mr. Hickman's chest was heavily bandaged. One by one, carefully, Dr. Judd removed the bandages and dressings and placed them on the nearby table. Then I looked into Mr. Hickman's open wound and saw that, exposed and vulnerable, nestled in the hollow that the surgeons had created, was Mr. Hickman's beating heart.

It was extraordinary.

I could see the fine, delicate film of the pericardial sac glisten as it pulsed and caught the light. Woven through it—I could just make out—were tiny veins and arteries. It was so alive, that beating heart! It was as alive as Mr. Baker's body at my first autopsy had been dead. For a minute or so Dr. Judd and I stood there and watched the heart beat, pink and oblivious to us, while Mr. Hickman stared up at the ceiling. Then Dr. Judd repacked the lung cavity with fresh, white four-by-fours. He covered up the heart with a new dressing, taped the chest closed, and pulled the sheet back around Mr. Hickman's neck. We walked back together to the doctors' office at the front of the ward, and he left me with my index cards and my patients.

I t was Dr. Rachman who showed me the ropes, which were refreshingly few.

Dr. Rachman was Italian from New York, and she was quick, funny, warm, and talkative. I was to have the rickety wooden desk in the corner next to the window. It looked out onto the green hill across the parking lot, and, hence, onto all the comings and goings of patients, staff, and ambulances. Crammed into the room were also a computer, Dr. Rachman's desk, Dr. Romero's desk, a hat rack, and extra chairs for family and visiting doctors.

Dr. Romero and Dr. Fintner were the other two doctors on the admitting ward, Dr. Rachman explained, and they were job-sharing; that is, they shared a desk and shared their patients. I would get to know them both very well. Dr. Romero was from Cuba but grew up in Florida; and she'd been the first in her family to go to college. She'd gone to Ivy League schools, trained in the best medical program in the country, and married well. She was ambitious and incisive, Dr. Rachman said, but her two upbringings—first as younger Cuban daughter and then as brilliant American student—were not perfectly melded together. So she was a little like those plastic figures whose left and right sides do not quite match up. Outside our tiny office, Dr. Romero was sweet and patient; inside it, she was sardonic and witty, and did not tolerate fools gladly.

Dr. Fintner, on the other hand, was melded together perfectly well. The daughter of a doctor, she was gentle and kind, both inside and outside the office; and, though she laughed at jokes, she did not make them. Dr. Fintner knew almost everything there was to know about medicine, Dr. Rachman went on, but she was modest and I would have to ask, because she never volunteered. It was a good thing that Dr. Fintner knew everything, since she could never find anything in the desk she shared with Dr. Romero. Everything that came into her mailbox, Dr. Fintner saved, piling it in a corner of the desk, not wanting to hurt anyone's—not even mass-marketers'—feelings.

The four of us were responsible for the daily admissions to the hospital, which were limited to three or four. So I could expect a new patient every morning. There was a waiting list of more than two hundred patients, and patients were admitted based on their needs and the hospital's capabilities. They came from hospitals throughout the city, from their homes if they had them, or from the streets. The doctors took the admissions one after another in an ongoing queue that was strictly followed—a queue of destiny, as I would learn.

After rounds, I would spend the rest of the morning on my new admission. It took that long, Dr. Rachman said, to perform a full examination; contact family, friends, and former physicians; review the records and medications; and formulate a plan. She showed me a sample of her previous day's admission. Handwritten, with every *T* precisely crossed and every *I* precisely dotted, her five-page workup was inspiring. She'd combined the knowledge we'd accumulated in medical school, the arduous experience of our residencies, and added her own common sense to produce a thing of beauty and of art. As she flipped through the sections of the chart with me, went over the forms for each test and X-ray, showed me the computer and the dictating system, she also continued to chat about the doctors and nurses I'd soon be meeting.

Then she took me upstairs to the X-ray department and the laboratory. I would read my own X-rays, Dr. Rachman told me. True, we had radiologists from the County Hospital who came in the morning, but any X-rays taken after that I'd have to look at myself.

Like the doctors' office, the two rooms of the X-ray department were old-fashioned and plain. In the first room sat the X-ray machine, and in a corner, the film developer and darkroom. This meant that we did not have to be satisfied with standard X-ray views, Dr. Rachman pointed out, as we had to be at modern hospitals, where the X-ray machines were off-limits to everyone but registered technicians. Instead, we could participate in our patients' X-rays, and even suggest the positions and views we wanted to see.

The second room was where I would read my X-rays. Its windows were covered by blackout shades from the 1940s, and its bookshelves held dusty, ancient, but, of course, still-relevant examples of the X-rays I'd be reading. On one wall were the light boxes. On the opposite wall were the files of X-rays for all 1,178 of the hospital's patients. Once I'd learned the filing system, I would have access to all of the patients' X-rays—no filing clerk or computer system to go through.

Also, Dr. Rachman said, I could examine my patient's blood, urine, sputum, or skin in the laboratory across from the X-ray department. She opened its door, and I saw the three rooms of the laboratory, lined with black-topped counters. There was a Bunsen burner, a centrifuge, and, best of all, a microscope, with boxes of slides and delicate slide covers, lens papers, and little bottles of chemicals. Then she closed the doors of the laboratory and the X-ray department, and we walked back together to the doctors' office.

I marveled, and I was thankful. Laguna Honda was off the radar screen. Tucked away in that tiny office, over the hill and far away from HMOs and insurance companies, I was going to be able to practice medicine the way I'd been taught, the way I'd learned, and the way I wanted.

Q uickly my habits were set.

In the early morning I'd make rounds on my patients on the ward; in the late morning I'd receive my new patient; in the afternoon I'd review lab tests, talk to families, and do procedures. In the late afternoon, doctors from the rest of the hospital would visit us on the admitting ward to talk over puzzling cases. We'd look at X-rays together, examine patients, and discuss diagnoses. Before going home, I'd round again on my patients. This was the time, as the sun got low in the sky, that I'd sit on their beds and listen to their stories.

For my first years, until I started working on my PhD, I was at the hospital full time, eight to five, five days a week; only after hours did I pursue my scholarly investigation of premodern medicine. The patients were always very sick, but on Mondays and Fridays they were even sicker. Mondays, because over the weekend they didn't have the concentrated doctor time they had during the week and were seen only for emergencies by the house physician. Fridays, because the sickest patients arrived on Friday afternoons—rejects from acute hospitals all over the city, who were clearing their decks for their weekends.

But the patients were very sick during the week, too. Since there were three of us (Drs. Romero and Fintner counting as one), we divided the thirty-six patients of the admitting ward into thirds. So I usually had about twelve patients, the same number I'd had as an intern in the acute hospital. And most were about as sick as the patients I'd had as an intern, as I'd learned from Dr. Judd on my first day.

So the admitting ward was comfortable, and it was also collegial and satisfying. It was comfortable because it was so familiar physically—the small office, the wooden desks, the open window, and the books. And mentally—the number of patients, the morning excitement, the resolution of that excitement during the afternoon, and the peaceful, social ending of the day.

It was collegial in the Latin sense of the word. The admitting ward had collected together a group of experienced doctors in a small space; we got along well and helped one another out. Put together, the four of us had more than sixty years of medical experience, and it was a very rare disease that one of us didn't recognize. But the patients did have very rare diseases. Instead of the usual medical adage that "common things occur commonly," at Laguna Honda the adage was "uncommon things occur commonly."

Above all, the admitting ward was satisfying. Without utilization-review managers hovering over us in their immaculate white coats, we could do a proper physician's job—that is, discover what was wrong with a patient and begin appropriate therapy. Often all it took was having enough time to do a thorough workup.

The workup, we'd been taught in medical school, was the rock upon which the diagnosis should be built. It had three parts. The first part was the "history." This was the patient's story, as told by the patient, and as elicited by the physician, with hundreds of potential queries regarding every possible symptom, from head (neurologic) to toe (orthopedic).

The second part of the workup was the physical examination: the methodical examination of the patient, also from head to toe. Over the centuries physicians had observed that it was possible to diagnose many diseases simply by observing the signs they left on the body. There were thousands of such signs—small and subtle, or striking and obvious—that could point to or even reveal particular diseases. In the mid-1960s they had been brought together in *DeGowin & DeGowin's Bedside Diagnostic Examination,* which was, therefore, a kind of bible of the physical examination. Each of us—Dr. Romero, Dr. Fintner, Dr. Rachman, and myself—had one; and it looked like a Bible, too, with a red leather cover and crepe pages.

The third part of the workup consisted of the results of blood tests and X-rays. Originally, it had been the shortest part, almost an afterthought, but as medical technology invented more and more blood tests, and more and more ways to visualize the inside of the body, this third part gradually superseded the physical examination. Which was understandable. Most patients seen in most settings are early in their illness, before the physical signs appear on the body, and most physicians do not have the hour it takes to perform a complete physical examination. But at Laguna Honda it was different. Patients were far along in their diseases, and we did have the time—lots and lots of time—to examine them carefully. And, although I'd always respected the art of the physical examination, now I learned just how often the physical examination, or its neglect, could lead to, or miss, the diagnosis.

I t was late afternoon, and I was up in the X-ray department when Dr. Romero came in to look at the X-ray of her newly admitted patient. She hadn't examined him yet, but had rushed to get the X-ray taken before the department closed at four PM.

Did I want to look at it with her?

Sure.

She snapped the film up on the light box, and we both stepped back and scanned it. It was an X-ray of a chest—lungs, heart, ribs. The lungs looked normal, and the heart looked normal, but coming out of the ribs on the left was some huge thing that seemed to be a mass of bone fragments and tissue.

"Wow. That's not good," I said. "What is it?"

"I don't know. I haven't seen the patient yet."

"Well, what does it say in the records?"

"It doesn't say anything about a mass. All I know is that he's been at the County Hospital for two months because he was weak and losing weight. They never figured out what was wrong with him, but since he was homeless, they sent him here."

So we went downstairs to find the patient and take a look. We found Mr. Jackson in bed, pale, thin, and surprisingly scruffy, given how long he'd been at the County Hospital. Dr. Romero introduced herself and me and then pulled back the sheets. Mr. Jackson's chest was thin, unwashed, and bony, and neither of us could see a mass. But then Dr. Romero rolled him onto his right side. And there it was, a stony lump as big as a clenched fist, growing right out of his back. It was obvious. Mr. Jackson had cancer, probably lung or kidney cancer. That was the reason for his unexplained weight loss and weakness.

Dr. Romero sighed. "The nurses must hate the interns at the County," she said.

And what she meant was that, even if the interns and residents and attending physicians had never rolled Mr. Jackson onto his right side as we just had, the nurses must have done so, many times. They must have seen that lump. Did they never tell the interns about it, because they were angry, sullen, and felt abused? Or did they tell the interns—many times and many interns—but in the new system that protected the interns from sleep-deprivation by assigning them shifts instead of patients, did each intern just pass along the news of the lump to the next?

That same afternoon, Dr. Romero sent Mr. Jackson back to the County Hospital, and he never returned. Most likely that was a good thing. Probably the surgeons biopsied or even removed the lump, and the oncologists, with the marvelous miracles of modern medicine, successfully treated his cancer with chemotherapy and radiation. Mr. Jackson was probably discharged from the County Hospital, improved or even cured.

Regardless, Mr. Jackson had taught me something important. It was not that all patients should have X-rays, and that the X-rays should be personally looked at by the physician, although that was one lesson to be learned from his story. Nor was it that communication between nursing assistant and intern, doctor and nurse, was crucial for patient care, although that, too, was a lesson. What I took away from Mr. Jackson was: The diagnosis is written on the body—look for it. Turn the patient on his side; examine him thoroughly. Don't miss the obvious.

This lesson proved its value to me many times. At Laguna Honda I would admit hundreds of patients for whom the key to diagnosis, and often to effective treatment, was just as easy to find as it had been with Mr. Jackson, if you knew where to look for it and did look for it. All those details of the physical examination in *DeGowin &* *DeGowin*: all those shadings of color; those patterns; those subtle sounds; the presence of abnormality; the absence of normality; and sometimes even the presence of normality, could, I learned in those first few years, save a life. Which is the most satisfying, doctorly thing of all.

There was the case of Mr. Grenz, for instance.

Lev Grenz was a young Polish man from Gdansk who'd taken to drink. And I mean taken—quarts and quarts of vodka every day. He was lonely; his girlfriend left him; he lost his job; he had no family—for whatever reason, he drank a good deal. During one exceptionally lonely time, he drank so much that the alcohol ate through his pancreas. This is often fatal, because the pancreas then spills its digestive enzymes into the belly, where they begin to digest the other organs—liver, spleen, intestines.

Mr. Grenz spent many weeks near death in the intensive care unit at the County Hospital. He had hundreds of blood tests, scores of X-rays and CT scans, and numerous tubes inserted not only into his natural orifices but into artificial orifices as well. A tube was inserted into his belly to drain it of its poisons. Another tube was put in to feed him. A tube was put into his arm, so that he could be given blood and antibiotics; and still another tube was placed inside his heart, so that the doctors could continuously measure its pressures. During that particular procedure, the tube punctured the great vein going into the heart, and there was bleeding into Mr. Grenz's lung, and so another tube had to be inserted, this one into his chest to drain the blood and reexpand his lung.

But, finally, he stabilized. Modern medical technology had saved him, and, though he was still quite ill, he was no longer ICU material; he was Laguna Honda material. Or so the doctors at County believed. And here he was, my new patient for the day, for rest, recuperation, and rehabilitation.

When I went over to meet and examine him, however, Mr. Grenz surprised me. What surprised me was his tongue. His tongue had not been mentioned in his records.

Mr. Grenz's tongue was very large. It was so large that it stuck halfway out of his mouth. It was beefy-red and dry, thick as well as long, and no matter how he tried, it would not, could not be fit back into his mouth.

Otherwise, Mr. Lev Grenz looked pretty good, all considered. He was only twenty-eight, but balding, with pale blue eyes and a short Polish nose. His neck was thick with many healed scars, and his body was flabby, an ex-muscular workman's body. His face did seem rather too large for his body, and it was a bit dusky. But it was the tongue that took me aback.

"How long has your tongue been like that?" I asked him.

It was hard to understand his response.

"Ip peen dike dat por a monpth," he replied, in a Polish accent mixed with tongue.

It had been like that for a month? That was strange. I'd never seen anything like it before. Did they miss it at the County? Had the team of doctors changed so frequently that no one realized that this appearance was not the appearance that belonged to young Mr. Grenz? Did no one in the ICU step back and look at their patient as they were inserting those lifesaving tubes and monitors? Or did they know Mr. Grenz's unusual tongue very well and simply leave it out of their records?

The large and dusky face, swollen tongue, and thick neck jogged something in my mind—a rare syndrome I'd learned about in medical school, called the "superior vena cava syndrome." The superior vena cava is the large vein that brings venous blood, dusky and depleted of oxygen, from the upper part of the body—arms, neck, head, face—back to the heart. If it gets blocked by a tumor or an abscess or even by scarring, then the depleted blood builds up, and the face and upper part of the body get dusky and swollen. I wasn't sure whether that would cause a tongue to swell, but it would certainly explain his swollen and dusky face.

I'd learned to put away such thoughts while I examined a patient, however; and so I continued to go over Mr. Grenz's body. He still had the hole in his neck from the breathing tube that had kept him alive for weeks; and there was the scar on his chest from the tube that had drained his lungs of blood. The sounds of his heart were muffled. His belly was swollen and also scarred, with a feeding tube still in place. His skin was doughy, and his life force diminished; he was pretty sick, I concluded, but definitely alive.

Still the swollen, dusky face and the large tongue bothered me. Why would a tongue swell that much and stay swollen? I felt the tongue. It was thick, muscular, and firm, not doughy; it was a physiologic swelling, and not an allergic reaction.

It had to be the superior vena cava syndrome. If so, what was the cause? Scar tissue from one of his many procedures? An abscess? A tumor? Laguna Honda was not fancy; we had no CT scan and no emergency room, but I wondered if I might see something helpful with a simple X-ray. So I sent Mr. Grenz upstairs and followed right away to take a look myself.

Now, an X-ray is pretty limiting as to what you can see, which is why CT scans were invented. An X-ray only shows shadows. The shadows of Mr. Grenz's lungs, I saw, were small; he wasn't taking much of a breath, but his lungs were clear of infection, abscess, and tumor. The shadow of his superior vena cava did seem wider than it should have been; but it was the shadow of his heart that I didn't expect. Mr. Grenz's heart was very large, and it was oddly shaped—globular, kind of like an old-fashioned hot-water bottle.

It was one of those times that I didn't know what I was seeing, but I knew that what I was seeing wasn't normal. So I went downstairs to the doctors' office to get some help.

Dr. Fintner was sitting at the little desk she shared with Dr. Romero. She was sorting through the patients' records she'd piled on top of all the mail she saved, and she looked a bit frayed.

"Hey, Julie, come up and look at an X-ray with me. I don't know what it is, but it's something."

She jumped at the chance.

On the way upstairs I told her about Mr. Grenz's face and tongue, and she studied his X-ray for quite a while. Finally she said, "Victoria, it's a pericardial effusion."

Ah. Yes. Of course.

Now, a pericardial effusion means that there is fluid between the heart and the pericardial sac, which is that shiny cellophane I'd seen around Mr. Hickman's heart. Normally there is only a small amount of fluid between them, just enough to lubricate the heart as it expands and contracts. A pericardial effusion means there is a lot of fluid in the sac; for a heart to be as large as it was on Mr. Grenz's X-ray, there had to be a huge amount of fluid.

That extra fluid would put pressure against the heart and, in turn, on the superior vena cava, causing blood to back up into Mr. Grenz's neck, face, and tongue. This would explain, perhaps, his superior vena cava obstruction. If so, I was possibly looking at an emergency, because whatever was filling up the pericardial sac might keep on filling it up until it put so much pressure on the heart that the heart could no longer beat. This is called "cardiac tamponade," and it can be fatal.

The key question was: How fast was this happening? How long had Mr. Grenz's heart been this big? A week, a month? Or a day?

It was never easy to track down a discharging doctor, and it took me a while, but, eventually, I did get hold of Mr. Grenz's doctor. He was pretty sure that Mr. Grenz's heart had been that big for some time.

How sure?

Pretty sure.

And the tongue?

"Oh, he's had that large tongue for a month."

That was reassuring. That made it less likely that I was looking at an emergent pericardial effusion, though it didn't negate the possibility. It did, however, make it harder to rationalize sending Mr. Grenz back to the County for a large tongue and big heart that he'd had for a month. On the other hand, if I ignored those signs while Mr. Grenz's pericardial effusion continued to increase . . .

Suddenly I remembered. There was a way to tell how much of an emergency Mr. Grenz was. It wasn't fancy, either. It was simple and nontechnical, and described in *DeGowin & DeGowin*. Because of the relationship between the beating heart and the expanding and contracting lungs, the blood pressure is not the simple measurement it has become. Before the steady beat called "systole," there is a higher pressure at which a few beats first get through the inflated blood pressure cuff. The difference between that higher pressure and the pressure of systole is called the "paradoxical pulse." It is easy to measure; all you have to do is take a blood pressure and listen for those first few

beats. According to *DeGowin & DeGowin*, the normal paradoxical
pulse was less than ten points. The higher over ten it was, the more
likely that the heart was about to stop.

Now, it used to be that doctors themselves took the blood pressure of their patients. The first thing a physician would do when he
saw a patient was take the "vital signs"—the blood pressure and pulse,
the temperature and the respiratory rate. In fact, the vital signs were
considered to be the most important, the most vital body signs of all.
They measured *vita*—life—and taking them provided numbers for
the beating of the heart, the heat of the body, and the vivifying breath.
But by the late twentieth century, the prestige of the vital signs had
tumbled down the slope, from doctor to nurse, to nursing assistant, to
machine, and today they are rarely taken by a human. Instead, when a
patient first arrives, a nursing assistant wheels the vital-sign machine
out, attaches a plastic pincer to the patient's finger, and reads off its
face precise numbers for the blood pressure, pulse, temperature, and
respiratory rate. The machine readings are instant and repeatable.
But the machine is not programmed to take the paradoxical pulse. So
the paradoxical pulse is never taken.

Dr. Fintner and I left the X-ray department and went back to the
admitting ward. I found a blood pressure cuff and went over to Mr.
Grenz, who was back in bed, looking exhausted and wan. I took his
blood pressure. At 170 I heard the first few beats—that was the first
measurement. At 140 I heard the rest of the beats of systole. Mr.
Grenz had a paradoxical pulse of thirty points. His pericardial sac
was filling up rapidly. It would soon cause cardiac tamponade, and his
heart would stop.

When I told Mr. Grenz he was going back to the County Hospital, he was not happy. Neither was the County. Nevertheless, two
hours later he was in the cardiac catheterization laboratory, where,

under video monitoring and with the full luxury of modern medical technology, two quarts of blood were drained from his pericardial sac. This freed up his heart and allowed it to start beating normally.

As a matter of fact, it saved his life.

What the surgeon later speculated was that Mr. Grenz must have had a slow leak of blood into his pericardial sac for weeks, probably because of the procedure that had punctured and collapsed his lung. That slow buildup of pressure gradually obstructed his superior vena cava and caused his face and tongue to swell. Now that the blood was removed, the surgeon thought that the pericardial sac would stick to the heart and not bleed again. Mr. Grenz's face would return to normal, though he couldn't say about the tongue.

Two days later, Mr. Grenz came back to me. He did look better. His color was pinker; his face not quite so big, although his tongue was about the same. He still had the open hole from his breathing tube and the tube in his stomach for feeding; and he still had that shocked look in his eyes that said: What happened to me? What is all this?

But he was young. Gradually his body reconstituted and repaired itself. The hole in his neck scarred down and closed. Then he was able to talk a bit around the tongue and eat. So his feeding tube could be removed. His strength returned, and he was able first to sit in a chair and then to walk. His eyes brightened, and his movements quickened. His tongue shrank, though never did it fit entirely back in his mouth. His girlfriend came back, and, after several months, I wrote Mr. Grenz's discharge order.

I can't say that he thanked us when he left. He was still angry and stunned; and he put the few possessions he'd acquired—a couple of folded shirts and slacks—into a paper bag and left without saying anything at all. He was still, I believe, angry about the tongue. Later I heard he'd found himself a lawyer and was suing the County for malpractice, though I don't know whether he won his suit or lost, or whatever happened to his tongue.

He did leave me with something, however. What I've always kept in mind since Mr. Grenz is that even the most subtle physical finding—something as minor, as simple, and as rare as the paradoxical pulse—can save a life.

从2次实石头.到拍 Xray 再到诊断 治疗

M eanwhile I was learning Latin.

It used to be that all doctors knew Latin. For centuries, medical books were written in Latin; medical terms were derived from Latin; and, most important, in the days before science, the knowledge of Latin differentiated the physician from the traditional healer. Even at Laguna Honda, all the doctors on the admitting ward, except for me, knew Latin, although each for a different reason. Dr. Fintner knew Latin because she went to medical school when Latin was still required. Dr. Rachman knew Latin because she'd been educated by nuns; and Dr. Romero knew Latin because she went, on scholarship, to elite Eastern private schools. But I had never learned it, Latin having been replaced by the time I went to medical school with physics, calculus, and biochemistry.

But Hildegard wrote in Latin, and I knew that reading her own words in her own language would be crucial for understanding her medicine. Finding a way to learn Latin, however, was not easy. The community colleges did not offer it, and even at the university the operator connected me through to Latin American Studies. So I got a tutor, and in the evenings after I'd taken care of my patients, I studied Latin. It was a provocative and rich study—not so much the military exploits of Caesar or the rhetoric of Cicero, but the language, the words themselves.

Next I went looking for a way to learn Hildegard's Latin in

particular. Because it turned out that Hildegard wrote Medieval Latin, not Classical Latin, and they differed. Medieval Latin was more colloquial than Classical; it was the language that the Middle Ages spoke, as well as wrote. It was also even more obscure a subject than Classical Latin. It took me a while, but, eventually, I found that the university near where I lived offered a seminar in Medieval Latin.

Dr. Major allowed me one morning a week at the university, and there I met and was mentored by that quintessential medieval scholar George Brown.

Professor Brown had not one but two PhDs, and before he'd become a professor, he'd been in a Jesuit seminary. Naturally tonsured by hair loss, he wore a beard, and looked surprisingly like the subject of his many monographs, the Venerable Bede. Small and fit, Professor Brown set the standard for medieval scholarship as much by the pressed shirt, precisely tied cravat, and wool blazer he wore, no matter how hot the day, as he did by his careful studies. He was as soft-spoken, modest, and quietly intelligent a scholar as Dr. Fintner was a doctor.

Classes were held in one of the tawny stone and red-roofed buildings of the university. It gave me a start, sometimes, as I walked past the fountains, the Romanesque church, and down the cloistered walk to class, to realize how similar were the institutions of university and hospital. Both had come into their own during the twelfth century. Both expressed the nonmonetary values that the West placed on learning and healing. Both professor and doctor were in service to ideals that went beyond themselves.

There were also profound differences. Around me, as I walked to class were youth and wealth. Society was spending its resources on its future—a long, productive life lay ahead of those students, not like the patients at my hospital. Also, education, unlike medicine, had not yet been commodified. The university was not yet an "information provider," and Professor Brown not only looked and acted but was treated like the scholarly knight he was.

I learned not only Medieval Latin from him but also paleography—that is, how to read the handwriting of the preprint Middle Ages. I learned about glosses—the notes written next to or between the lines of a manuscript that commented on the text. And I learned about palimpsest, shadow texts that could sometimes be discerned beneath another text. Parchment—the sheepskin on which everyone wrote during the Middle Ages—had been expensive, and it was sometimes reused by scraping ink off old pages. This wiped the page clean, but not completely. The erased text could still be seen as a faint shadow beneath the new.

Palimpsest seemed to be a perfect way of describing what I was beginning to learn at Laguna Honda: That underneath our scientific modern medicine was an earlier way of understanding the body—erased, to be sure, just a faint shadow on our consciousness, but active in our thoughts and desires, nonetheless.

The two months I'd promised Dr. Major were long gone, and she had not queried me about my plans. I was comfortable on the admitting ward, seeing patients with Dr. Rachman, Dr. Romero, and Dr. Fintner, and I was more and more intrigued by the hospital. I was beginning to learn something special from my patients, something that would take me all my years at Laguna Honda to grasp, and that was the experience of being a patient.

It happened because I saw my patients twice or even three times a day, usually for months; I got to know them, and they, of course, me. Toward the end of those first years, there was one patient in particular, a terrible patient. She wasn't even my patient. She was

Dr. Romero's patient, but her bed was between two of my patients, and I passed her every day. She had a horrible disease, and a horrible disease at Laguna Honda was really horrible.

Miss Tod was thirty-five years old. She had cancer. Her cancer was brain cancer, and what made it horrible was that it was just behind her right eye, and it had grown, in spite of surgery and radiation, right out of her eye. The surgeon had removed the eye and sewn the eyelid down over the cancer, but the cancer was still growing.

Miss Tod had never been beautiful, but, what with the radiation, which had caused her hair to fall out; the steroids, which had caused her face to balloon; and the sewn eyelid, which had started to bulge, she was now very hard to look at. Yet she was pleasant and quiet. She always smiled as I passed her by. Eventually we were on speaking terms, with a quick hello and a how-are-you from me to her, and from her to me. I got used to her deformity, although only by blocking out, in some way, my experience of her experience.

One day I finally braved my reluctance and stopped by her bed. Full stop. We looked at each other. She at me, white-coated, rushed, a bit disheveled. I looked only at her left eye.

"Is there anything I can do for you?" I asked her, after we talked a bit.

"Yes," she replied, "there is. I really don't like the food they're giving me. It's all cut up and bland. Do you think it could be changed? And another thing. Could you arrange for me to visit the eye doctor? I need a new pair of glasses."

I was, and am to this day, floored by her response. I was, and am, awestruck by such equanimity. She wanted—not euthanasia or a miraculous cure, stronger pain medications or a second opinion but—different food. A pair of glasses. She said nothing about her terrible misfortune. She was calm, matter-of-fact. Somehow she'd accepted her fate, and it was the small things, the little daily things, that were important to her.

We did change her diet, and we did get her new glasses. Not long after, she moved to another ward, and there she died peacefully, eighteen months later. But her lesson, which I was taught over and over again by so many patients, took me much longer to assimilate. Bravery. A core, a rock of self, radiating courage.

It's a quality that most young doctors, even most middle-aged doctors, can't understand, having had the good fortune to never have been a patient, at least not a patient like Miss Tod. Doctors, after all, start out as young students, healthy, curious, hardworking. What do we know of misfortune and the hand of God?

One medical school tried to remedy this lack with a preadmittance program: Medical students were required to check themselves in as patients, incognito, to the hospital where they'd be working in the near future. This was so that they could gain some idea of what it felt like to be a patient—your watch and belt given over, and a backless gown put on, to wait exposed and vulnerable on a gurney in the hall, a luckless anonymity. It was a good idea, but it didn't work too well. Long about June, when those young and handsome men checked into area hospitals, hair and face and eyes intact, the nurses and doctors knew who they were, of course. They winked; they smiled and even flirted with these "patients" admitted for "abdominal pain."

Still, it was a good idea, a good thought.

Miss Tod capped my experience of those first years at Laguna Honda. She summarized it and hinted at what I would be learning later. Even when there is nothing to do for a patient—no cancer to discover, no paradoxical pulse to take—there is still something to do. It doesn't have to be lifesaving, grandiose, and heroic. It can be as simple as a pair of glasses or a different diet. In fact, it usually is.

She taught me that I didn't have to be afraid of the possibly conta-
gious bad luck of my patients. That they would manage by themselves.
What I had to do was ask them what I could do for them and then do
it, if I could. For those who couldn't answer for themselves, there were
other ways of learning what they needed: their neighbor-patients
across the way, the nurses, the nursing assistants, the volunteers.

Before I came to Laguna Honda, I'd been convinced of the
importance of scientific medicine; Miss Tod convinced me of the importance of the little things.

She also convinced me of the corollary: It's not the big thing. The
big thing—the hand of God, fate—can be accepted, perhaps because it
is so big and fateful, so unchangeable. But the small things are correctable, or should be, if people only cared to notice. The thrice-daily
arrival of an unpalatable diet, the broken glasses—these are constant
reminders that we are not cared about. Perhaps we can accept that God
has it in for us for reasons of His own, or reasons (in the case of Laguna
Honda's patients) that we know very well. But that our fellow human
beings don't care enough to change our diet or repair our glasses . . .

Which is why the cute medical students who went incognito to
their hospitals-to-be, waited in admitting, gave up their watches,
belts, and clothes, even lay in a gurney for the elevator, couldn't have
learned about the real small things. Because the winks, the nudges,
the tender flirtations of the staff reassured them that they were worth
caring for, and were cared for.

Not too long after my experience with Miss Tod, I met Professor
Brown, by accident, in the library.

He was impressed by my project for his paleography class, he told
me. But I had come to the end of what I could do without formal

training in history. I knew Latin well enough to read Hildegard, and I knew enough paleography. Still, if I wanted to go further, I needed to go to graduate school, and not in medieval history but in the history of medicine. There were only a few such graduate programs in the country; however, there was a good one just around the corner from Laguna Honda. He advised me to contact its chief—Professor Doctor Gerhard Weitz, MD, PhD.

So I did. On the phone, Professor Doctor Gerhard Weitz was rather cool. His was a small graduate program, he said, and a PhD in medieval medicine would be difficult, perhaps impossible, for him to supervise.

Would he be willing to meet me for an interview, anyway?

He would. So we arranged to have lunch together at a restaurant near the hospital the very next week.

Two

THE LOVE OF HER LIFE

RECOGNIZED Professor Doctor Gerhard Weitz right away.

He was almost exactly what I'd imagined from our phone conversation—white-haired, clean-shaven, blue-eyed, the very model of the German medical scholar. He was dressed less formally than I'd expected, though, in slacks and a white open-collared shirt. We met at the South American restaurant he'd recommended, found an out-of-the-way table, and sat down. He ordered a roasted-red-pepper dish and a small glass of wine, and I chose the same.

As soon as he opened his mouth to speak—a full mouth with red, moist lips—I understood the dissonance between his German appearance and his un-German manner. He was Latin. Though born in Germany, Dr. Weitz had been raised in Argentina, and his accent was a mix of German and Spanish. Just so, beneath his German exterior there beat a hot-blooded, cayenne-loving heart. To his detriment, I would learn over the years. Like the gender misfit—a woman in a man's body—Professor Doctor Weitz, MD, PhD, was a Latin in a German body, ever mis-taken and ever mis-understood.

He began the interview by telling me about his graduate program in medical history, which was tiny, he said, with only two professors, and focused on American medicine. It was not equipped to take on premodern medicine or Hildegard. If he accepted me, I would have to take classes and organize advisors at other universities, although, frankly, he had no idea how that might be arranged. First I would complete a master's degree, and then—perhaps—go on to the PhD, which had formal orals at the end of the third year and two required languages. As a practicing physician, I would not find his program easy. But . . . here he sat back in his chair and looked at me. My project interested him. A medieval German nun who'd written a practical medical text . . .

His own project was hospitals. As a matter of fact, he was writing the definitive history, he hoped, of hospitals. With this, he brightened and leaned across the small table, trespassing on the arm's-length distance decreed by German etiquette.

What was interesting about hospitals, he said, was that they were specifically Western and Christian institutions, not Greek or Roman. The closest thing the Greeks had to hospitals had been their healing temples—which were beautiful places near healing springs, but staffed by priests, not by doctors. The Romans did have something like hospitals, but only for their soldiers; nothing like a hospital system for their sick citizenry. Instead it was the Christian monastery of the Middle Ages that originated the hospital system we know today. In the monastery, caring for the sick was the foremost Christian duty, and each monastery had, therefore, a hospice for taking care of the sick poor and an infirmary for taking care of the sick monks. A monk infirmarian or, Dr. Weitz supposed, even a nun infirmarian, would be in charge of both the hospice and the infirmary, but no one knew much about what they did or how the system worked. Yet these monastic hospices and infirmaries had been the models for Europe's hospitals and almshouses. Sometimes even their direct ancestors; today's Hôtel-Dieu in Paris was founded by monks in the seventh century, and it still functioned as Paris's hospital for the poor. The West's unique and, when you thought about it, surprising ideal—that a society should take care of its sick poor—had originated in those monastic hospices and infirmaries of the Middle Ages.

But that was pretty much all we knew about them, which was why my project intrigued him. Perhaps Hildegard of Bingen had been the infirmarian for her monastery, and that was why she wrote her medical text, Dr. Weitz said. Then I could use it to find out what went on inside the infirmary and hospice: how diseases were diagnosed and treated; what medications were used and why; even how premodern medicine actually worked. I could use what we already knew about medieval medicine as the background for my research. It was an extraordinary opportunity and would be very helpful to him for his book.

Dr. Weitz leaned back in his chair, wiped his mouth, and looked directly at me.

"It's going to be a long and complicated project, though. You will have to learn German, as well as Latin, and you will spend a lot of time in libraries, looking at medieval manuscripts. You must cut your medical practice down to half-time. The department has a small fellowship, and I will award it to you."

With this generous if abrupt offer, Dr. Weitz stood up, and so did I. We walked out of the restaurant together and down to the corner, where he stopped. Then he gave me an intense but shuttered look, turned up the street, and walked back to his university.

When I told Dr. Major about my plans to start graduate school in medical history, she was supportive and flexible. As it turned out, Dr. Romero was taking a leave of absence, so I could cut back to half-time by taking her place, job-sharing with Dr. Fintner. Dr. Isaiah Jeffers would take my full-time position.

Up to then I'd known Dr. Jeffers only slightly; we would get to know each other very well over the next years. He was tall, dark, and handsome—black, as a matter of fact, and a success story of affirmative action, as he told me one day. He grew up in Florida, and his grandmother raised him out in the country. Jim Crow laws were still in force, and at his school they'd studied with the previous year's used textbooks. Which were okay, he pointed out with his signature smile; they weren't any less accurate than the new ones. He won a scholarship to Morehouse College in Atlanta, and then he was "affirmative-actioned" into medical school. The system had worked for him, he said; and by "worked" he meant that his two children, who were in private schools, would not need affirmative action when it was time for them to go to college.

Dr. Jeffers took over the desk opposite mine. It was not really a desk but a narrow counter that ran along the wall. Over the years it would always be the desk of the lankiest male physician, perhaps because, lacking drawers, it had a natural place to wrap and store those long legs.

Unlike Dr. Fintner, Dr. Jeffers did not know just about everything about medicine. He knew just what was necessary. And unlike Dr. Rachman, his workups were not long and elegant, but short; his scrawl transgressed the lines of the paper and went right to the point. What interested him was not so much what the patient might have—he was usually satisfied with the conclusions of others—but where the patient was from and what kind of life he'd lived.

Dr. Jeffers also knew a good thing when he saw it, as he said to me one slow afternoon. Pushing back his chair from his counter desk, he looked around the walls of our office, which were just as bare as when I'd arrived. He glanced at our lone, uncomplicated computer, at the books on our bookshelf, and at our single, barred window. He tilted back in his chair and then said in his low-pitched drawl, "You know, Victoria, we'll never have it this good."

And what he meant was—this peaceful, this unhassled, this left-alone-to-do-what-we-needed-to-do for our patients. No one paid any attention to us. The pharmacists left us alone to use medications the way we wanted, for their side effects or their off-label use; insurance companies didn't bother to manage us; outside hospitals were simply delighted when we took their complicated patients. Above all, Dr. Major trusted us to do what was right for our patients. Which, for a doctor, is a wonderful thing.

With Dr. Jeffers at the counter desk full-time, I began to job-share with Dr. Fintner.

I knew Dr. Fintner pretty well by this time, but it still took some adjustment. There was her corner of our common desk, piled high with everything she saved to look at later: drug companies' invitations for free dinners, administrative memos on asbestos, patients' X-ray reports and laboratory tests. Each morning when I came in, I went through the pile, tossing out and tidying up; and every few weeks Dr. Fintner arrived with a new system of organization—colored folders, numbered binders, labeled pads of paper.

Slowly the two of us came to understand that Dr. Fintner had the temperament of the physician and I, although I was an internist, the temperament of the surgeon. I was interested in action, or not; she was interested in the most precise action and would spend quite a bit of time to get it right. It took us a while to work it out, to use our differences as double strengths and not as double weaknesses. Truth to tell, both strategies worked well. Especially when applied to the right patient at the right time.

One day of the week we overlapped; that is, we were both in the doctors' office at the same time. On those days we would see patients together, walking around the ward at the end of the day, discussing cases. One late afternoon we came to the bed of Mrs. Georges, who'd been admitted by Dr. Fintner with the diagnosis of, well, old age. She didn't have Alzheimer's disease or another dementia or any fatal disease. She was a widow, with no children, no family, no friends. Her life, as far as Dr. Fintner could tell, was the dash between the date of her birth and the not-yet-established date of her death.

It was late-afternoon quiet, and when we got to her bed, Mrs. Georges was sleeping, or so I thought. Nevertheless, Dr. Fintner went over and stood at the left of her bed, and I went to the right, and for a while we both stood there in silence. After a time, I realized that Mrs. Georges wasn't sleeping. Although her eyes were closed, they fluttered a bit, and her breathing was not the even breathing of the sleeper, but the active breathing of the dreamer or the thinker.

Dr. Fintner was looking down at her, not saying anything. Then softly, she asked, "Mrs. Georges, what are you doing?"

Mrs. Georges's eyes opened, and she looked up at us.

"I was at my high school prom, and I was waiting to be asked to dance. . . . The boys were so handsome! And the girls were so pretty!"

"Is there anything you need? Can we get you something?"

"No, no . . . I'm fine, thank you."

We left her bed then and continued on our rounds, but I never forgot that moment. I was surprised when Dr. Fintner bothered to stop at Mrs. Georges, who seemed to be sleeping. But as we stood there, waiting or maybe just watching, I gradually became aware of a quality I'd felt before with patients, though never consciously—the quality of shared, peaceful silence. It was a healing space, I realized at that moment, and not only for the patient. For the doctor, too, a quiet space of non-asking and non-answering, of non-doing.

Then there was Dr. Fintner's voice, tentative but persistent, which pierced that quiet space and crossed the distance between herself and Mrs. Georges. And there was Mrs. Georges's answer to the questions that hang in the air of the dementia ward, of the coma ward: What are you doing? Are you still here? Are you someplace else?

"I was at my high school prom, and I was waiting to be asked to dance. . . . The boys were so handsome! And the girls were so pretty!"

It was a hint from behind the curtain, about where those patients might be in their muteness. Perhaps not all of them, and not all the time, but some of them, much of the time. They were not dead, Mrs. Georges showed me, but lived in that other world we all know so well: the inner world that has everything this world has—anxiety and anticipation and appreciation; dances and dresses and decorated gyms—that kingdom within.

Dr. Fintner and I worked out our job-sharing, both for ourselves and our patients, as we learned what each was best at. The aged and the feeble, those who had retired after a lifetime of work, of duty; these were the patients that Dr. Fintner appreciated and understood. The Bad Boys and Bad Girls were mine. Dr. Fintner just couldn't quite understand or appreciate them. Their choices, their actions, made no sense to her.

Early in this process, she admitted Jim Jay, and he was a problem. Hair long and uncombed, unwashed and unshaven, with decayed teeth, he had come to the hospital in order to recover from still another bout with alcohol that had ended in a draw. His liver was regenerating; and his mind was clearing; his balance was steadying. In fact, he'd improved enough to walk himself out to the large hall, where he sat at the little round tables with other patients, sipping coffee from a paper cup and sometimes staring into space, but still—recovering.

He came back to the ward after one such outing, however, smelling a little—not much, but a little—like alcohol. We had a long meeting to discuss the matter, with nurses, social worker, doctors, and Jim Jay himself. He hadn't had anything to drink, he assured us. Absolutely not. He knew that drink would kill him; he could not understand why we thought he smelled like alcohol. Perhaps it was his aftershave lotion.

Since she'd admitted him, Dr. Fintner was his main doctor, and she ran the meeting.

"But Mr. Jay," she said, in her soft voice, "you understand how bad alcohol is for you, don't you? It damages your liver cells, and you don't have many left. You remember how you were when you first got here? You don't want that to happen again, do you?"

"No, ma'am, I do remember, and I don't want that to happen again. But ma'am, I've made a vow not to touch the stuff ever again, not ever; and I'm hoping once I get well I can go and live with my sister in Akron."

Dr. Fintner looked satisfied.

"Well, I'm relieved to hear that, Mr. Jay. We're all here to help you do just that, and we will help you, won't we?" she said, looking around.

Everyone nodded cheerily.

But a few days later, when I telephoned in to see how our patients were faring, Dr. Fintner had some bad news.

"Mr. Jay has disappeared."

Humph, I let out, under my breath.

"What did you say, Victoria?"

"Nothing. What happened?"

"Well, you're going to laugh at me. Don't be mad, but yesterday Mr. Jay stopped me in the hall, and he looked so nice, Victoria, all cleaned up. His hair was slicked back, he'd shaved really well, and the nurses had found him a nice sports coat in the clothing department. And, well, he told me that he needed fifteen dollars to mail a package to his sister. He'd lost the money the social worker had given him. Someone had stolen it from him, Victoria, while he was sleeping!"

"You didn't give it to him?"

"I did."

"Oh, Julie!"

"He went to Reno, Victoria; that's what we found out; and he hasn't come back."

And he never did come back. But after that, Dr. Fintner and I took pains to sort our patients or, perhaps more accurately, to choose the proper instrument for the case. When gentleness, forgiveness, and patience were needed—long meetings with angry family members, demented patients, and officious bureaucrats, for instance— Dr. Fintner was on. But when a firm disciplinary hand and an ironic frame of mind were needed, well, we sent me out. It was better for both of us and undoubtedly better for our patients.

By this time, I was well into my first year in Dr. Weitz's History of Medicine program.

It met in a small seminar room on the fourth floor of the University Hospital's oldest wing. I'd walk into the new hospital building and then through the lobby, splashed with news of the hospital's latest nanotechnological discoveries. I'd go through research departments and past well-appointed clinics, and then up three flights of concrete stairs with their old-fashioned iron banisters. The history department was hidden away upstairs, as if modern medicine, like a second wife, did not want to know about or even have a past.

There were six of us graduate students, three physicians and three nonphysicians, and in a few months Dr. Weitz marched us through the medicine of Ancient Greece, Rome, the Middle Ages, the Renaissance, and the Enlightenment, on our way to Modernity, where we would dwell for many weeks. During those 2,400 years, we learned, premodern medicine had been the only medical system in the West. It was how everyone understood health and disease; the way all physicians practiced; and how all patients expected to be treated. Then suddenly, in only a few decades toward the end of the nineteenth century, premodern medicine was abruptly replaced by modern medicine and forgotten.

Dr. Weitz explained its theory to us. For premodern medicine, he said, the cosmos was made up of four abstract elements—Earth, Water, Air, and Fire. Each of the four elements, in turn, was made up of four qualities—hot and cold, and wet and dry. Thus Earth was cold and dry; Water, cold and wet; Air was hot and wet; Fire, hot and dry. Everything in the universe was made up of a mixture of these four elements and four qualities, but in various proportions, and this included the building blocks of the body, which were the four humors—blood, bile (or choler), phlegm, and melancholia. Blood was hot and wet; and bile, hot and dry; phlegm was cold and wet; and melancholia, cold and dry. Health was thought to be the proper balance of these four bodily humors, and disease was an imbalance. The job of the physician was to diagnose his patient's humoral imbalance and correct it by prescribing a "regime." For diagnosis, the physician took the pulse of the patient and examined the urine. The prescribed regime was made up of diet, herbal medicines, bleeding, moxibustion, and bathing. It also included prescriptions for changes of climate, sexual activity, rest, sleep, and exercise.

This system, Dr. Weitz told us, was usually known as the "humoral system," but, because there were four elements, four qualities, and four humors, it was also called the "System of the Fours." Sometimes other "fours" were included in it: the four seasons—spring, summer, fall, winter; the four directions—east, west, north, south; even the four evangelists—Matthew, Mark, Luke, and John. Then he showed us a medieval drawing in which the entire theory was portrayed. The human body was in the center; arrayed around it, top and bottom, left and right, were the four seasons, directions, elements, humors, and qualities.

Humoral medicine was a beautiful and long-lived medical system, Dr. Weitz ended, but how it actually worked to explain the body was pretty much a mystery.

Naturally the physician graduate students among us had many questions. Why did premodern medicine last so long, and why did it end so abruptly? Why was it so similar to the Chinese and Indian systems, which were also based on elements, qualities, and humors, and yet so different?

Dr. Weitz didn't know. He couldn't say. He looked over at me. That would be Dr. S.'s project, he said.

The second year of the program prepared us for writing our master's theses, teaching us the many ways to write history. Toward the end of that year, I started my thesis. I would use the medical text of Hildegard of Bingen, the twelfth-century Benedictine nun, to explore how humoral medicine worked. I would approach it, I decided, as if I were her student—and as if I had her text, and only her text, to guide me.

I can't say that I learned how to practice humoral medicine from Hildegard, but I did learn quite a lot. I learned that it was not just an elegant philosophical system, but a real medicine for real patients with real diseases, although the diseases were understood differently from how modern medicine understood them.

I learned that the System of the Fours was useful as a heuristic device—that is, as a way of imagining how the environment outside the body could affect the inside of the body. And there was a trick to it. The trick was that the four elements were not imagined as abstractions but as real material substances. Earth meant land or dirt; Water, rain; Air was wind; and Fire was the sun. The "elements" of the humoral system were not the elements of the philosopher, but the natural elements of the farmer and the gardener.

I began to understand that the premodern system was based on the gardener's understanding of the world, and that Hildegard took a gardener's approach to the body, not a mechanic's or a computer programmer's. She did not focus down to the cellular level of the body; instead, she stood back from her patient and looked around. She calculated in her mind not just the internal balance of the four humors, but the whole balance of her patient within and as a part of his environment. With that numberless measure, she manipulated and rebalanced the environment inside of and outside her patient. She did so slowly, like a gardener, by fussing and fiddling, doing a little of this and a little of that. Then she waited to see what would happen. Which is to say that she followed the patient's body; she did not lead.

There seemed to be something in it, to me. And while I did not start giving my patients complex medieval concoctions, I did bake some of Hildegard's antidepressant cookies; I did brew some of her medicinal beers; and now and then, with a difficult, puzzling patient, I asked myself: Now, how would humoral medicine understand this? What would Hildegard do?

The first patient I tried this with was Mrs. Maria McCoy.

She was sent to us to die, but I didn't know that at first because, ever since Lev Grenz and his tongue, I'd changed the order of my workup. I'd try to see the patient right away, before I looked at the records, and I didn't spend much time on asking the patient for his history, either. The histories of the patients who came to us were just too complicated for anyone to remember. Instead, I'd follow the ambulance drivers into the ward and watch as they moved my new patient into bed. Then I'd take the vital signs myself and begin my examination. I'd see how much I could deduce about the patient and his life from my examination alone—which medications he was taking, which diseases he had, his line of work, and something of the course of his life. It was amazing how much I could learn.

For instance, some blood-pressure medications cause distinctive physical signs, as do certain neurological medications, and I could often figure out which medications the patients were on and why by noticing those signs. Then there are the physical signs of diabetes, and those of high blood pressure, and both can reveal how long-standing those diagnoses are. There are the patient's scars—from surgeries forgotten or remembered, from stab wounds, war wounds, childhood accidents. And there are the tattoos. Many of the patients who came to us had tattoos, and they are informative. For instance, there are specific tattoos acquired in prison; others obtained when someone is high on hallucinogens; there are schizophrenic tattoos; tattoos from a drunken high school night on the town; and tattoos of the merchant seaman. Sometimes a patient had all kinds of tattoos, and his history was really written on his body: first the drunken night on the town, then the LSD, then the time in prison, the schizophrenic break, and the flight to sea.

So I followed as the ambulance drivers wheeled Maria McCoy into one of the semiprivate rooms at the front of the ward. This in itself was a bad sign, because the nurses reserved those rooms for the sickest patients. I watched as the drivers transferred her from the gurney into the bed in the corner, next to the window. She was bundled up in a coat as if she were a package being delivered, and they grabbed the sheet on which she was lying by its top and bottom, and heaved her onto the bed. She didn't move. Then they handed me her records, maneuvered the gurney around me, and left.

I began to look over my new patient.

Her eyes were half closed, glazed, and almost empty, and she did not seem to realize I was there. Her face was yellow, and her hands, which the drivers had placed outside the bedclothes, were puffy. Then I went over to her right side and looked down. It was not a pretty sight, or, to be precise, it was not a pretty feeling. Mrs. McCoy had almost no life force left.

"Life force" is not a medical term. In the more than one hundred thousand words of *Stedman's Medical Dictionary,* there is no word that names what I didn't feel from Mrs. McCoy that day—there was almost nothing coming from her to meet my presence. She was alive, to be sure; she was breathing, and I could sense the faint warmth that emanates from the living body. But there sure wasn't much to work with.

I introduced myself, and her yellowed eyes turned toward my voice. Her hair was thin and unwashed; her face swollen; her lips cracked; and her mouth dry. The rest of her body was swollen, too, especially her belly. It was as big as a beach ball, and when I lifted up the sheets, I saw that her skin was covered with the death marks called "spiders"—red spots that signified, as did her yellow skin and eyes, and the swelling of her face, arms, legs, and belly, that her liver was no longer working.

Her records made it clear that Mrs. McCoy was not expected to live. She was expected to die of liver failure, and soon. Her crime was alcohol. Now, the liver can tolerate many years of drinking; unlike the brain, heart, or limbs, under the right conditions the liver can regenerate and reconstruct itself. And that's a good thing, because, as Mrs. McCoy's body demonstrated, without a functioning liver, the body fails. The liver makes protein—the protein that clots our blood; without that protein we bleed to death from nose, mouth, lungs. It makes the protein that holds serum—the yellow fluid of our blood—inside our blood vessels; without that protein, the serum moves out of the blood vessels and swells the face, arms, legs, and belly. The liver also removes toxins from the blood; without it, they poison the brain, putting it into the state of Mrs. McCoy's brain—first dull, then confused, sleepy, and, ultimately, dead. We don't need that much liver, though, only 5 percent of what we're born with. *With* 5 percent, our liver can clot our blood, make proteins, filter toxins, and even regenerate itself. *Without* that 5 percent, we die. And Mrs. McCoy was going to die.

She would bleed to death, suddenly and without warning. She

would sit up in her bed and vomit blood—all her blood—and then fall back in a minute or two with a puzzled look on her gray, dead face. Or she would get agitated and combative, with a fever and infection that confused her further, and she would die in twenty-four hours. Or, lacking fluid in her veins, and, therefore, lacking enough blood pressure to adequately irrigate her kidneys and brain, her belly would get bigger and bigger; her face, yellower and yellower; and her spirit, quieter and quieter, until her lungs stopped breathing and her heart stopped beating.

That's what would happen to Mrs. McCoy. And there wasn't much we could do about it. Which is not to say that we wouldn't try, or that we hadn't tried, as was evident when I sat down to go over her records in detail.

Between January and June of that year, she'd had thirty visits to the emergency room, and two long admissions to the County, the most recent being, presumably, her last. She was fifty years old and a widow with four children, but only two sons were still in contact with her. She lived, when she wasn't in the emergency room, in an SRO, or what used to be called a cold-water walk-up flat, and Mrs. McCoy's was in the Tenderloin. If it was like all the other SROs, it would be a room with a dusty twill bedspread on a single bed, the smell of mildewed carpet, a scuffed chest of drawers, and a shared bathroom down the hall.

All thirty of her emergency-room visits had been for alcohol. During visit number fifteen, she had almost died from a blood infection; and during number thirty, she'd gone into a coma from the alcohol. It had taken the County a month to sort things out. They dried her out, and she woke up, but because her liver wasn't working, she was still confused. It was during this visit that her sons had agreed with the doctors that, in view of her terminal condition, "a natural death should be allowed," and so the doctors sent her over to us to die. Although not without exercising their best efforts to improve her medical condition. They had put her on thirteen different medications—medications to dry her out, medications to support her blood pressure, medications to calm her, to stimulate her, and to treat the diabetes from alcohol's toxic effects on the pancreas. They'd done a good job. She was, after all, still alive.

I sighed. I wrote her orders, handed the complex list of medications to the nurses, and went about the rest of my afternoon.

By the next day, Mrs. McCoy was not dead, although she wasn't any better. In fact, she was worse. She was yellower and nearly comatose; her belly was bigger and tight as a drum; and she was beginning to moan. Her belly was so big from fluid that I would have to drain it.

Now, I don't like to do this much, although it isn't a difficult procedure. A thin tube with a needle at either end is used. After the skin of the belly is numbed, one of the needles is inserted into a vacuum bottle, and then the other needle is put into the belly; a vacuum is created, and the liquid inside the belly is drawn into the bottle. The belly decreases in size, and the patient is more comfortable, but only for a few days, because, since nothing else has changed, the belly fills right back up again. So the procedure has to be repeated within a week.

But there was nothing else to do. I walked over to Central Supply, which was a Dutch door behind which were the wooden shelves of the hospital's supplies. Leaning on the shelf of the open door, I filled out the two-line request form, and the attendant gave me the two quart bottles, the needles, the catheter, and the bottle of numbing medication I'd asked for. I took everything back to Mrs. McCoy's room. By this time she was moaning and nearly unconscious. I cleansed her belly, numbed the skin, inserted the needle, and, sure enough, honey-colored fluid began to flow. The first bottle filled, and then the second. Her belly deflated quite a bit, and she stopped moaning. I withdrew the needle, bandaged the site, cleaned up, and made ready to leave. But I didn't leave, not immediately. I sat for a while.

I sat next to Mrs. McCoy, who was now sleeping, and I looked at the yellow liquid in the bottle. The afternoon light was coming through the window, and it came through the liquid, making evident by the swirls that this liquid was not just yellow water. It was not nothing—something to be thrown away, as I would do shortly. This yellow liquid was life. I could see that its consistency, as well as its color, was like honey from all those important proteins. It would taste like honey, too, sweet from the sugar in the blood; and it would be sticky, like honey, from the clotting factors wasted, and the enzymes needed for life. It was just too bad, I thought, that we couldn't, some-how, put this fluid back into Mrs. McCoy's veins. But, even if we could, it wouldn't stay in her veins. There was not enough pressure inside the veins, and the fluid would flow right back into her belly. What Mrs. McCoy needed, I mused, was some way to *push* this magic yellow fluid of life out of her belly and back into her veins.

I wondered, as I sat there, how Hildegard would have thought of Mrs. McCoy's disease, and what she would have done. Clearly, the element, Water, was in the wrong place. Then I recalled that humoral medicine had used physical techniques more often than we do today. One of its techniques was wrapping an abdominal binder, a kind of girdle, around the belly, in order to press fluid from a swollen belly back into the veins.

It was worth a try. If any place would still have an abdominal binder somewhere on its shelves, it would be our central supply. So I ordered one up, and, sure enough, it came. It looked like a wide ACE bandage—its only modern touch a Velcro closure. The nurse helped me wrap it around Mrs. McCoy's somewhat deflated belly. It didn't seem to make her uncomfortable. She continued to sleep, and I left the room.

The next day when I went by to see her, Mrs. McCoy was still not dead.

She wasn't even worse. She was the same or, perhaps, a bit better. The abdominal binder was still around her, and her belly was no bigger than right after the procedure. That was significant. Although the liver cannot perform its functions if less than 5 percent of it remains, if just a little more than 5 percent is working, then the downward spiral begins to reverse. With just a little more, the liver can produce just enough more protein to increase the blood pressure a bit, and this allows the kidneys to start excreting excess fluid and toxins. The doctor can then start to use more medication for stimulating the kidneys, and fluid will start to go out of the face, arms, legs, and belly, which revert to their normal size. Because the patient is more comfortable, pain medications can be decreased, and the patient will wake up and start to move around, mobilizing still more fluid.

And this was what was happening with Mrs. McCoy. She wasn't worse. That meant she was better—she had a chance.

By the end of that week, she was opening her eyes at the sound of my voice and even at the sound of my footsteps. The abdominal binder was still on, but it was loose; her face was beginning to acquire a shape, and when I sat down in the chair by her bed, she looked at me. Not only did she look at me; her eyes looked into mine with recognition and love—a particular kind of love. Not the love of a parent for a child or a lover for the beloved, but of a subject for his ruler—trusting, all will resigned. I recognized the look. It was the transference.

The transference is the name that the psychiatric profession, Sigmund Freud in particular, gave to the emotions that the patient transfers to the doctor during treatment. It is the love that he or she felt for his or her parents—not the rational love, but the irrational love for the all-powerful father/mother in a three-year-old's life. This transference was the key to psychic healing, the key to psychic change, Freud wrote, because it made the doctor what the doctor was not—all-powerful. After the transference, the words, the nod, the blink of the doctor's eyes would be all-important to the patient, would mean acceptance or rejection, pride or guilt, self-love or self-hate. And Mrs. McCoy, I saw by that flicker in her eyes, had fallen in love—which is what the transference really is—with me, her doctor. Not, of course, with me, the person; but with Me, the doctor-being sitting in the chair by her bed.

It's a lot of power, the transference. Mrs. McCoy's transference to me meant she would wait, during the day, for my footsteps; she would stay alive for that reason. Her transference to me meant she would hang on my every word and try to please me. If I asked her, she would bestir herself; she would make an effort. She would sit up in bed and feed herself; she would exert herself and get stronger. She would go without complaint to rehabilitation; she would take her first steps, to please me. She would be pleasant to the nurses; and, if her sons came to visit, she would impress them, she would smile and talk to them. She would participate in the life of the ward. Her transference to me meant she would live and not die.

And that is what happened. After two weeks the abdominal binder was no longer necessary. The fluid in her belly had just about disappeared, as had the swelling in her face and arms. She had had no infections and no bleeding; and she had woken up. Her liver was improving. So the nurses moved her out of the quiet semiprivate room into the noisy communal open ward, and there she stayed for weeks. I saw her almost every day.

One day I noticed that she had a photo—one photo, saved from the wreckage of her life—above her bed. Black and white, yellowed and faded, shiny and creased. It was the photo of a dog. Who was the dog?

"That's my dog, Spreckles," she told me. "I had him for a long time, but when I moved into the SRO, they didn't take dogs so I had to give him away." She fell silent and then added, "Dogs are just like people, only they have four senses instead of five. They can't talk, that's all. They understand everything, though, everything. They just can't talk."

"Even politics and religion?" I teased.

"Everything!"

Not too long after that conversation, she appeared at the door of the doctors' office. Our door was always open, partly because it was such a small office, but mainly because that way we were an integral part of the ward. We could see and hear the scene: the comings and goings of ambulance drivers and family members, nurses and volunteers, and, especially, patients—shuffling, wheeling, lurching, occasionally falling, occasionally running—as well as the crashes, shouts, spills, giggles, whispers, and, once in a while, the silence of the ward. Nevertheless, the custom was to knock on the open door, which Mrs. McCoy did.

"Dr. S., are you busy?" she asked.

I looked up from my desk. It was the first time I'd seen Mrs. McCoy standing. She was short and square. Her hair was dark brown and straight; her skin beneath the resolving jaundice was also brown; and she had the warm brown eyes of her Mexican heritage. There was a cane in her right hand and a potted plant in her left.

"I have a present for you, Dr. S. I potted this plant for you, on Saturday, in the greenhouse."

I walked over and took the plant. There wasn't much of it. Two leaves in newly potted dirt. "Thanks." I put the plant on my desk.

"Make sure you keep it moist," she said. "It's easy to care for; you'll see. Just make sure it's watered."

A week or so later, Mrs. McCoy was transferred off the admitting ward. I didn't see her again for almost a year. But one day, as I was making my way through the smokers and poker players in the large hall, she limped up to me, cane in hand. She looked quite good, quite normal, quite like a stocky fifty-year-old Mexican woman.

"Dr. S., they want to discharge me. They want to send me back to the SRO."

I looked at her. I looked at her cane, and I looked at her. I thought about the thirty emergency-room visits and the two monthlong hospitalizations she'd had in the six months before she came to us. I thought about the abdominal binder and the two bottles of honey-colored fluid I'd taken from her belly. I thought about the spark in her eyes.

"You know," I said, "they can't discharge you if you can't walk, if you are in a wheelchair because of that bad knee." (She had a bad left knee, which is why she used the cane.)

She looked at me, and I looked back at her. Message sent, and message received.

It was almost a year before I saw her again. She came to my office, this time in a wheelchair.

"They're discharging me tomorrow," she told me.

"How can they discharge you if you can't walk?"

"They know I can walk."

We both sighed, and we shook hands. For form's sake I went over to talk to the social worker who was discharging her. Mrs. McCoy no longer had a physical need for hospital care, she explained, and hospital care was expensive, so she had to go.

But what about all the emergency-room visits, the expensive ICU hospitalizations that she hadn't had during the years she'd been with us? I asked. The social worker agreed. It was a pity; it was just too bad; it would be more expensive in the long run; but there was nothing she could do about it.

never saw Mrs. McCoy again. But I did watch the computer for her next admission to the emergency room at the County Hospital.

For months there was nothing. And then, about six months after she left, there it was. An emergency-room visit, but—ominously—only one. She was not admitted to the County Hospital, and there were no subsequent emergency-room visits. Was it her last emergency-room visit because the paramedics had found her dead on the streets? Or was she doing well, and it had been an emergency-room visit that anyone might make for something trivial—a hangnail, a cough, a cold? Or was it the emergency-room visit that convinced her not to drink again?

I never found out.

But I've thought of her often since. Because the plant she gave me did survive, though not thanks to me. Although I was in the midst of discovering that premodern medicine had the garden as its main metaphor, where the patient was plant and the doctor was gardener, I had a difficult time remembering to water that plant. It did not, in my hands, do well.

But it did do well in the hands of Larissa Russof, our Russian nurse who'd been a pediatric neurologist in the USSR. She was a good nurse, and the struggle of Mrs. McCoy's plant in my forgetful hands pained her. One day, standing at the open door of the office, she offered, "Dr. S., that plant is dying. It needs to be watered."

"I know."

"I'm going to take it and help the poor thing."

"Okay."

So she took the plant away. I don't know where she took it, maybe home for a few days, and when it returned, it was better, much better—green again and cheerful.

Over the next many years, Larissa continued to take care of Mrs. McCoy's plant. It stayed green, and it grew very well—up over my desk and along the wall above my desk, then over the top of the window and down along the side of our computer. It was just beginning to grow around the corner and up along the wall of Dr. Jeffers's counter desk when one day, unexpectedly, the consulting firm of Dee and Tee, Health-Care Efficiency Experts, arrived.

Three

THE VISIT OF DEE AND TEE, HEALTH-CARE EFFICIENCY EXPERTS

T HE CONSULTING FIRM of Dee and Tee, Health-Care Efficiency Experts, did not, however, knock on the door of the admitting ward or on the door of the doctors' office. Nor did administration, not even Dr. Major, announce their visit to the staff. Instead, we learned of it from Larissa, whose information came from her extensive network at the hospital, which was made up mostly of her Russian connections.

Although we had hundreds of staff from all over the world, only a few were from Russia, and the Russians were particular. In Russia they'd been professionals, and they brought their skills and knowledge, prejudices and irony, with them when they came to America. There was Head Nurse Raisa, for example, who in Russia had been an oncologist, and there was Fedorov, the electrician, who'd owned a factory. Although they were few, the Russians knew when to listen and when to hold their tongues; and they knew an evolving secretive bureaucracy when they saw one. So they were useful to Larissa up to a point. But it was the mafia of Russian ambulance drivers who were her best informants because they went all over the city, delivering patients, pizza, and clandestine goods—and picking up gossip and rumor.

However, Larissa did not limit her network of intelligence to the Russians. One day we ran into each other. Being herself doctor and nurse, Russian and American, Russian Orthodox and Jewish, she excelled at crossing boundaries, and almost everyone liked her and passed information to her—doctors, nurses, therapists, janitors. It didn't hurt that she was intelligent and charming, humorous and well-groomed, with a touch always of something European—a thin gold bracelet, an Italian scarf—to show that she had not given in completely to American ways. Larissa, consequently, knew just about everything at the hospital and would divulge some of what she knew in exchange for what she didn't know, or sometimes just to oil the wheels of her machine.

She knew all about Dee and Tee's visit, and, standing in the doorway of our doctors' office, she told us with a satisfied air not all but some of what she'd heard.

The city had hired Dee and Tee to help solve its health-care budget problems, she said, and they were expected to be at the hospital for months. They would be paid 10 percent of any cost savings they came up with, although—here she smiled—they would not be responsible for any cost increases their recommendations might create.

How would they go about their mission? we asked.

She hadn't yet heard. So far they were talking to senior management and looking at the payroll, especially at the laundry and the nursing department. At this, she gave us that meaningful look I'd come to know from all the Russians, told me that my Mr. B. had a bladder infection and needed antibiotics, smiled again, and went back to her job as nurse. We—Dr. Jeffers, Dr. Fintner, Dr. Romero, and I—looked at one another and then we, too, went back to our work.

B y this time, Dr. Romero had finished her second residency, this one in internal medicine, and she had returned to the admitting ward. She took the place of Dr. Rachman, who'd finally paid off her hundreds of thousands of dollars in student loans and left to start a family.

Dr. Romero moved into Dr. Rachman's chair at our rickety wooden desk, and there she would stay for many years. And it was true, what Dr. Rachman had told me on my first day, Dr. Romero did have two sides: witty and cynical inside our little office; openhearted and even unctuous—adjusting bedclothes, chucking the homeless under their chins—outside it.

Other than the change from Dr. Rachman to Dr. Romero, and the knowledge that somewhere out in the vast, unpatrolled spaces of the hospital were consultants inspecting, life on the admitting ward went on about the same. It was even busier, with ever-increasing numbers of patients without insurance who depended on the city's fraying safety net. Now we were admitting four or five new patients each day. Usually they were from the County Hospital, though more and more often they were from hospitals around the city, or even, sometimes, directly from the streets—patients who'd been picked up, delirious, infected, and lice-ridden, by the police or the paramedics.

Not only were there more patients, but they were sicker—with complex medical problems more appropriate for an intensive care unit than an almshouse. Now and again a patient came to us directly from the ICU, not even passing through the chimerical reassurance of a day or two on the step-down unit of the acute hospital.

This increase in the number and acuity of the sick was unexpected, although it was the predictable outcome of the health-care policy decisions made in the 1980s. There'd been the shutting down of most of the almshouses in the country; then the phasing out of most of the free county hospitals; and, last but not least, the closing of the state mental hospitals. The closing of the state mental hospitals was particularly disastrous, the result of an unwitting but agreeable collusion of Left and Right; the Left being convinced that institutionalization of any kind was harmful, and the Right, that institutionalization of any kind was expensive.

A trade-off had been arranged. Most of the state mental hospitals would be closed, and part of the money saved would be used for halfway houses, so that the previously institutionalized could be slowly reintroduced to society. Each halfway house would serve five or six patients; its live-in staff would be psychiatrically trained; and a psychiatrist would visit weekly to ensure that the newly released schizophrenic, manic-depressive, or brain-injured would get the medications he needed. A more humane, less costly solution for all concerned, and both Left and Right signed on.

But shortly after the state mental hospitals closed, there was a budget crisis, and then another and another, and the money for this careful outpatient treatment was trimmed, pared, and finally excised. Many of the halfway houses were shut down, and their formerly institutionalized patients put out onto the streets without medication, supervision, or shelter.

Some patients did well for a while, especially after they discovered that drugs—heroin, marijuana, cocaine, and alcohol—were pretty good medications for their schizophrenia, mania, depression, and anxiety. But in the decade that followed, many started to get ill—physically ill like everyone else—with high blood pressure, diabetes, cancer. Since they were homeless and unemployed; since Medicaid—the health insurance formerly provided to the "indigent adult"—had been taken away, and since most of the free county hospitals had been closed, these former psychiatric patients received medical care only at the last moment. Moreover, once their medical condition stabilized, they were discharged from the hospital, often without their psychiatric medication, which in the 1980s they'd won the right to refuse.

So they got physically sick and stayed sick. They lost their legs or their sight to their untreated diabetes; they had strokes at an early age from their cocaine use or their untreated hypertension. They got infections that, undiagnosed, migrated into their hearts, bones, and brains. They broke their legs, their arms, their spines, and their skulls in fights, in car accidents, or in suicidal or drug-related jumps out of buildings. They wandered the city streets, physically ill and often psychotic.

Eventually they would be picked up and brought, or would find their way—at least in our city—to the County Hospital, where they would be treated and stabilized. And then, because our city still had its almshouse, they would be sent to us. At the time of Dee and Tee's visit, about one-third of our patients were these so-called "triple diagnosis" patients—with their three diagnoses of untreated complex medical illness, florid mental illness, and drug abuse.

O f all these patients—and there were many—it was Jimmy Turner whom I most regret.

He was the skinniest patient I ever admitted and one of the

craziest. I use the term *crazy* as fitting in his case; no complicated DSM-IV diagnosis was needed: Jimmy was crazy, and he thought he was a vending machine. Like so many of the failures from the well-meaning policy changes of the 1980s, he'd taken up residence in our city's beautiful park not far north of the hospital. He slept in a clearing, in a sleeping bag under his own tree, and there he'd been eating coins—quarters, dimes, nickels, and pennies. Someone—perhaps another ex-patient, a thief, or even the pleasant bicycle patrol—noted that Jimmy had been asleep under his tree for a very long time. The paramedics were called and found him alive but unarousable—that is, comatose—and they took him over to the County.

At the County tests revealed that Mr. Turner had a life-threatening anemia (low red cell count)—an anemia so profound that he couldn't stand up without passing out. But his anemia was not due to the usual causes, such as blood loss from an ulcer or a cancer, or iron deficiency from malnutrition. Rather, on X-ray Mr. Turner was found to have $1.26 in change scattered through his gastrointestinal tract. And, since coins are no longer made of silver, nickel, or copper but mostly of zinc, it turned out that Mr. Turner was severely zinc-toxic, his blood level being more than ten times normal. The zinc in the coins had seeped into his blood and interfered with his body's ability to utilize copper. Since copper is needed to make blood, he was profoundly anemic.

The doctors at the County Hospital went to work. They cleaned out his gastrointestinal tract with laxatives and enemas; and they made sure that they recovered all the coins—two quarters, five dimes, three nickels, and eleven pennies—from his stool. They transfused Mr. Turner, and they investigated him for other possible, though rare, errors of copper metabolism. They even treated him with an expensive drug, penicillamine, just in case he did. Nevertheless, even after all their work, Mr. Turner was still too weak to stand; he wasn't eating enough to stay alive; and he was looking for coins. So they sent him over to us, for rest, relaxation, and rehabilitation.

When I first saw Jimmy, sitting in the chair by his bed, I was shocked.

He looked like a concentration camp victim. His temples were hollow; his cheekbones jutted out beyond his chin; his color, despite the transfusions he'd had, was sickly and sallow; and his scanty hair was the dry, reddish hair of protein deficiency. I could make out every vertebra in his spine, and his ribs were so prominent that I couldn't get my stethoscope to sit right on his chest. Through his sunken belly I could see the edges of his beating aorta, and his arms and legs were just skin-covered bones.

His main problem, it seemed, was that he wasn't eating. He wasn't talking either, so it was difficult to learn his side of the story—about the coins, I mean—and he had no family or friends to ask. Fortunately, the County Hospital had obtained a court order that let us give Mr. Turner the antipsychotic medications he needed, and I expected that soon he would begin to eat as well as to talk.

It took longer than I thought it would. Even after the psychiatric medications began to work, and Mr. Turner became more sociable, he was never loquacious. Moreover, even though he seemed to try to eat, he couldn't or wouldn't. He was nauseated, he told me, and after a time, he began to vomit. I adjusted his medications, ran quite a few tests, and discovered that he had a second side effect from his elevated zinc level, decreased copper level, and severe anemia. He had an obstruction in his esophagus, the muscular tube that takes food from mouth to stomach. This obstruction was not another coin but a web— a weird shelf of tissue that sometimes grows when patients have a severe anemia, though no one knows why—and that web was preventing nutrition from reaching his stomach. Jimmy needed, therefore, to be fed for a while with a tube. So we got another court order and placed a feeding tube past the obstructing web into his stomach. And with that, Jimmy began to improve.

Significantly. What with the absence of coins in his gastrointestinal tract, and the nutrition and vitamins from the feeding tube; with a roof over his head, a bed to sleep in, and antipsychotic medications, Jimmy improved a lot. His body excreted the excess zinc; his copper level normalized; and his anemia resolved. The web in his esophagus dissolved, and we removed the tube. He began to eat quite a bit on his own. In fact, Jimmy was not only the skinniest patient I ever had, he was also the patient who gained the most weight, so that at the end of three months he was looking quite normal, quite presentable. At 140 pounds, with his reddish hair now shiny and combed, and his frame filled in, he looked even a little younger than his age, which was thirty-one. I was pretty proud and happy with his progress.

So was he. Indeed, he told me one day about four months after his admission, he was ready to leave. No, he didn't need a place to stay; he'd find some place to live himself. It wasn't a big deal; he'd done it before. No, he didn't need food stamps or General Assistance or a caseworker. He was strong; he'd find work. And no, he didn't need any medications. Vitamins? No. What about his nerve medicines? The ones that kept him anchored to Planet Earth? No. Thanks. He didn't think he'd need those either. No, really not. He didn't like them. When he took them he couldn't think properly.

And, according to our psychiatrist—and I knew this already— Mr. Turner was quite within his rights. He had the right to refuse psychiatric medications, even if he was crazy, as long as he wasn't so crazy as to be a danger to himself or to others at the time he refused

them—even if the only reason that he wasn't thinking he was a vending machine and eating coins was because he was being given his
antipsychotic medications by court order. We could try to get a per-
manent conservator for him, our psychiatrist told me—that is, a legal
guardian who would be awarded the right to consent to psychiatric
treatment on Jimmy's behalf. But, he said, good luck. It was almost
impossible to get a conservator in our city. They were few, and they
rarely took our patients, who, they knew, were well cared for. Besides,
Jimmy looked and sounded great. No judge would take away his right
to refuse medications.

I was disappointed but not surprised by his assessment.

Because I knew about the second, equally well-meaning and
equally disastrous health-care policy decision made in the 1980s,
around the same time as the closure of the state mental hospitals.
This was the decision to give psychiatric patients the right to consent
to, or refuse, psychiatric care. It had been a reaction to the excesses of
the twentieth century: to the involuntary commitment of homosexu-
als; to electric shock therapy for anxiety, depression, or just plain
orneriness; to lobotomy—that is, brain surgery—for what sometimes
seemed, in retrospect, to be nothing more than a refusal to conform.
That policy, of making involuntary psychiatric commitment difficult
to obtain and of requiring consent for psychiatric medications, had
not been wrong. It had been necessary. I knew that from Mrs.
Lantos.

I met her one day while I was taking care of the patients of a vacationing doctor. Although "met" would be an exaggeration. Rather, I
passed her bed on my way to see another patient. But she stopped
me cold.

Mrs. Lantos was tiny; she was old; she was wizened; she looked
like the witch in a Grimm's fairy tale. Her legs and arms were

contracted up so that she was even tinier. She took up less than a third of her narrow bed, and when I stopped, I saw that, although her eyes were open, she didn't turn to look at me. She was staring into space and saying over and over and over again, in an anguished and desperate voice: "My cat, my cat, my cat, my cat."

That's what stopped me.

Who was she? Why was she here?

What I learned from the fifty-year-old admission report still in her chart—one page, typed and yellowed—was that she'd been transferred to Laguna Honda from a state mental hospital in 1958. She'd initially been admitted to the state mental hospital in the 1940s at the request of her husband because, so the record quoted, "She wouldn't keep house properly; she wouldn't act like a good wife." Back then, in the 1940s, there were essentially no effective treatments for psychiatric conditions. Patients were mostly hospitalized—committed—to back wards indefinitely, and, if necessary, they were restrained. And so, apparently, was Mrs. Lantos.

When the first effective treatment for mental illness was discovered, it was considered a miracle, and its discoverer was awarded a Nobel Prize. The treatment was based on the observation that severing the connections between the frontal lobes and the rest of the brain calmed schizophrenics and even cured them. The operation was called lobotomy, and until 1952, when the first psychiatric medicine, Thorazine, was synthesized, thousands of lobotomies were done. Some were successful, and the patient was cured, or, at least, improved, and discharged.

Many, though, did not improve, and some even worsened, and this is what happened to Mrs. Lantos. In the early 1950s she'd had a lobotomy, and it had not been successful. Whether she had or had not been schizophrenic, after her lobotomy she did not return home and start cleaning the house or being a proper wife. Rather, she shriveled up and contracted. And after that particular state mental hospital was closed, she was sent to Laguna Honda, where she was placed in a bed and turned every two hours to prevent bedsores and called out all day long in a high-pitched and distressed voice, "My cat, my cat, my cat, my cat."

It was because of patients like Mrs. Lantos that Jimmy Turner had won the right to refuse psychiatric medications unless he was psychotic—even though the reason he was no longer psychotic was that he was involuntarily taking them.

In many ways it had been the right decision, but, like so many of our society's decisions that end up as laws, it was intractable. It was a law. And, while medicating people because they don't conform to our ideas of rationality had been incorrect, the more I saw of people like Jimmy—of the acutely psychotic, the real schizophrenic—the more inclined I was to believe that schizophrenia was not primarily a mental affliction, but a physical disease with mental concomitants.

When I'd first read Jung and decided to become a Jungian psychiatrist, I'd accepted the idea that schizophrenia was a mental disease with philosophical significance. Then, during my year as a psychiatric intern, I'd been impressed by the success of the antipsychotic medications, though not entirely sure of the ethics of using them to change someone's worldview.

But at Laguna Honda I'd seen many more schizophrenic patients, for a much longer period of time, and I'd been struck by how stereotypic their symptoms were. The Chinese schizophrenic, the Filipino schizophrenic, the English schizophrenic, the Jewish, Greek Orthodox, Muslim schizophrenic, all had the same fear: that someone—the FBI, the KGB, the Grand Order of the Saints, the Kabala, the

Devil—was following them, listening to them, talking to them, commanding them. Then, when given psychiatric medications, which block the brain chemicals of dopamine, serotonin, and other still-unknown compounds, they improved. The volume of their voices diminished; their fears lessened and even disappeared.

Gradually I became convinced that schizophrenia is not primarily a mental disease, but a physical disease with a good, if not perfect, treatment. It is probably a chemical deficiency of some kind and, therefore, just as medical a problem as any other chemical deficiency— of insulin, of thyroid hormone, of cortisone—that also has mental effects. I also learned that it is a painful disease, a disease of solitude and terror, of waking nightmares, and of fear, a disease I would want treated if I had it. And it is a disease such that those who have it cannot know they have it and need treatment, any more than a patient hallucinating because of low blood sugar, too much thyroid hormone, or too little cortisone knows what is wrong and what is needed.

So letting Jimmy sign himself out of the hospital without his medications was, to my mind, as mistaken, as wrong, as letting a delirious patient sign himself out without treatment. Our psychiatrist emphasized this when he observed that if we declared Jimmy's delusions due to a medical condition—AIDS, syphilis, or Wilson's disease—we could treat him without his consent. But a schizophrenic like Jimmy? No.

So one fine spring day at the beginning of April, Mr. Jimmy Turner, resuscitated crazy person, untreated schizophrenic, left the hospital. He took nothing with him but ambled out, wearing the Levi's and the plaid shirt he'd picked up in our clothing department. Several weeks later the social worker told me that Jimmy had been spotted in a clearing in the park. He was dead.

And this is a death I regret to this day. Because it was a prevent-able death, as preventable as a death from pneumonia. And also, in a manner of speaking, it was a preventable life.

n the meantime, my studies of Hildegard and humoral medicine were coming along. I had taken all the courses that Professor Brown gave and all the classes that Dr. Weitz's Department of Medical History offered, and I was well into my master's thesis.

As Dr. Weitz had warned me at my interview, his department was a very small department, beset by a modernity that did not believe in the value of history. Medical history, anyway, only really began at the end of the nineteenth century, when humoral medicine gave way to modern medicine. Before this, although there had been a kind of history of the Great Doctors, such as Hippocrates and Galen, and of new medicines, such as quinine and caffeine, medical history didn't really exist. It had been the discontinuity between premodern and modern medicine that had created the need to understand the now-incomprehensible past.

But by the time Dr. Weitz arrived, the department was at the end of its flush period, and during his tenure, as modern medicine became ever more successful, the past became ever less compelling. Every year his budget was cut, his endowments raided, and his tiny depart-ment threatened. He did what he could; every year he presented himself to the budget committee and pleaded the case for medical history. He opened his department up to the study of health care and changed its name from History of Medicine to History of Health Sci-ences. He gave free lectures and held fund-raisers and succeeded, amazingly enough, in building the department with new postdoctoral fellows, with PhD students, and even with a second professor, Jack Pressman.

Unlike Professor Doctor Weitz, however, Jack was not a physician. Instead of going to medical school, he'd gone straight to graduate school for a PhD in the history of science. This was no longer unusual; there was a whole new generation of medical historians who had PhDs but not MDs. They were scholars, but not doctors, and they studied medicine from the point of view of the patient, not the doctor. Indeed, they were skeptical of the doctor's point of view. They interpreted medical professionalization as simple power politics, and, though few, they had an outsized effect on the health-care policy decisions of the 1980s and 1990s. The closure of the state mental hospitals, for instance, was based on research by a PhD graduate student about the negative effects of institutionalization on mental patients. Jack was young and energetic, and we became friends instantly. He talked fast and laughed often, and was Professor Doctor Weitz's polar opposite. Together the two of them made a good, if truncated, team for my research.

My master's thesis was to be a prelude to my PhD, and the question Jack and Dr. Weitz wanted me to answer with it was: What was the context of Hildegard's medicine? That is, who else was practicing medicine in the twelfth century? How were they trained? What medications did they use? What theories did they hold? Their idea was that I would apply what we already knew about premodern medicine to Hildegard, and then apply what I learned about Hildegard's medicine to fill out our understanding of premodern medicine. No one had ever done that. Instead, Hildegard's medicine was dismissed by historians as simply an example of saintly medicine, based only on faith and prayer. No one had tried to use it as a way to understand premodern medicine, or use premodern medicine as a way to understand it.

I started by researching the kind of medicine practiced around Hildegard in twelfth-century Germany. I learned that there were many kinds of practitioners—monks, university-educated doctors, herbalists, and Jewish doctors. Each had a different way of learning medicine—as an apprentice, at a university, through family and friends—and each had his own medical texts, in German, Latin, or Hebrew. Many of these texts survived, and I studied them. All of them, I was surprised to discover, although written in different languages and coming from different traditions, were similar. Each had a simple, practical structure. First, a short explanation of the System of the Fours; next, an explanation of the humoral body; last, a series of herbal prescriptions for the maladies of the body, in order, from head to toe.

When I compared Hildegard's text, *Causae et Curae,* to them, it was not different. It was structured just like the others, and was practical, relying on medications, not on prayer. Hildegard did have her own way of looking at things, and she did include some things that the other texts did not include—a technique for bleeding a patient; a method for moxibustion. She even had a section on taking care of farm animals, which I found rather whimsical, particularly her herbal prescription for headache in mules. But on the whole, Hildegard's medicine simply reflected the usual practice of medicine in the twelfth century.

I wrote up my thesis; Jack and Dr. Weitz approved it, and they advanced me to the doctoral level.

My PhD, I decided, would be a much deeper exploration of Hildegard's medicine. I would immerse myself into her life, education and medical training, into her context, and, finally, into her practice of medicine, which I wanted to understand thoroughly, as if it were mine.

Dr. Weitz advised me that my plan was quite ambitious. It would take me years. I might even have to spend some time in Europe, studying medieval medical manuscripts in the old libraries.

That would be fine with me, I told him. I enjoyed my every-other-day alternation between practicing medicine in the hospital and exploring Hildegard's medicine in the library. Each illuminated the other. It would be good for me to have an alternative world anyway, since, with the report of Dee and Tee, the going at Laguna Honda was beginning, but just beginning, to get the tiniest bit rocky.

t was Kathleen who told me that Dee and Tee had finished their investigation and, after six months, were leaving.

Kathleen was one of our Irish-Catholic nurses. Redheaded with pale, delicate skin and clear blue eyes, she had an honest, almost naive face. As an Irish-Catholic, she belonged to the oldest sect of the hospital's nurses, which reached back in a continuous line to the nurses of the city's almshouse of 1862, and further back to the nuns who took care of the almshouse patient before it was called an almshouse, when it was still the hospice of the Middle Ages.

I liked Kathleen. She was a good nurse—attentive and careful, with a strong work ethic and a willing pair of hands. Also, conforming to two out of the three of the traditional requirements for a nun, she was obedient and stable, though, being married, not chaste. She had trained as a student nurse with us; and then, after her RN degree, stayed on in the admitting ward. Over the years she would rise in the nursing hierarchy from floor nurse to charge nurse to head nurse, and finally to nursing supervisor, although never into the august region of assistant nursing director.

We ran into each other in the hallway, and Kathleen pulled me into the linen closet and shut the door.

There was a reason for this: The director of nursing, Miss Lester, did not approve of fraternization between nurse and doctor. Evolving friendships, confidences, even the usual caretaking of nurse for doctor—making coffee, hanging up white coats—she viewed askance. Nurses seen to be too friendly with the doctors would find themselves mysteriously transferred to a different ward and a nighttime schedule, and all the nurses except for Larissa took account of this.

Consequently, I got to know the linen closets on many of the wards quite well. I liked them, especially the linen closet on the admitting ward. It was a little smaller than the doctors' office, and it, too, had a long window at its far end. Wooden shelves lined its walls, on which were stacked the white towels, white sheets, and white cotton blankets our patients used. The linen closet was always sweet-smelling and heated, so that the towels, sheets, and blankets started out, at least, warm and clean. The linen closet was also private.

"Did you hear?" Kathleen asked. "Dee and Tee left yesterday."

"Really! You know, they never talked to us doctors," I told her.

"Well, they never talked to us nurses either."

"What have you heard?"

"Well. They didn't like us very much. They didn't like the building—the open wards, the open windows, the open spaces. But they know they can't do much about that until it's replaced. So their main recommendation is going to be to cut the number of head nurses in half."

"How are they going to do that?" I asked.

"They're going to change the title of head nurse to nurse manager and give each nurse manager two wards instead of one. She'll carry a beeper and have to supervise both!"

She looked to me for indignation. I didn't know what to say. It didn't seem like such a bad idea. Cutting one-half of the head nurses would save a lot of money, and, at the time, I didn't know much about what the head nurses actually did. On the admitting ward, our head nurse was certainly very busy, what with our thirty-six sick patients, our four or five daily admissions, and our four or five daily discharges, and I couldn't imagine her with two wards to run.

I also knew that the head nurses made up the caring structure of the hospital, just as the wards made up its physical structure. Each head nurse was responsible for her own ward, and this went all the way back to the medieval monastery. The earliest monastic infirmary was built like a church, with an altar at the end and patients in beds along the walls, under windows; a monk or nun infirmarian was in charge.

After the Middle Ages, other organizational structures for the hospital and the almshouse were tried, but when Florence Nightingale wrote her *Notes on Hospitals* in the middle of the nineteenth century, she favored the medieval. Hospitals should be made up of individual wards she called "pavilions." Each ward, she advised, should have thirty or so patients, with beds set up along the long walls and a solarium at its far end. Each ward should be independent of all the others and capable of acting like a small hospital within the larger. Most important, each ward should have its own head nurse; she would sit at the front, observing and being observed by all thirty patients at once. The head nurse would be in charge of the ward; one head nurse, one ward.

Nightingale's recommendations were why our wards were structured as they were, each with about thirty beds, a solarium at the far end, and a head nurse at the other; and they were why the head nurse was in charge of her own ward, which was architecturally and in fact a minihospital inside the larger one.

In my visits to other wards I was always struck by how, despite their architectural similarity, each ward had its own character—cheerful or somber, quiet or noisy, social or lonely. Each ward was decorated individually and had its own kind of patient, too; each seemed like its own neighborhood within the village of the hospital. But, until that conversation with Kathleen in the linen closet, I'd never stopped to think about how much, or whether, this individuality depended on the head nurse. All I knew for sure is that when I went to a ward, the head nurse was always sitting in her chair at the glassed-in nursing station, and from there she monitored her ward, both patients and staff. She also answered the phones, tidied the charts, talked to the families, and helped the nurses, if they were busy, with whatever they had to do. Still, cutting the number of head nurses by 50 percent would save a lot of money, and, though I didn't tell Kathleen, I wasn't sure whether it was a good idea or not.

When Dee and Tee's report came out some months later, Kathleen turned out to be right.

Dee and Tee had been taken aback by their time at Laguna Honda, the report said. They'd been stunned by the immensity of the aged facility and its inefficiencies of space; by its wide, tiled corridors and its long, open windows; by its legless smokers congregating in the hall and drinking out of brown paper bags. They'd been appalled by the time the therapists wasted in taking care of the aviary, the greenhouse, and the barnyard; by the live-in priest, by the resident nun, and by the podiatry students who lived in an unused wing.

Above all, the report said, they'd been amazed by the anachronistic presence of a head nurse on every one of the hospital's thirty-eight wards. As far as they could tell, this head nurse did nothing but sit most of the day in her chair in the nursing station. She answered the phone, to be sure, and kept the charts tidy; now and again she went out and inspected a patient with one of her nurses. Also, she made coffee, kept the TV room and lounge neat, organized patients' birthday parties, and, in general, did whatever needed to be done. It was a pleasant job, Dee and Tee observed, helpful, no doubt, but one hundred years after Frederick Taylor's description of scientific management, and in a time of tightening health-care budgets, such a use of a skilled RN was excessive. They'd even seen one head nurse whose only task was knitting. That's right, a head nurse who, as far as they could tell, spent all day in her chair at the head of her ward, doing nothing except knitting blankets and booties for her patients.

So their main recommendation was to change the nursing structure at Laguna Honda. The job of head nurse should be eliminated. Instead, a new nurse manager position should be created, where each nurse manager would be responsible for two wards instead of one. She would no longer answer the phones, tidy the charts, or help out with patient care. Rather she would manage the staff. And managing meant instituting the fastest, most efficient way of providing care.

This would require a significant use of resources in order to retrain the remaining head nurses—many hours and days would be spent in education and training meetings. But in the end, Dee and Tee were sure, this would produce a tighter ship. And, for certain, it would save a lot of money right away—nineteen salaries, amounting to about two million dollars a year, of which Dee and Tee, as per their contract, would receive 10 percent.

Although the full report was never released, a ripple of distur-

bance went through the hospital. Soon after, one-half of the head
nurses were cut. They weren't actually laid off, though, but simply
reassigned to other administrative positions. The other half were
given a beeper, two wards, a new title, and considerable training in the
principles of scientific management. As for their former duties—
those were not reassigned. They would be done by whoever had the
free time to do them.

I t was a lesson in the inefficiency of efficiency. And the best way to
explain that is to tell you about the head nurse who knit. Because
Dee and Tee had been correct; there was a head nurse who sat at the
head of her ward and knit all day.

I'd first run into the results of her industry on one of my days covering the hospital when, on the way through the wide hall to another
ward, I passed two little ladies sitting outside of their ward. They had
been wheeled there so that they could have a porchlike view of the
passing world, and they looked almost identical, with white hair,
small bodies, and quiet manner. What made me stop were their blankets. The lady on the left was wrapped in a thick, hand-knit white and
blue blanket; and the lady on the right had a hand-knit white and
purple blanket tucked around her.

When I got back to the admitting ward, I asked Larissa about the
blankets, and she told me that the head nurse of their ward had vowed
to knit blankets and booties for each of her thirty-six charges. I
should go take a look. So I walked back to that ward.

It was a little-old-lady ward, with thirty-six little old ladies—
white-haired, tiny, and old—and sure enough, almost every one was
wrapped in or had on her bed a hand-knit blanket: white and green,
white and red, white and yellow. And there was the head nurse, sitting

in her chair in the nursing station, answering the phone, fussing with the charts, observing her charges, and knitting one of the few blankets remaining to be done.

I've thought a lot about those blankets since the disappearance of the head nurses and their well-run neighborhoods of wards. About what the blankets meant and what they signified. And here's the thing: The blankets made me sit up and take notice. Made me pay attention. Marked out that head nurse as especially attentive, especially present, especially caring. It put me and everyone else on notice.

It's not that the ladies for whom they were knitted appreciated them or even noticed them. Who did notice was—everyone else. Visiting family noticed. Looking down the center aisle, they saw two rows of little white-haired ladies—their mothers, great-aunts, and sisters—each lady bundled up in a bright, many-colored, hand-knit blanket. They also saw that each had makeup on, and her hair done and her nails polished, by the nurses who knew that, down at the end of the ward, was the head nurse, knitting. The Russian ambulance drivers noticed, when they rushed onto the ward to pick up one of the ladies, that each was wrapped in a colorful identifying blanket. They also noticed the head nurse, sitting in the nursing station, answering the phones, arranging the charts, and directing them to the correct patient. Even the doctors noticed. The blankets put us all on notice that this was a head nurse who cared.

Those knitted blankets lasted for years, through many other investigations, and every time I passed a little lady wrapped in one, I thought about that head nurse, about her vow, and about Dee and Tee. And about efficiency. Because those blankets signified even more than attention and caring. The click of that head nurse's knitting needles was the meditative click of—nothing more to be done. Although it had seemed to Dee and Tee that the head nurse did nothing except knit, that nothing was the nothing that, as the Tao says, the Superior Man does when everything that was supposed to be done has been done.

We did get used to the new system eventually. The remaining staff learned to answer the phones, tidy the charts, talk to families, help the doctors, survey the ward, and support one another at the same time as they were looking on the computer or filling out the forms that the new nurse managers created. But the new system had a cost. It was stressful. After the head nurses were cut in half, there were more illnesses and more sick days among the staff; there were more injuries, more disabilities, and earlier retirements. Among the patients, there were more falls, more bedsores, more fights, and more tears. And this, in the broader scheme of things—even of economics—is not efficient.

It was not unlike the closing of the state mental hospitals, which had also seemed at the time so efficient and so cost-effective on paper. And was efficient and cost-effective—on paper. Just not in the real world, where good budgeting intentions will be cut; ideals will be compromised; and where, sometimes, what has no place in the Excel spreadsheet is the key to what makes a system, even a hospital, work.

The report of Dee and Tee taught me not only the lesson of the inefficiency of efficiency. It also taught me the lesson of the efficiency of inefficiency.

Because it wasn't just the tasks of the head nurse that fell by the wayside with Dee and Tee's recommendations. It wasn't even their watchful re-creation of neighborhoods within the village of the hospital. It was the time they had, the unassigned time, that not only belonged to them but spread itself to all the staff—doctors included. That unassigned time, as inefficient as it seemed to Dee and Tee, turned out to be one of the secret ingredients of Laguna Honda. With the elimination of the head nurses, so economical on paper, some of that extra time was also eliminated, and with it, some of the mental space to focus and to care. There was, I discovered, a connection between inefficiency and good care, and it was epitomized by one of my heroes, the handsome Dr. Curtis.

Four

THE MIRACULOUS HEALING
OF TERRY BECKER

DR. CURTIS WAS HANDSOME as soon as I saw him, which isn't always the case. Many of my friends and even patients seem pretty ordinary at first, and only as I get to know them do they become attractive. But Dr. Curtis was handsome right away. In fact, he was the handsomest of the physicians in a group of rather good-looking doctors. Dr. Major had a penchant for good-looking people.

I met Dr. Curtis during my first week, while I was standing in the wide hall with the vending machines, looking at the scene. The hall was filled with cigarette smoke and patients in wheelchairs, who were gathered at the round tables, with cigarettes at the corner of their mouths, intently playing poker. The vending machines dispensed candy, ice cream, and coffee in paper cups printed with playing cards, and the patients were also betting on them, I saw, as the coffee came out of the machine.

Dr. Curtis suddenly appeared next to me, and stood with me looking at the patients. Up until then, I'd seen him only from a distance as a trim, quick-moving figure. I knew that he was the assistant medical director and that he was leaving the hospital the next day to join a private practice on the coast. I also knew that when he wasn't being a doctor he was being a surfer, and as he stood next to me, I noticed that he had a kind of surfer stance, holding himself from the center of his body, perfectly balanced. He was wearing a Hawaiian shirt. His hair was black and curly, and when he turned to talk to me I saw that his face was square and clean-shaven, his blue eyes warm and attentive.

But it was his manner and smile that were arresting. His manner was quiet and poised; he seemed light on his feet and ready for anything. And his smile was particular. He didn't show his teeth; rather, the corners of his mouth turned slightly up—exactly the smile of ancient Etruria—in a benign gaze that seemed to see just a bit into the distance. Standing next to me, Dr. Curtis was also looking at the scene, amused more than bemused. Then, out of nowhere, he said in a solemn tone and without any introduction, "You may not realize it, Victoria, but you should know that Laguna Honda is a special place."

It was an odd thing to say, and I looked at him more closely. "What do you mean?"

He smiled. "Laguna Honda is a gift. You'll see."

And with that he drifted off.

It was clearly a message, but what he meant by it and why he delivered it to me, I didn't know. Nevertheless, I remembered what he said; I tucked it away and took it out, now and again, when something remarkable, touching, or strange happened at the hospital.

I didn't see Dr. Curtis again for a number of years. He joined a private clinic on the coast and threw himself into creating the kind of medical practice that attended to what mattered to him: the way patients felt, the way the staff felt, and the preventative measures he believed in—exercise, diet, happiness.

But like so many of the staff who left, to the accompaniment of parties and thank-yous and presents and plaques, after a few years, Dr. Curtis returned. He preferred the city. The surfing wasn't that much better on the coast; city schools were better for his children; and he liked Laguna Honda. So he took up his duties as assistant medical director once again. This meant that while Dr. Major was at her ever-more-frequent meetings, Dr. Curtis was minding the store. He took care of the patients and covered the wards of doctors who were sick or on vacation; he interviewed prospective new doctors; he wrote procedures and protocols; and he provided a sympathetic ear for angry, stressed, or divorcing physicians—or sometimes just an ear.

Since the admitting ward pretty much took care of itself, I saw him only rarely—up in the X-ray department or in the hallways. Still, I got to know him and discover that Dr. Curtis was a serious as well as a handsome man. What he was serious about was living his life well. After college he had not gone directly to medical school but to India, and there he studied yoga and Sanskrit and the lute. Then he decided to become a physician; he wanted to put yoga and Indian spirituality and Indian medicine into practice, so he strummed his way back to the United States and went to medical school. He came to Laguna Honda after he discovered the hospice movement and decided to set up the first hospice in the city.

He set about doing so lucidly, harmoniously, and with integrity; and within a year he had pulled in not only Dr. Major, who was easy, but also Miss Lester, director of nursing, who was not. Like

Manjusri, the Indian god whose sword of discrimination cuts through difficulties, Dr. Curtis cut through knots and charmed away intransigence. He obtained grants for his hospice project and the service of all kinds of volunteers—Zen meditators, hippie harpists, volunteer gardeners. Then, once his new hospice unit was up and running, settled and operating smoothly, he handed it off, along with its glory, to Dr. Kay. Dr. Curtis wasn't just enthusiastic, he was an enthusiast, in the ancient Greek sense of *entheos*—"having a god within"—and, as with the rest of us, his strengths were his weaknesses. He did not take root. He stayed where he stayed as long as was needed and then went on to his next project, his next enthusiasm.

Dr. Curtis was one of my heroes at the hospital because, with his keen eyes, free of the spectacles the rest of us wore, he not only seemed to see farther and deeper than the rest of us but did, in fact, see farther and deeper. So while Dr. Romero's and Dr. Fintner's admitting notes were detailed and elegant, and Dr. Jeffers's scrawly and to the point, Dr. Curtis's were often no more than a page, neatly printed. I saw one once that was no more than a few sentences: Mr. Gates was terminal; he was to have hospice care; his family had been contacted; he was at peace.

I learned a lot from Dr. Curtis, but it was with the case of the missing shoes that he taught me the most about care and caring, time and inefficiency.

On this particular day, I met him by accident in the wide, windowed corridor that ran the length of the hospital and connected all the wards. He was in a hurry.

Where was he going? I asked.

Back to the rehabilitation ward, he said, where he was covering for a few weeks.

The rehabilitation ward, like the admitting ward, was its own minihospital within Laguna Honda. It admitted the patients with the milder strokes and the less traumatic head injuries, most of whom would recover and be discharged back to their homes, if they had them, although its patients, too, were often without friends, money, or health insurance. Like the admitting ward, it had its own physicians to admit, examine, and discharge its patients, and this month, Dr. Curtis was one of them.

He'd just returned from outside the hospital, he told me, and was headed back to a patient who, having been rehabilitated after a stroke, had been ready for discharge for months. But every day when Dr. Curtis made his rounds, checking on the thirty-six patients on the ward, this patient was still there, still zipping around in his wheelchair, still going to therapy.

"Finally," Dr. Curtis said, "I asked him why, since he was able to walk, he was still here. Why was he still in a wheelchair? Why hadn't he been discharged?"

"No shoes, doc. They ordered me special shoes, but they're waiting for Medicaid to approve them."

"How long have they been waiting?" Dr. Curtis asked.

"Three months."

Dr. Curtis thought a bit. "What size shoe do you wear?"

"Size nine."

Dr. Curtis reflected for a while. He thought about his duties, his other patients, the charts he had to dictate, the quality-assurance forms he had to fill out. And then he left the hospital, got in his car, and drove to Walmart, where he bought a pair of size-nine running shoes for $16.99. He'd just come back with the shoes and was going over to the ward to put them on the patient and write the discharge orders.

Was he planning to submit his receipt for reimbursement? I asked.

He laughed.

As I watched him hurry back to the rehabilitation ward, I wondered: Why had Dr. Curtis done this? And why hadn't anyone else?

It was a simple thing to do, but it never would have occurred to me to do it. I would have been frustrated with the shoe delay, of course, and I would have filled out a second or even a third Medicaid request. I might even have written Medicaid or braved its phone tree to complain about the time that pair of shoes was taking. But it would never have occurred to me to go to Walmart and buy the patient's shoes. I had too much to do, too many forms to fill out, too many other patients to see. It would have meant crossing a kind of inefficiency boundary. And yet Dr. Curtis got in his car without much questioning; and he was hurrying back to the ward with the shoes to put them on the patient—himself.

He reminded me of an aphorism I loved but had never understood: "The secret in the care of the patient is in caring for the patient." I'd always assumed that it meant caring about the patient—loving or at least liking the patient—but when I saw Dr. Curtis rushing off to put shoes on a patient he barely knew, I thought there must be more to it than that. So I tracked down the quote and found it in a talk by Dr. Francis Peabody to the graduating medical class of Harvard in 1927. It turned out that Dr. Peabody didn't mean caring about a patient but caring for a patient, which, he explained, meant doing the little things, the little personal things that nurses usually do—adjusting a patient's bedclothes or giving him sips of water. That took time, Dr. Peabody admitted, and wasn't, perhaps, the most efficient way for doctors to spend their time. But it was worth it, he told his students, because that kind of time-costly caring was what created the personal relationship between patient and doctor. And that relationship was the secret of healing.

So what Dr. Peabody really was saying was that the secret in the care of the patient was—inefficiency.

It was ironic. And it was also ironic that, while Dee and Tee were examining just about everything about the hospital (except its patients)—the books, protocols, costs, and revenues—Dr. Curtis had been providing the most efficient health care of all, leaving his ostensible duties to perform his real duty. He must have saved the healthcare system many thousands of dollars by buying those shoes, and yet Dee and Tee would not have thought his action efficient. They would have thought it very inefficient—wasteful of the time of a highly paid, highly trained physician.

Dr. Curtis also reminded me of the Indian description of the good, the better, and the best doctor. The good doctor makes the right diagnosis and prescribes the proper treatment. But the better doctor also walks with his patient to the pharmacy. And the best doctor waits in the pharmacy until his patient swallows the medicine. Going to Walmart to buy shoes was exactly what the best doctor would do.

Before Dr. Curtis and the shoes, I'd striven to be a good doctor—to make the right diagnosis and prescribe the right treatment. Dr. Curtis raised the bar. Miss Tod taught me the importance of the little things—a changed diet, a prescription for new glasses; Dr. Curtis taught me that I might consider, now and then, fetching the food or fixing the eyeglasses myself.

Afterward, I did that sometimes, as did many of the doctors at the hospital. Once in a while I would cook special food for an anorexic patient or fix the eyeglasses of a desperate reader—downstairs in the clinic with the beautiful tools in their shabby velvet case and the huge jar of ancient eyeglass screws. Such inefficient care often was efficient, in the sense that it solved a problem quickly and definitively. And I wondered for the first time whether Laguna Honda's care, with all of its inefficiencies, might not actually be more efficient than Dee and Tee's cost-effective health care. Even from a monetary, Excel-spreadsheet point of view.

We did have many inefficiencies at Laguna Honda, and I had my favorites. There was Christmas, for instance, which was particularly inefficient, especially the Christmas presents.

Every year, the morning before Christmas—and I mean real Christmas, not Happy-Holidays-Hanukkah-Kwanzaa Christmas—with its dusty trees and resuscitated ornaments, the police department would deliver 2,356 wrapped presents. To the women's wards, presents for women; to the men's wards, presents for men. Every patient in the hospital would receive two wrapped presents, and talk about inefficient! That entire morning nothing else happened. I'm not even sure that patients got all their morning medications, although, knowing the head nurses, they probably did. The activity therapist of each ward would place the two presents, one small and one large, at each patient's bedside, and then the rest of the staff would gather around to watch, or often help, the patients open them.

There would be plaid shirts for the men (red, blue, green; small, medium, large) and cardigan sweaters for the women (pink, blue, beige). In the small packages, watches (steel, gold, silver). And for the rest of the morning there would be the trading of shirts and watches; the collecting of wrapping paper, ribbons, and boxes; the fitting of batteries to watches; the donning and doffing of clothes; the swapping of colors and sizes. It was extremely inefficient, and it wasn't even health care.

Later, after the head nurses were eliminated, the new nurse managers, busier and more efficient, changed the system. The packages were still delivered to the wards, but written on them were size, color, and style; and days before Christmas, the activity therapists would take orders from the patients. A steel watch or silver? A blue cardigan or pink? The day before Christmas, presents would be passed out appropriately. It was quieter; it took less time; and the patients did still receive their new shirt, sweater, watch. But it was not as much fun, neither for staff nor for patients. It was subdued and a little sad. And it made me wonder whether fun, although inefficient, might actually be therapeutic and, therefore, efficient.

Even Christmas was not my favorite inefficiency, however. My favorite inefficiency was the barnyard, the greenhouse, and the aviary. I only got out to the aviary once, but once was enough.

The aviary was next to the barnyard, and it was enormous: long and tall and made out of large panes of glass set into a wooden frame. Its walls were lined with homemade wooden worktables, whose surfaces were covered with droppings from the doves and pigeons roosting in the nests above the tables. There were also finches and sparrows, who, like the hospital's homeless but healthy patients, had somehow sneaked in. On the left of the entrance were incubators with chicken eggs and, in a box on the right, chicks.

The activity therapists were in charge of the aviary, the greenhouse, and the barnyard. On Saturdays they brought patients out from the hospital to the greenhouse to pot little bent plants, which was how Mrs. McCoy got the plant she gave me. During the week they sometimes brought patients to the barnyard to visit the rabbits in their hutches, the little black potbellied pigs who foraged in the lawn, and the birds in the aviary.

One day an activity therapist took an incubator and some eggs to the AIDS ward, and a few weeks later one of the eggs hatched into a chicken. This was before effective treatment for AIDS, and Dr. Curtis had set up the AIDS ward as an extension of hospice, so that AIDS patients could die in peace. And they did die, almost every day, usually after becoming demented. Demented or not, the AIDS patients loved that AIDS chicken, who turned into the AIDS hen and roamed through the open ward, pecking at the bread the patients saved her from their meals. Also at the potato chips (which she didn't much like), the soft green peas (ditto), and the limp lettuce. She preferred bread. Still, she did quite well; she survived many patients.

Of course she was messy, being no less than the demented men with AIDS, untrainable and incontinent, and she left bits of lettuce and chicken droppings around, but the nurses cleaned up after her. Which was inefficient, not to speak of unhygienic, as the investigating nurse from the State Licensing Bureau noted in one of her reports. Although, as a matter of fact, in the months when the AIDS hen roamed the open AIDS ward, she did keep her diseases to herself, as the AIDS patients did for her.

Nevertheless, it was deemed unhygienic to have an AIDS hen wandering about the ward, and one day she was gone.

As for inefficient, she was that, too, but there was therapy in her inefficiency. I can't document the numbers, but it was worth my while to walk to the AIDS ward just to see the spark of interest in those cachectic faces when lunch was served and the AIDS hen began her strut down the ward. It was a spark of life, an extra spark and sparkle that must have extended a life or two by a day or two, which, when you only have a few days left, is worth something.

I wasn't sure whether all of the hospital's inefficiencies were therapeutic, but I did begin to wonder how it would come out if they were all added up. Correct diagnoses instead of incorrect ones. Visits to the emergency room avoided because doctors had enough time to spend with their patients. Feelings soothed, glasses fixed, free avian entertainment. Would the money saved on unnecessary hospital days by a doctor who runs out and buys shoes at Walmart balance out or even pay for luxuries like the best food and drink, massages, fresh flowers, alternative medicine? I began to think that perhaps, in this new day of evidence-based medicine, the Laguna Honda model of inefficient health care deserved a trial.

During all this time, I was working on my PhD on Hildegard and premodern medicine. I had completed all the requirements, including German, Latin, and French, and put together my thesis committee; now I began sketching out my dissertation. I wanted it to show how premodern medicine could work as a way for conceptualizing the body, once its underlying horticultural metaphor was understood.

I would explain Hildegard's medicine and the System of the Fours using her text and those other medical texts in Latin, German, and Hebrew that I'd unearthed in my master's thesis. I would show that the four elements, four qualities, and four humors were not the abstractions of the philosopher, as most writers had assumed, but the practical concerns of the gardener. It was ambitious. I would start small, I decided. I would start by condensing my master's thesis into an article for publication.

It was not unlike condensing everything I knew about a patient into that essence: the history of present illness. And right away I ran into something I'd missed in my master's thesis—Hildegard's remark-able concept of *viriditas*. *Viriditas* comes from the Latin word for green, *viridis*—which also gives the French *vert,* and the Italian and Spanish *verde*. *Viriditas* meant greenness. So usually it referred to the color of plants or of gems like emerald, although it was also used met-aphorically to mean vigor or youthfulness.

But Hildegard used *viriditas*—greening or greenness—in a broader sense, I learned as I wrote my article. She used it to mean the power of plants to put forth leaves, flowers, and fruits; and she also used it for the analogous power of human beings to grow, to give birth, and to heal. I didn't know how I'd missed it in my thesis. But there it was—greenness—a medical or perhaps spiritual concept that supported the gardening analogy I saw at the basis of premodern medicine. Had Hildegard invented the concept? I wondered. Was there a precedent in older medical texts for a power related to plants that also stood for the body's ability to heal?

I spent the next year investigating those two questions, and in the meantime I met Terry Becker, who would show me what *viriditas* really meant.

I f Jimmy was my skinniest patient and my patient who gained the most weight, then Terry was my longest and most miraculous patient. I had her for the longest time, she teetered the most on the edge of disaster, and she ended up by surprising me the most.

And the best way to tell you about Terry, about what she meant for me—the first time I admitted her, the second, the third, and now, when I look at her paid obituary in the *River City Times*—is to start with the photograph attached to that obituary.

You wouldn't call her pretty, but her face, at least through the medical retrospectoscope, is arresting; it is the face of a robust, barely smiling Native American. Hair thick, dark, and flowing down her back; full face with broad cheekbones, dangling beaded earrings, beaded necklaces, and beaded armbands. Behind the glasses we gave her on the day she left the hospital, her eyes are dark and Indian.

That picture tells it all; it shows just what Laguna Honda could do in its time and with its time. Whether it was efficient or inefficient, I'll leave you to decide, but I think you'll agree that only death is truly efficient. Life is very inefficient and not cost-effective at all, from a health-care efficiency point of view.

met Terry for the first time while taking care of the rehabilitation ward. Its usual doctor was on vacation; Dr. Curtis was elsewhere; and the admitting ward was temporarily closed due to the budget crisis, which occurred annually. No matter whether the economy was good, great, or a disaster, our city's budget was always in crisis and the hospital's budget especially so. When it came down to it, why did our city need an almshouse? No other city still had its almshouse. In other cities, patients somehow found elsewhere to go, and though that was more expensive in the long run, in the short run it was way less expensive. So there was always a money crisis and always attempts to cut Laguna Honda's budget.

Dr. Major took this particular budget crisis as a challenge, however, and she decided to make a point by shutting down the admitting ward. This meant that no new patients could be admitted, except for patients for rehabilitation who could go to the rehabilitation ward and terminal patients who could go to the hospice ward. All the other patients in the city who normally would have come to us, could not; instead they stayed on at the County Hospital and at other hospitals around the city, waiting for someplace to go. Since hospitals did not get paid for patients who no longer needed acute care, this meant that hospitals around the city were losing money and pressure was, therefore, being applied to approve Laguna Honda's usual budget as soon as possible. In the meantime, Dr. Fintner and I were taking care of the patients on the rehabilitation ward.

That was how I met Terry Becker the first time. She was transferred from the County Hospital for rehabilitation, and I admitted her.

She was a street person, I read in her records, a heroin addict, and a prostitute; she had a boyfriend; and they lived on the streets. She'd been fine—at any rate, in her usual health—until twelve days before, when she woke up to find that she could no longer move her arms or her legs. So her boyfriend took her over to the emergency room and there the diagnosis was made: she had transverse myelitis, which is an inflammation of the spinal cord that, in just a few hours, can cause a section of the spinal cord to swell against the inner bony sides of the spinal column. This swelling is devastating to the body's ability to move because the spinal cord is made up of nerves that act like wires, transmitting messages and impulses between the brain and the rest of the body. When the spinal cord swells, the nerves stop working, and everything past the swelling can't function. Terry's swelling was in her neck. So she couldn't move anything past her neck—not her arms or legs, bowel or bladder. Transverse myelitis is a rare disease, one in a hundred thousand, but Laguna Honda being what it was, Terry was my third case.

The County Hospital admitted her, and its doctors made sure that there was no other cause for her paralysis, such as AIDS, syphilis, or multiple sclerosis. Then they waited to see if she would get better, which is often the case. She did get better, but not enough better to go back on the streets, and so they sent her over to us for rehabilitation. The nurses assigned her to one of the double-bedded semiprivate rooms at the entrance to the rehabilitation ward, and after I'd reviewed her records, I went over to her room to see her. When I got to her room, I stopped in the doorway and looked in.

She was sitting in her wheelchair with her back to me, staring out the window; an uncovered urine bag was hanging from her chair. No one else was in the room—no friends or family—and nothing of her was in the room either—not even the usual plastic bag of clothes, framed photos, and cigarette packs left in a lump by the Russian ambulance drivers. Then I knocked on the open door, walked in, and went around the wheelchair to take a closer look.

She was worn, like so many of the drug users and street people, and looked to be in her fifties, though I knew from her records that she was only thirty-seven. She was very thin. Her long, colorless hair was stringy and unwashed; her face was tired and drawn, and there were dark circles under her dark eyes. Her teeth were decayed; her nails dirty, untrimmed, and stained with nicotine; and she was positioned uncomfortably in the chair, with her neck awry. Her eyes, when she looked up at me, were slightly out of focus.

"Can I sit on the bed?" I asked.

"Can I have a cigarette?" she replied.

I sat down. "After I talk to you for a bit and examine you; how about that?"

She sized me up. I wasn't very big, but I was determined, and she couldn't move.

"Okay."

I commenced my exam. On the whole, the news was good. She was able to move her right shoulder and her right foot, a bit. Also she was able to feel her limbs, somewhat. Even though there is no treatment for transverse myelitis, most patients do get some recovery, and this improvement meant that Ms. Becker was likely to regain a considerable amount of her movement and her independence.

"Do you have anybody to take care of you when you leave?" I asked.

"My boyfriend. Mike. He'll be here soon."

After my examination and her cigarette, the nurses took Ms. Becker away to bathe her, shampoo her, and cut her nails. Then she started our program of rehabilitation.

Soon after her admission, though, the first of the month rolled around. Now, in our city this is "payday" for the homeless, because anyone who shows up at City Hall on the first of the month receives $360, no questions asked, as part of General Assistance. And right on schedule—that is, on the first of the month—Mike the boyfriend did show up. He was blond, cute, and in his twenties; and he wore tight and not-entirely-clean Levi's and a denim jacket. He was not unkempt, and he was polite, but he was not kempt, either.

He wanted to take her out, he told me, just for a few hours, down to South of Market, where she could sign her check over to him.

I watched as he wheeled her off in the wheelchair with the bag of urine, now covered, at her side. She was somewhat better than when she arrived. Her hair was washed and brushed; her clothes were clean; and she could move both shoulders. Mike put a cigarette in her mouth and off they went.

She didn't come back as promised, though. At least not right away. What I learned through the doctor grapevine was that a few days after she left, she'd been found alone on the streets in her (actually our) wheelchair, with a blocked urine catheter, a swollen bladder, and, consequently, a rip-roaring kidney infection that had infected her blood. So she was admitted to the County Hospital, stabilized, and then sent back to rehabilitation.

By this time I was back on the reopened admitting ward, but I kept track of her progress anyway, which was good and bad. Good because she continued to improve: her arms strengthened, and she was able to stand. Bad because Mike, her cute blond boyfriend, continued to roll her out and bring her back intoxicated and high. After three such misadventures, Dr. Major gave up and discharged Terry, in her wheelchair, to the Baxter Hotel and into the care of her boyfriend.

Over the next several months, Terry was admitted to the County Hospital many times—mostly for kidney infections and once after Mike beat her up and robbed her. Finally, in the middle of winter, she was found sitting in her wheelchair on the streets, cold, unarousable, and without a heartbeat. Someone called the paramedics. Even though she was clinically dead, they began resuscitation efforts and also warmed her body. It took them a while, but once she warmed up, her heart resumed its steady beat; her pulse returned; and she began to breathe. After two hours, she woke up.

The paramedics took her to the County Hospital, and a few days later, she came back to us.

This was the second time I'd seen her. She'd lost quite a bit of function. She could still move her arms, but not her legs, and she couldn't stand anymore. The rehabilitation staff went to work. After a few months, she was back to her baseline; she could stand again. And again, after a time, Mike appeared with alcohol and drugs, and Terry left the hospital.

But not for long.

Mike did not do a good job of taking care of his patient, and Terry did not do a good job of taking care of herself. They drank; they smoked; they took cocaine; sometimes she stayed for days in her wheelchair. Eventually she developed an open wound on her sit bones from sitting so long—a bedsore—and it became infected. So she was admitted back to the County Hospital, where the plastic surgeons spent many hours covering the open wound with a graft of skin from her thighs—an expensive operation needing weeks of careful nursing to heal properly. But after the surgery, the first of the month rolled around, and Mike turned up.

The County Hospital taught him how to take care of Terry's graft, dressings, and bladder catheter. Although, since they were homeless, he never was able to change the dressings, not even once. It must have been frustrating for Mike, who was a kind of mystery man, anyway. What tied him to Terry? Money? Love? At any rate, a week after that particular discharge, he took a two-by-four to her, fracturing her skull and breaking her left leg.

When she showed up in the emergency room for this, the twenty-eighth time, even the ER doctors were dismayed. The expensive surgical flap that covered her wound had deteriorated; it was no more than a mass of rotten flesh; and there were two new open sores on either side of her sit bones. They called in the surgeons to take a look.

The surgeons were appalled at the damage to their handiwork. The beautiful piece of skin that they had, over so many operating hours, detached, rotated, and then affixed with meticulous sutures to the open wound on her back had turned gangrenous. It had to be removed—picked out of her open, infected wound in tiny pieces.

Would the surgeons consider, the ER doctors asked, trying again?

They declined. Perhaps in several months, if Terry complied with their orders. In the meantime she should have the old-fashioned treatment of thrice-daily dressing changes laid in the wound and removed when dry. This would clean the infected wound, and it could be done at Laguna Honda.

And so I admitted Terry for the third and last time, four and a half months after her second flight from us.

Those four and a half months had not been good to her, I saw when she rolled into the admitting ward. She was thinner and more wan than she'd been at the beginning of the year. There was an IV going; there was a cast on her left leg; and the circles under her eyes were darker. She looked even older than she had the first time I admitted her. But—and this was a change—when she saw me, she smiled.

We knew each other pretty well by this time, so I waited for her to have her smoke and for the nurses to bathe and shampoo her, and change her clothes. Then I went over to examine her. This time the nurses had placed her at the far end of the ward, next to the wall and nearest the bathroom, which was good, but far from the smoking room, which was bad. Best of all, she was under the care of Connie, the nursing assistant whose patients, I'd noticed, always improved.

Terry's physical exam was much as I'd expected from her records and not much different from the last time I'd seen her, except more so. Although this time she seemed played out, her spirit tired, given up. Her flesh—the tone of her skin, the absence of muscle—told the same story; it, too, lacked that vital force, that *vis vitalis* that is the essence of health and the substance of life.

I looked at the soiled cast on her left leg, and from the rest of the exam it was clear that whatever gains she'd made on her previous admission had been lost.

Then Connie turned Terry on her left side, and I saw the open wound on her back. The description from the County Hospital had not done it justice.

Terry's bedsore was the worst I'd ever seen. It was huge, enormous, and deep. It went from the middle of her back all the way down to her tailbone, and it spanned both of her sit bones. The skin was completely gone, of course, but so were the fat and the muscles that cover the spine. In their place was an unidentifiable mass of decayed and decaying and infected tissue from the failed skin graft, and at the bottom of this wide, deep hole I could see bone—Terry's spine.

Now, before I came to Laguna Honda, and even for a while after, I didn't understand the importance of a bedsore. It doesn't sound that bad—a sore from lying in bed. In fact, though, bedsores are a disaster both in what they mean and in what they signify. They mean that someone has not been paying attention to the difficult problem of a patient like Terry, who no longer feels the lower part of her body and so does not make the unconscious, fidgety movements the rest of us make to relieve pressure on the parts of our body pressed against shoes, chair, bedclothes.

What bedsores signify is even worse. They signify that the body has lost its integrity. Normally the body is covered with skin, which is impermeable to fluids and to germs. Slather healthy skin with any amount of germs, and nothing will happen—no infection—unless there's a break in the skin. As extra protection there is the fat under the skin, which cushions the muscles, and the muscles under the fat, which protect the bones, and the bones, which protect the spinal cord.

So Terry's bedsore was scary. She had no protection. Everything delicate and crucial in her body—bones, kidneys, spinal cord—was exposed and vulnerable to an environment full of danger, full of germs—to bacteria of all sorts and from every source, even the bacteria that live on and within our bodies. Giving antibiotics to try to prevent infection wouldn't protect her, I knew, because germs would rapidly become resistant to them. And the bedsore was too big to graft, even if the surgeons agreed. It would have to heal on its own, and that would take years. In the meantime, what chance did Terry have of not getting an overwhelming infection that would kill her? I walked back to our little doctors' office and sat down at my rickety desk. I stared for quite a while at the wooden shelf on which was Mrs. McCoy's robust plant, now grown all over the wall. This bedsore was a catastrophe, and possibly the end of Ms. Terry Becker.

For the second time with a patient, I thought about Hildegard, and I asked myself: What would Hildegard do? How would she treat Terry Becker's huge and open wound? And as I did so, I stared into Mrs. McCoy's green plant.

What she would do, I suddenly saw, was remove obstructions to Terry's *viriditas,* to Terry's natural ability to heal. Because if nothing was in its way, then *viriditas* would heal her wound as surely as a plant will grow green.

What was in its way? I asked myself.

The mass of dead tissue was in its way, and every bit of it had to be removed.

Any pressure on Terry's body, from wrinkled bedclothes to hard mattresses, was also in its way and had to be removed. Anything that interfered with the circulation of her blood—nicotine, for instance—was in the way of *viriditas.* Dirt, unkemptness, stale clothes. Unnecessary medications. Fear, depression, hopelessness. All were in its way.

My first job, therefore, as gardener-doctor, was not to make a brilliant diagnosis or give any magical medication, but to remove obstructions to Terry's own *viriditas*.

What else?

To see what else was needed, I had to start with a vision of Terry whole, complete, and healthy, in a future when all that was missing from her complete health was a pair of glasses. And walk my way back from that. Which I did. I walked past the repair of her teeth, the strengthening of her body, the strengthening of her will, the resolution of her depression, and the healing of her bedsore. I walked all the way back from the perfect future to the imperfect now, and then I organized my strategy forward.

What my strategy would be, I understood from Hildegard, was that, in addition to removing obstructions to *viriditas,* I would fortify Terry's *viriditas* with Earth, Water, Air, and Fire. That is, with good nutrition—tasty food, vitamins, liquids—deep sleep, fresh air, and sunlight.

After that? Peace. Rest. Safety.

Not much else. It might be just that simple. Oh, and time. As much time as Terry needed.

I t was quite amazing how fast Hildegard's prescription worked.

Within a few weeks I began to see signs of healing deep within Terry's wound. There was no infection, and deep down, at the base of the wound—was it my imagination?—there was a smooth and pink glistening, which was starting to cover and protect her spine.

But then the first of the month rolled around, and Mike showed up.

He was still pretty cute, still wearing his tight Levi's, still walking with a flirtatious, though constrained, strut. The nurses made him wait in the smoking room, and Terry wheeled herself on her gurney, facedown, back covered, the whole length of the ward. Then she rolled into the smoking room. They were there a long time. Then the door opened, and Mike came out and left.

Terry had thrown him out. She told him never to come back.

Then she stopped smoking. So her appetite improved, and she gained weight. Without nicotine constricting her blood vessels, the tiny new arteries and veins at the base of her bedsore could absorb the vitamins and protein she was eating, and the hole in her backside began to fill in.

Since I did not check the bedsore daily but only once a week, its progress seemed as magical to me as one of those time-lapse movies they showed us in school, where a plant grows from a seed in a matter of minutes. Dirt falls on either side of the sprout as it pushes its way up through the earth; then a minute later tiny leaves unfurl; buds appear and then expand until their sides split open and the first petals uncurl.

Just so, Terry's bedsore seemed to heal. There was her back filleted open, with a huge, deep wound over half of it. Then the base of it began to shine as endothelial cells spun blood vessels and connective tissue. The bones began to glisten, and then muscle, fat, and subcutaneous tissue appeared. This week, a few new blood vessels over the spine; at the edges of the wound, a few millimeters of new skin. Next week, nothing in particular, except that the bedsore was a little shallower.

Terry's wound began to look like a huge scab. The scab thickened until it was even with the rest of the skin, and then, just as petals push against the constriction of the bud and open it, so the scab flaked off, and there was pink skin underneath. That awful crater filled in from bottom to top and from side to side.

It took a long time. It took two and a half years. But we were in no hurry, and neither was she.

After two and a half years the bedsore had healed. Also Terry's teeth had been repaired by our dentist, and eyeglasses prescribed by our optometrist. She'd gained a considerable amount of weight. The crevices in her face had filled in; her hair grew in thick and dark; and behind her new eyeglasses, makeup appeared.

One day toward the end of the two and a half years, the social worker found her brother, who still lived back in Arkansas with his wife and two children. He asked whether his sister could come and live with him. He was not rich; he didn't have the money to send for her; but if the hospital would send her out to Arkansas, he would do the rest. Since we did have the Patient Gift Fund, donated by families for just this kind of situation, the social worker bought an airplane ticket and made arrangements for Terry to be cared for in a hospital in Arkansas.

With Terry Becker I got a glimmer of what Dr. Curtis meant when he told me that Laguna Honda was a gift. Laguna Honda was a once-in-a-lifetime opportunity not only to see cases that no one any longer got to see, but to observe processes that no one any longer got to observe. With Terry, I witnessed healing from the inside out.

It was a long, ironic, and miraculous process.

I was impressed by how long it took. Two and a half years. And it did take two and a half years; I can't imagine her healing in any less time. The general rule of thumb in premodern medicine was that it took as long to heal an illness as it took for the illness to develop. Depending on how we label Terry's illness, as transverse myelitis, as a bedsore, as drug abuse, as a poor self-image, or—what I really believe it was—as some deep spiritual wound, two and a half years was just about right.

Not only did her healing take a long time and need a long time, but time was the most important ingredient in her treatment. Premodern medicine knew about that special ingredient; it was called "tincture of time." Almost everything, it had observed, healed in time under the right conditions. And the most valuable thing that Terry received at the hospital was just that: enough—that is, the right amount of—time, the right amount of time being time without pressure and without end.

What was ironic was how difficult it was for her to get it. Our much-criticized health-care system provided every medication, no matter how expensive, and every necessary procedure; and yet, after each of her fifty-thousand-dollar hospitalizations, she was discharged in a wheelchair to the streets or the Baxter Hotel. The value of Laguna Honda, where time was not at a premium, struck me. Patients like Terry should, I decided, be tucked away at our hotel, out of sight of the administrators and out of the mind of budgeters, so the tincture of time could do its work.

But it was watching her healing that was miraculous, that transformed my practice of medicine. In this day of efficient health care, no one ever gets to see such a process. It seemed to me more than mechanical; it seemed magical, a sleight of hand.

Of course, modern medicine can readily explain the mechanism of Terry's healing. Once the breeding tissue for microbes had been removed by our plastic surgeon and nutrients provided, healthy cells at the base of the wound dedifferentiated—that is, they lost various inhibitive structures on their DNA. They turned into pluripotential stem cells, and then, by means of a complex but explainable process of membrane receptors, enzymes, and transcriptases, they began to produce first the RNA and then the proteins necessary for reconstituting the muscle cell, the endothelial cell, the cartilage cell, the collagen. There was nothing magical about it. Once this process was set in motion, it happened mechanically.

And yet it felt like something different, as if I were watching an invisible artist fill in his vision of Terry Becker's perfect body. I wouldn't say that modern medicine was wrong in its explanation, but the process seemed more than mechanical; it seemed deliberate, as if there were a perfecting force, clear about its purpose and its final form. But, just like the absence of the little black box at Mr. Baker's autopsy, I had no word for it.

Although, as I researched Hildegard's concept of *viriditas* for my PhD and tried to understand what she meant by it, I discovered that premodern medicine did have a name for this magical act that the body performs. It was called the *vis medicatrix naturae*, usually translated as "the healing power of nature." But this is not a great translation. *Vis* is related to *vim* and *vigor* and means the force of life, of youth, of newness. *Medicatrix* is related to *remedy* and *medication*. And *naturae* does not mean nature as in "Mother Nature," but rather your nature, my nature, Terry Becker's nature. It means the nature of us to be ourselves. So the *vis medicatrix naturae* is really "the remedying force of your own nature to be itself," to turn back into itself when it has been wounded.

The idea goes all the way back to Hippocrates, who wrote that "what heals disease is nature [*physis*]." And what did he mean by *physis*? *Physis* comes from *phuo,* which means to grow, and signifies the observation that a seed grows into the only plant it can: a mustard seed into a mustard plant, a seed of wheat into a sheaf of wheat. By *physis* Hippocrates meant the "nature" of a being to grow into itself; and it was, in part, what Hildegard meant by *viriditas.*

Physis—the individual nature of each person—also gives us the word *physician.* The physician is the person who studies *physis,* the individual nature of his patient, who understands it and follows its lead.

But like *anima* and *spiritus*, *physis* and the healing power of nature were exiled from medicine more than one hundred years ago. They were victims in the battle between two completely different conceptions of health, disease, and healing—mechanism and vitalism.

The mechanists believed that life was mechanical, simply a series of processes that science could eventually understand and duplicate; the body was a machine that could be fixed. For the vitalists, the body was not a machine. They believed that life had something special about it that science could never duplicate. The vitalists were the romantics of medicine, and in the last decades of the nineteenth century they lost their battle with the mechanists. By the early twentieth century, any reference to vitalism or the healing power of nature was considered heretical. Yet vitalism did not disappear. Instead, it dived down into the subterranean rivers of Western medicine and reappeared in the many side streams of alternative medicine.

Whether there is such a thing as the healing power of nature is, perhaps, beside the point. What I do know for sure is that it is a useful way of looking at my patients' bodies; it gives me a way of imagining that the body's natural state is to be whole, perfect, and without blemish. And it is what differentiates the living body from a machine: because if nothing interferes, the body, unlike a machine, will heal itself.

Watching Terry heal from Hildegard's perspective of *viriditas* changed my point of view from figure to ground. Forever after, instead of focusing on my patient vaguely surrounded by his environment, I also did the opposite—I stepped back and focused on the environment surrounding my patient. And asked myself: Is anything interfering with *viriditas*? What can I do to remove it?

There was still one more insight that I got from Terry Becker.

And that was the other—and just as impressive—healing process that went on, beginning with her throwing out her boyfriend, then giving up smoking, alcohol, and drugs; and then moving on to a remarkable change in temperament, from irritable and angry to pleasant, grateful, and even, I think, happy. Some fundamental change gelled and became irreversible just when she wheeled herself into the smoking room to meet Mike that last time.

I don't know when it started or how. It wasn't when he abandoned her, quadriplegic and wheelchair-bound on the streets of our city, because she let him check her out of the hospital two or three more times after that. I don't think it had started even when she was admitted with that huge and terrible bedsore. I think it happened after she got to us, before Mike turned up at the first of the month, while she was lying there at the far end of the ward with the window open above her, facedown, for weeks.

After two and a half years, Terry was discharged.

Her social worker drove her to the airport, and her brother, whom she hadn't seen in years, was waiting at the airport in Arkansas to pick her up. After that, I don't know what happened to her or how she lived. I only know what I read in her obituary, eleven years later, which mentions children and grandchildren but nothing about her long stay in our city; nothing about Mike or living on the streets or the big bedsore. Or the effort of will that saved her life, that reaching down for a sense of self she'd forgotten or didn't know she had, or didn't have until that moment on the gurney in the smoking room.

Perhaps she never spoke to her family of those lost years; perhaps they never asked. Perhaps she spoke of them often, and her children and grandchildren knew all those stories. From the narrowed eyes and high cheekbones in the obituary photo, the proud lift to her head with its traditional beads and the firmly closed mouth, I think not. Although—who knows?—in the photo she is still wearing our glasses.

Five

SLOW MEDICINE

NOT LONG AFTER Terry Becker went back to Arkansas, Laguna Honda was notified that it was under investigation by the Department of Justice. Someone at the hospital had contacted the DOJ with a tip, although what the tip was and who contacted them were never divulged—to the satisfaction of Larissa, I might add.

But everyone had his favorite suspect. Some thought it was Dr. Kay, our hospice director; others that it was Sister Miriam, our resident nun. Larissa guessed Miss Lester, the director of nursing, who'd protested the halving of her head nurses all the way up to the director of public health. Larissa thought Miss Lester might have done it as a last resort, a way of stopping the destruction of the nursing system she'd spent her life creating. That seemed unlikely to me, at first. From what I knew of Miss Lester, she was not the kind to turn in her own people, though from what I later learned, she was a possible, even probable, informant.

By the time I arrived at Laguna Honda, Miss Lester had been director of nursing for thirty-six years and would be director of nursing for another eight. She'd been at the hospital longer than almost anyone else—longer than the chief of our institutional police, longer than the baker in the kitchen, longer even than Mrs. Lantos with her lobotomy, although just barely. Miss Lester had accepted the position right after she got out of the army, and so far she'd survived five executive administrators, six medical directors, and eight directors of public health.

As soon as she arrived, she took over the two-room office between the entrance door for ambulances and the large hall where patients smoked and played cards. In the first room she stationed her second in command, Donnie McFarland, and for the next forty-four years Donnie stood sentinel at the open Dutch door of that first room, where nurses hovered to ask about sick leave and problem patients. Anything that went wrong in the hospital during the day was taken to that Dutch door and vetted by Donnie.

Miss Lester herself moved into the second room, which could be reached only through an inside door in the first office, so she was mostly undisturbed in her work. Larissa told me that she'd been in Miss Lester's office only once. Donnie being gone for a minute, she'd stepped inside and found Miss Lester's door open.

"I looked inside," she told me in her Russian accent. "The room was dark, and Miss Lester was sitting at her desk, smoking. There were two piles of white papers on each side of the desk, and two cats sitting on them, one on each pile. She asked me what I wanted; and I was scared; but I was asking for vacation so I told her. She said just make sure that my request was written on yellow paper because she only looked at the yellow paper. If I wrote it on white paper, it would get thrown out."

Larissa was quiet for a moment. "She was tough, that one, but fair."

Miss Lester was short, stocky, and squarely built, and though she no longer wore a white uniform or a nursing cap, she might as well have. She ran the hospital with a firm hand, which, I gradually realized, was what gave the hospital its stability. Also, perhaps, its hidden softness. Miss Lester's nursing structure was simple: She was at the top; underneath her was the assistant director of nursing, then the nursing supervisors and the head nurses for each ward. From her little office she ran the hospital or, at least, the nursing part of it. She did so without a computer, a secretary, or an answering machine. If something needed to be typed, she typed it; if a call needed to be made, she made it; and she answered the telephone herself. Unhappy family members got the director of nursing right away; so did patients and so did staff—which minimized the number of sick days requested.

Miss Lester stayed in that office for decades. She stayed in it through the hospital's transition from premodern nursing to modern medicine; and during its transition from modern medicine to health care. Through all the changes Miss Lester kept her staff—many hundreds of nurses and orderlies—as organized and disciplined as an army, or at least a battalion. More disciplined, really.

Each morning at six-thirty AM, she was met at her office by the nursing supervisor of the night and the nursing supervisor of the morn, and the three of them went to see every patient in the hospital, all 1,178 of them.

I knew this because every day at eight AM they came through the double doors of the admitting ward and sailed past the open door of the doctors' office. They would stop at the nursing station, and the head nurse would join them. Then, with Miss Lester, top lip clamped firmly on the lower, at their head, the group would walk the ward. Miss Lester would stop at each bed. Her eyes would latch for a moment on the patient and then scan the area. Any evidence of commotion, anything out of place, but also any sign of unmet suffering—of moaning, dirty bedclothes, twisted limbs—would be noted and questioned. And then the procession would sail on to the next patient.

Before leaving the ward, Miss Lester would give her orders to the head nurse and then walk to the next of the thirty-eight wards. It took her the good part of the first three hours of her day, but by the end, Miss Lester knew just about everything about her army and had a plan. She would return to her dark, cool office, light up a cigarette, and set to work.

Her plan, however, did not include the doctors. Rather, it precisely excluded them. In fact, for all my years on the admitting ward, Miss Lester marched past the open door of our office, surrounded by her officers, and never once looked in. Once and once only did we meet face-to-face, and she didn't have time to glance away. But she did have time to glaze her eyes and stare just past me, not acknowledging my presence or position in any way.

I didn't mind, though. For one thing, even with the disadvantages of her system—with doctors and nurses meeting in stairwells and linen closets—it worked pretty well. With so little in the way of modernity, Miss Lester nonetheless provided what is necessary for the best care of the patient—a gentle and reliable staff. The peculiar softness underneath her system—the kindness woven like an invisible thread through the decrepit fabric of the place—may or may not have been due to her, but it was not hindered by her. It wasn't dismantled, removed, or teased out.

For another thing, I didn't take it personally. Miss Lester was right to be suspicious of the medical profession; I knew this from Dr. Weitz's class on the history of the hospital. Ever since the duties of the monk infirmarian had been split between doctor and nurse, and the Latin *curare* split into cure and care, there'd been a battle going on for control. Who would be in command of the hospital? Doctor or nurse? Whose model of *curare* would triumph? Cure or care? And this battle was joined at the French Revolution, when the doctors tried to wrest control of the Hôtel-Dieu in Paris from its nursing nuns.

For more than a thousand years the nuns ran the Hôtel-Dieu: Caring for the sick poor defined their monastic vocation. They provided food, shelter, and spiritual care; they nursed the sick; and only when necessary did they call in a physician. Until the end of the eighteenth century that was just fine with the doctors, because the sick poor at the Hôtel-Dieu did not offer them a pecuniary or any other reward.

But around the time of the French Revolution, medicine, like so much else, was changing. Doctors were beginning to believe that the best way to understand the body was to correlate their treatments with what happened to their patients. They started to keep careful records and perform autopsies on patients who died. Their records and their autopsies allowed them to relate the course of a disease to the dysfunction of internal organs, and to connect their physical examination of the living body to the pathophysiology they found inside the corpse. These were powerful innovations; they would provide much of the data for our bible, *DeGowin & DeGowin.* And the reason that the doctors of Revolutionary France suddenly wanted control of the Hôtel-Dieu in Paris was that the best "material" for their new approach was at the Hôtel-Dieu—the most varied patients, the most multitudinous, and the most compliant.

The doctors convinced the Revolution's administration to remove control of the Hôtel-Dieu from the nuns and give it to them.

The nuns protested. They refused to serve under the doctors. The head nun at the Hôtel-Dieu had always come before the physician, they argued. The idea of using patients—Christ's charges—as experimental objects was a murderous, a disastrous idea, they said. They were turned down, but step by step they went up the levels of administration. Finally they were ordered to leave the Hôtel-Dieu if they remained unwilling to obey the doctors. They did remain unwilling, and they also refused to leave. They declared that should workmen attempt to enter their wards to begin any alterations of the old structure, they would stand fast and prevent them.

With this, the administration buckled and rescinded its order, returning control of the Hôtel-Dieu to the nursing nuns. And there they remained for the next one hundred and fifty years, taking care of their patients until France secularized the institution in the early 1900s. Then the nuns left.

I don't know if Miss Lester knew this story. Perhaps they teach it in nursing school. But I do know that she embodied the stubborn and passionate caring of those nuns at the Hôtel-Dieu, and that her suspicion of the medical profession in general, and modern medicine in particular, was to some extent justified.

The main thing was that Miss Lester was certain that good nursing was crucial for the healing of the patient. And good nursing meant nurses, especially a head nurse for each ward. She'd done everything she could to get her head nurses back. She'd gone all the way up the chain of command to the director of public health and then to the board of supervisors, complaining about the cuts. The director of public health defended his decision to follow Dee and Tee's recommendations, and when asked he reassured the board that there'd been no cutbacks in bedside nursing; the staffing patterns were still above the standards in the industry.

So perhaps it was Miss Lester who called in the DOJ. The nuns of the Hôtel-Dieu certainly would have.

f it was Miss Lester who turned the hospital in to the Department of Justice and if her intention had been to reach past the new director of public health and get her head nurses back, then her plan went completely awry.

The Department of Justice arrived, and in its wake, still a second investigative agency, the Health Care Financing Administration, and suddenly there were teams of DOJ and HCFA doctors, nurses, and lawyers poring over our patients' records. They questioned Dr. Major, the executive administrator, and Miss Lester in detail about everything, and perhaps it was those interrogations that convinced Miss Lester to resign. Or perhaps she realized that her head nurses were never coming back. At any rate, midway during the eighteen-month investigation, Miss Lester quit—in protest, she told the newspapers. She protested the cutting of her head nurses, with the consequent decline in nursing and inevitable danger to patients.

The city's Health Commission accepted her resignation with regret. They issued a certificate of commendation and voted that the little animal farm be named after her, and so it was. And Miss Lester left Laguna Honda, six years shy of half a century of service.

It was just as well that she resigned before the eighteen-page letter of the Department of Justice appeared. Because the report blamed her nursing department for almost everything that the DOJ didn't like about the hospital, except for its old-fashioned wards, which they didn't like either. Their biggest issue was the physical facility. It didn't meet the fire codes, the ventilation codes, or the earthquake codes; worst of all were the open wards, which violated patients' right to privacy.

Now, most of us liked the open wards. The nurses liked them because in an open ward they could see all the patients all the time. If a patient fell, if a patient was in pain, if a patient was doing something dangerous, the nurse would see it immediately. We doctors liked the open wards because they were so inviting to stroll around, and they made it easy to talk to and evaluate patients. And patients liked them because the open wards were interesting and social, especially if a patient was bedbound. There was even a 1986 study done at the hospital in which 88 percent of the patients said they preferred the open ward to a private room.

Now and then, I did have a patient who suffered from the lack of privacy. But I had many more who turned down a private room with "Doc, don't send me there; it's too lonely." And it was true: On an open ward it was easy for patients to make friends. There were many people to choose from, and they saw one another every day. Patients gossiped and traded information on the open wards; cliques formed. Occasionally the visiting family of one patient would adopt an orphan patient and bring in food for him, too. The privacy so valuable to the middle-aged and stressed, to the harassed investigator and the harried doctor, was not so valuable, it turned out, and even harmful to the bedridden and disabled.

But the DOJ would have none of it. There was no way the investigators could be convinced that the open wards were not "thirty-six-bed rooms" but big, open spaces, with lots of windows, sunlight, and fresh air. Or that the community the open wards fostered was more important than the privacy they lacked. The city must do something about the old hospital, the DOJ demanded: Either rebuild it according to twenty-first-century codes or close it down.

But the building was not their only problem with us. They'd discovered patients in the hospital who didn't have to be there, who could be managed in the community, and this violated their civil right to be cared for in the least restrictive environment. So their second demand was that Laguna Honda immediately evaluate every patient and discharge any who could be managed outside the institution, whether the patient wanted to be discharged or not.

Last, the DOJ found numerous problems with the nursing department. Even while its investigators had been on-site, patients had wandered away without their nurses realizing they were gone. Other patients had smuggled in alcohol and drugs. When the nurses became aware of such incidents, the DOJ noted, they dealt with them on an ad hoc basis; there'd been no monitoring tools, no investigations, no committees. In general, the nurses lacked training; they did not always know the side effects of the medications they gave; some did not know what to do during resuscitation attempts, and the nursing policy-and-procedure manual was more than three years old.

All these problems had to be resolved, the eighteen-page DOJ letter ended, and quickly.

The mayor read their report and passed it to Dr. Stein, our new director of public health.

Dr. Stein was from New York, and he was young, energetic, and swarthy, with a five o'clock shadow even at seven AM. He wore a suit and tie to funerals and ribbon cuttings; otherwise he wore open-collared plaid shirts and Levi's, with one cuff rolled up because he had no car and rode a bicycle. Dr. Stein was a problem solver, an optimist, and a good listener. He listened with an open face, a curved smile, and narrowed eyes. Later in his reign he was not quite as good a listener, although he was still optimistic.

The first thing he did with the DOJ report was to have us reevaluate every one of our 1,178 patients for discharge. It took us several weeks, and the DOJ turned out to be correct: There were patients who could be discharged to the community. There were sixty. Twenty-five of them refused to be discharged, and another thirty had no place to go. But five patients were agreeable to discharge and did have a place to go and were discharged.

Next, Dr. Stein began studying his options for the old hospital. Should he close it down? Rebuild it? If a rebuild was in order, how big should it be and where should he put it? On the same hill where the city almshouse had always been? Or as many smaller facilities, scattered around the city? He spent the next year evaluating the different possibilities.

Last, he appointed a replacement for Miss Lester—Ellen Mary Flanders, RN, MSN, PhD-to-be—and he bicycled over to make the announcement. Ellen Mary, he told us at the meeting, was an outstanding administrator, highly regarded for her commitment to consumer-focused care. We should all welcome her.

Scattered applause.

Ellen Mary got up for her acceptance speech. She could not have been more different from Miss Lester. She was petite and blond and dressed in a gray skirt-suit, stockings, and pumps. She wore a bouffant hairdo and expensive-looking earrings, and she smiled widely; she spoke in a warm Southern drawl. She was impressed by the hospital, she said, and excited at the prospect of bringing it into the twenty-first century. And then, perhaps to emphasize how very different her

New Nursing was going to be from Miss Lester's Old Nursing, she told us to call her Ellen Mary.

The first thing Ellen Mary did was to move the Department of Nursing out of Miss Lester's rooms in the back of the hospital into the administration wing at the front. It was quieter there, more peaceful, and completely out of the way of ambulances, doctors, and patients. She had the old-fashioned suites redecorated in taupes, with cream carpets, blond Danish desks, and new computers, and she brought over from the County many of her coworkers, who were also pleasant and ambitious nurses. Finally she sat down to analyze the DOJ report. What was needed, she concluded, were new forms, new committees, and new training for the nurses.

So she and her new staff began devising forms, creating committees, and setting up the new Nursing Department of Training and Education. They staffed the new committees with the best nurses from the wards and required everyone to attend their newly developed PowerPoint presentations and online training sessions. Since the budget was tight, they could make little provision for substitute nurses during these forced absences, however, and patients ended up getting less nursing care.

It took the new nursing administration quite a bit of time, but eventually they had a form for just about everything and a committee, too. Now when a patient disappeared from the hospital, there was an appropriate form to fill out—the patient disappearance form—and an appropriate committee—the patient disappearance committee—to send it to. When a patient fell, there was the fall form and the fall committee; when a patient got a bedsore, or was caught using drugs, there were specific forms. If bedrails had to be pulled up to prevent a patient from falling out of bed, there was a form, and there was a form whenever a psychiatric medication was instituted or even changed.

There were so many forms that the charts began to explode, and every six months all the doctors' notes were taken out of the charts to make room for the forms.

Despite the perennial budget crisis, Ellen Mary was even able to hire enough managers to oversee her new bureaucracy. We would see them sometimes in their dark suits and shiny shoes, looking through our patients' charts.

Unlike Miss Lester, Ellen Mary did not visit the wards daily, weekly, or even monthly. She didn't have to. There was a form for that also—the daily report, which listed all the rapscallion activities—the drinking, falling, and wandering away—that continued, of course, to take place. Although I didn't find the nurses any better trained or educated with all their new training and education, it didn't seem to hurt them. Mostly they kept their common sense. They did pay more attention to whatever required a form, and what with all the forms and committees, they did spend less time with their patients. That was all I noticed, except that I kind of missed Miss Lester and her early-morning parade.

I t was a time of change at the hospital, and I felt lucky to have my study of Hildegard and premodern medicine as a refuge and a bulwark.

By this time I'd finished the requirements for my PhD and condensed my master's thesis into an article, and I was exploring new ways of thinking about Hildegard's medicine. I spent months in libraries. Before those months, if I'd been asked how many medieval books had survived the Middle Ages, I would have guessed a few hundred. But there were thousands, I discovered.

All of them were originally published as handwritten manuscripts, the printing press not yet having been invented, and the important manuscripts were often "illuminated" with miniature paintings inside the initials that began each chapter. Despite their being painted with plant-derived inks—saffron, buckthorn, indigo— when I opened those manuscripts in the library, I was amazed to see that their thousand-year-old illuminations had not faded. The figures inside the tiny paintings were bright and lively; the red of a doctor's hat, the blue of a pilgrim's cloak, the yellow of a girl's hair popped right off the page. There were thousands of such illuminations, it turned out, and they portrayed just about everything: women in their kitchens, gardeners in their gardens, doctors with their patients. They were snapshots of life in the Middle Ages, and looking at them, I felt the chasm between us, the sense of otherness, disappear.

Hildegard did not have illuminations in her medical text, but she did have them in her three most important books, which were theological texts based on complex visions that Hildegard had had since she was a girl. We don't know what those visions were, physiologically speaking. Some physicians think they were the auras of migraines, auras being the scintillating visual images that sometimes precede the migraine headache. Other physicians speculate that her visions may have been epileptic phenomena. But whatever they were, they transformed Hildegard from a timid nun into a confident and determined woman, and in her theological books she had paintings made of each one. Copies of these illuminations still exist, and they are beautiful, complex, and odd, with the feeling tone of dreams. When I discovered them, I was amazed not only at their beauty, but at how much they could tell me about Hildegard and her world.

There was even a picture of Hildegard herself, painted while she was alive. It was not true to life, but it did reveal quite a bit about her—about how she saw herself, and wanted to be seen. Dressed in the black Benedictine habit, she was sitting inside her church at a writing table. Her feet rested on a stool, and she held a quill. Her long hair was covered; flames descended from the sky to her forehead, and her friend and secretary, the monk Volmar, looked at her in amazement.

But my favorite of her illuminations was Vision Three of her first book, *Scivias,* because it illustrated the System of the Fours. Painted in gold and blue, it was shaped like a pointed oval, with sun, moon, and planets all in a vertical line at the top. This signified their conjunction, and portrayed the moment that God created the world. Outside the oval were flames; inside the flames was the night sky with its stars; this illustrated the element of Fire. In the middle of the oval was the round earth, which illustrated the element of Earth. Between Fire and Earth was the element of Water, represented by wisps of rain clouds in the sky. Last was the fourth element, Air, represented by the North, South, East, and West winds at each corner of the painting. These winds were the motive power of the universe, Hildegard explained: They were how the four qualities of hot and cold and wet and dry changed into one another as the cosmos turned around the earth and created the seasons.

It was a beautiful, unifying image, and though I didn't know it at the time, it would be my key to Hildegard's medicine, and to premodern medicine, too.

The trove of medieval books I was discovering in the library protected me somewhat from the stress in the hospital, but outside the admitting ward it was tense; it was chaotic; I could tell by the fatigue in Dr. Major's face. Inside the admitting ward, however, things were going on about the same. Dr. Fintner and I continued to share patients; Dr. Romero continued to do her thorough workups; the well-tempered Dr. Jeffers continued to accept whatever happened with a smile. Not that the admitting ward was easy or peaceful, ever. What the admitting ward was, was hectic and a lot of work, but it was always interesting.

The day I met Mrs. Klara Muller, for example.

Since I'd admitted the last patient of the day before, Dr. Jeffers would be getting the first patient who came in. I'd already walked around the ward that morning and seen my patients, and I was sitting at my rickety desk when an ambulance pulled up. I watched as the drivers went round to the rear, opened up the double doors, climbed in, and wheeled out Dr. Jeffers's next patient. He was flat on his back, strapped to the gurney. A bit later the drivers trundled past the open door of our doctors' office with the gurney, and Dr. Jeffers unfurled his long legs, put on his white coat, and went out to greet his new patient. I went back to my work.

But a few minutes later I heard running, and then Dr. Jeffers popped his head into the office.

"Victoria! He's escaped! My new patient! He ran outside, and he's out in the parking lot. Help me get him back!"

I jumped up and we ran out together past Dr. Major, who joined us, and out into the parking lot. Then we stopped, and Dr. Jeffers scanned the area.

"What happened?" I asked.

"My new patient. He's got Huntington's disease, and his mother couldn't handle him anymore. He's demented, but still young and strong, and as soon as he was unstrapped from the ambulance gurney, he took off. There he is!"

And there in the trees on the forested hill across the parking lot was Mr. X.—tall and slim, trim and alert, arms flailing about, and alternating his weight from leg to leg in the characteristic dance of Huntington's disease. He was standing in the trees and looking around for some escape like, I am sorry to say, a hunted animal. Which he was.

The three of us split three ways to corral him before he ran down the hill and out onto the busy street. At the same time, our institutional police—big and slow-moving but unstoppable—showed up, and the four of us moved in on Mr. X., who looked around and made a dash down the hill. But the police had stationed someone there, too, and the five of us tightened our circle until Mr. X. was trapped. He looked around one last time, took a deep breath, and dropped his shoulders. The police surrounded him, and with the situation under control, Dr. Jeffers and I walked back to the doctors' office.

"What's the story?" I asked.

"Well," Dr. Jeffers began, with his drawl, looking over at me as we walked, "it's a sad one. David and his brother, Steve, both have Huntington's disease, and their mother has been taking care of them. They've gotten much worse, demented but still strong, and she can't manage them anymore. They've run away from the house, showed up in neighbors' beds, and fought with her. So a few months ago she brought Steve in, and we were hoping to put David on the same ward. Easier for their mother and better for both of them. But we can't manage that," he finished, as we sat down in our office. "He's too much for us these days, after the DOJ and the budget cuts. We don't have the staff, anymore. I'm calling the County. They're going to have to take him back until he agrees to stay here."

Huntington's disease is a good example of the miracles of modern medicine. An incurable brain disease, it is inherited in an autosomal dominant fashion, which means that if one parent has it, a child has a 50 percent chance of getting it. In David's family both his father and his grandfather had died of it. It destroys the brain in a characteristic way: first the areas of judgment, then those of perception, last of strength and vigor. It also destroys the part of the brain that modulates movement, so the movements of patients with Huntington's disease are the jerky, dancing movements I'd seen in him.

What makes the disease especially cruel and ironic is that it does not appear until middle age, and until a few years ago, there was no way to tell whether you had escaped the family curse or not. So family members went ahead and had a family of their own, and thus the disease was passed on. Then a predictive blood test was discovered, and now the irony has changed. One wants to know, of course, that one is free of a hereditable, dementing, and incurable disease, but one wants not to know that one has it. So taking that test is a kind of test of moral strength. It became available, however, only after the Gutierrez brothers—and David and Steve had been unlucky—scored 100 percent in the Huntington's disease lottery.

Before Dee and Tee and the DOJ, we would have tried to manage David at Laguna Honda, as Dr. Jeffers said. The head nurse would have placed him nearest her observation window and kept a full-time eye on him. We would have used vest restraints and tranquilizers to decrease the chance of his running off again; and if he did escape now and then, well, that was to be expected. But we no longer had the head nurses, with their extra time to knit and to watch; the use of vest restraints and tranquilizers was frowned upon; and the DOJ had little tolerance for even an occasional escape.

So Dr. Jeffers had to call the County Hospital and send David back for a long, unnecessary hospitalization. David could return to Laguna Honda, Dr. Jeffers told the County doctors, but only after his disease had progressed to the point where he was confined to his bed—self-restrained, as it were, by his encephalopathy.

That was the first admission of the day.

The second admission was mine, and it would be Mrs. Klara Muller, who was coming in from home. I looked over her records before she arrived, which were scanty but informative enough. What they told me was that Mrs. Muller, age seventy-eight, just couldn't manage anymore.

Until eight months before, she'd been doing fine. Fine meant managing her house and taking care of her forty-year-old retarded daughter. She was healthy and led a pretty ordinary life for a widow her age—playing cards, running errands, doing lunch in the little corner of the city where she lived. But then she fell and broke her hip.

Now, the treatment of hip fractures is another of the wonders of our modern medical system. Thirty years ago a hip fracture often meant the end. The surgery to fix a hip was time-consuming and followed by a long convalescence in bed, with many potential complications—blood clots to the lung; bedsores; pneumonia; loss of job, house, social position; boredom; depression; and expense. Nowadays a hip fracture means a forty-five-minute surgery, a few days in the hospital, and a new hip.

Which is what Mrs. Muller received. She fell and broke her hip; 911 was called; and the ambulance took her to the Best Hospital in the City. She had surgery the same day: The ball of her hip was excised and replaced with a titanium ball. She was given a wonder drug to prevent blood clots, and then, so as to prevent bedsores, depression, and boredom, she was encouraged to get up and start walking right away.

There were, however, a few unexpected complications.

First, Mrs. Muller became delirious after surgery. When her workup showed no acute medical problems, her doctors ascribed her delirium to a psychosis from undiagnosed Alzheimer's disease, and they started her on an antipsychotic medication. Also she was found to have diabetes, and it was difficult to control, with many highs and lows in her sugar levels. Then, even though she recovered physically from her surgery, she remained confused in spite of the antipsychotic medication, though now she was quiet and withdrawn. She was so confused that she couldn't learn to manage her new diagnosis of diabetes or give herself the daily injections to prevent blood clots or take her pain medications correctly.

Her doctors couldn't imagine how she would take care of her adult retarded daughter or her house; nevertheless, they agreed with the utilization reviewer that it would be better for Mrs. Muller to be at home than in the hospital. Better for the hospital, because it had already been paid whatever it was going to get for Mrs. Muller's hip fracture; it wouldn't receive any additional payment no matter how long she stayed. It would be better for Mrs. Muller, too. She would avoid the unusual germs that thrive in the hospital; home would be familiar; and perhaps her confusion would clear. It would be better for her daughter also. And it would be better for the health-care system. Because no matter how expensive it was to arrange for a visiting nurse to give her injections, pain medications, and check her sugars; for physical therapists to go to her home to exercise her hip; for home-care workers to help with the housework; for Meals on Wheels; a caseworker to manage the services; and a social worker, it was still less expensive than keeping Mrs. Muller in the acute hospital.

So it was all arranged, and Mrs. Muller went home.

Her discharge worked like clockwork. Every day the physical therapist came to the house to exercise her new hip. The visiting nurse gave her the necessary pain medications, checked her sugars, administered insulin, and even tried to teach her daughter to give the injections. Meals were delivered twice a day. The home-care workers came every day, too, and straightened the house, prepared her daughter for school, dressed Mrs. Muller, put her into her wheelchair, and returned in the evening to do it all in reverse.

Except that Mrs. Muller did not get better. Or so the social worker told me when I called about Mrs. Muller, who, in the meantime, had arrived. She did not improve. Her hip continued to hurt despite the narcotic pain medications she was getting, and they had to be increased. More and more often she refused to get out of bed; she wouldn't get into her wheelchair; and she wouldn't walk. Finally the physical therapist stopped going to the house. The diabetes was better because she wasn't eating much, but her dementia was the same or worse. Mrs. Muller lay in bed all day, and if she spoke at all, it was to ask for more pain medication.

So, the social worker told me, they'd finally given up. Mrs. Muller had failed their best efforts to keep her at home. She needed to be cared for in an institution, and with her complicated medical problems and on her widow's budget, Laguna Honda was the best place for her. As for her daughter, she would have to be placed somewhere, too.

I thanked the social worker and then left the doctors' office to find Mrs. Muller. I was looking for a frail, white-haired old lady, lying in bed, withdrawn and quiet, who would mumble in response to my questions. I found her, and she was white-haired; she was lying in bed with her eyes closed, and she did look feeble and weak.

But when I greeted her with "Good afternoon," Mrs. Muller surprised me. Though her voice was soft, she said "Good afternoon" back in a lilting Austrian accent. Not only that, she looked at me from the bed, and her blue eyes were cagier and more wary than her diagnoses allowed. She knew her name and where she was; she knew the date;

and she knew what was wrong with her. She couldn't walk, she told me clearly, though wearily, drowsily, and druggedly, because her hip hurt.

When I examined her, I couldn't find any of the subtle signs of diabetes, which was a little surprising. Her hip also surprised me. The surgical incision was healed, but when I checked the hip's range of movement, Mrs. Muller winced. This was unusual six months after a hip replacement. So as soon as I finished my exam, I sent her upstairs for an X-ray, and a few minutes later I ran up to take a look. The X-ray was not normal. Mrs. Muller's titanium hip was dislocated out of its socket and had done so months before. No wonder she couldn't walk.

I went back down to the office, called her surgeon, and told him about the X-ray. And to his credit, of all the doctors and surgeons I ever called about a missed diagnosis, he was the most embarrassed and apologetic. He offered to come over and examine the hip himself. After he realized that wasn't necessary, he volunteered to arrange remedial surgery for her at the Best Hospital in the City the next day. Which he did.

Mrs. Muller had her surgery without a problem, and three days later she came back, artificial hip now in its socket. She seemed about the same—quiet, still in bed, and still in pain—and yet different. Chronic pain, which is what the dislocated hip had caused her, is mysterious and debilitating, while postsurgical pain is expected, localized, and, above all, temporary; and Mrs. Muller had exchanged the one for the other. Her face had relaxed, her brow had unknit, and now I could appreciate that she was a pretty woman.

It's rare to be elderly and pretty. I've had only a few women patients and even fewer men who in their old age were beautiful or handsome, and they must have been extremely beautiful or handsome when they were young. Most of my patients did have something—a smile, a lift to their head, a flash in their eyes—that distinguished them, and the badder they were, the more attractive. But Mrs. Muller was just plain pretty. Her hair was white and thick; her eyes, lake blue; her skin, protected from the sun all her years, was almost unwrinkled, clear and milky.

Nothing else was different. Her medications were the same, and she was still weak, withdrawn, and drowsy.

Over the next few weeks the new incision healed, and Mrs. Muller's hip pain disappeared. Since she no longer needed pain medications, I discontinued them. With that, her mood brightened, her voice cleared, and she seemed stronger.

Then the nurses began moving her into a chair every morning, and when I made my rounds, I sat on her bed and practiced my German. She told me about her Austrian village, her arrival in America, and about the little neighborhood in the city that she and her husband had discovered. A few streets, but very Austrian. I would like it, she said. There I could find German books and magazines, German music and candy, bread, sausage, and cookies in the little store; there was an Austrian tailor; and I could even get a good German meal and good German beer in the restaurant on the corner. I should be sure to visit.

After a few more weeks, I began to wonder if Mrs. Muller really was demented and psychotic. She didn't seem demented. Her eyes were observant; sitting in her chair, she noted everything that was happening on the ward; and she could report on patients' and nurses' activities from the evening before. Nor did she seem psychotic. She didn't hallucinate; she had no delusions; she wasn't fearful, not even at dusk, when the paranoia of Alzheimer's increases. True, she was still on medications that would mask those symptoms, but they work only so well. It is usually possible to see a suppressed psychosis behind them. But Mrs. Muller was quite lively, quite sharp. It seemed worthwhile to try taking her off her antipsychotic medications.

So I did, over the next several weeks. This takes time because antipsychotic tranquilizers can last in the body for a long while. Patients can do well at first and then, weeks after their last pill, become irritable, then delusional, and then begin complaining that the nurses are poisoning them. But Mrs. Muller did well without them. It was a pleasure to watch. Her personality increased in proportion to the decrease in those medications; like a photograph developing, her self became more colorful and more definite with each day.

About three months after she arrived, she asked me if she could go to physical therapy and learn to walk again. She worked hard in therapy, and soon she was getting around the open ward with a walker and then with a cane. I began to wonder if she might even get home, although there was still the diabetes, the insulin, and the daughter.

I knew she could learn to give her own insulin, but on her first physical examination I hadn't seen signs of long-term diabetes—no nerve changes, no eye changes. What's more, in her three months on the admitting ward, her sugar tests had been normal. It seemed worthwhile to try to taper her off the insulin, and see what would happen.

Nothing happened. She was fine without the insulin. She didn't have diabetes.

How had she gotten the diagnosis? Hard to say. Perhaps during her first admission to the Best Hospital, a latent glucose intolerance was precipitated under stress. Or perhaps an intern had overinterpreted some lab values; or perhaps the diabetes diagnosis was simply a mistake, magnified by episodes of low blood sugar treated with intravenous glucose.

In any case, with her hip fixed, Mrs. Muller could walk without pain; without pain medication, she was no longer confused; without the antipsychotic medication for her confusion she was no longer lethargic; and without the diabetes diagnosis, she could go home.

We began to arrange her discharge. Her social worker was delighted to hear that Mrs. Muller was going home and wouldn't need visiting nurses to help with her medications, home-care workers to help with her house, physical therapists for walking, or a caretaker for her daughter. So six months after her admission, Mrs. Muller was discharged to her flat, her daughter, and her little piece of Austria in our city.

What struck me most about the case of Mrs. Muller was how much money I'd saved the health-care system and how little effort that had taken. It hadn't been a difficult diagnosis to make. Just about any doctor at Laguna Honda would have taken that X-ray eventually and made the diagnosis of a dislocated artificial hip.

Then why hadn't anyone else done that in the six months she'd been bedridden? I don't know, but I can guess. The visiting physical therapist let Mrs. Muller's doctor know that she wasn't improving, but there her responsibility ended. The visiting nurse, who was at the house to take care of her diabetes, did so. The home-care aides did their home care, and the social worker, her social work. It wasn't anyone's responsibility to put it all together.

What about her doctor? Didn't she have a doctor, and shouldn't the doctor have made the diagnosis?

I don't know as Mrs. Muller did. Bedridden upstairs in a flat, she may not have seen a physician during those six months. She hadn't seen her surgeon. He'd received reports from the visiting nurse and physical therapist, but he told me that he hadn't thought to have Mrs.

Muller come in for an examination. It was just too difficult. At Laguna Honda, by contrast, it was easy to examine her and get an X-ray, and once the X-ray was done, easy to run upstairs and look at it myself.

Most of the doctors at Laguna Honda would also have stopped Mrs. Muller's pain medications once she was no longer in pain. We had a kind of corporate culture about that. Outside the hospital it was different. I'd admitted many patients whose pain medications had never been discontinued even though their pain had resolved. Why not? Inertia, but also the difficulty of assessing a patient during those short, infrequent outpatient visits. Safer not to rock the boat by taking a medication away from a stable patient.

Fewer of the physicians at Laguna Honda would have tapered her off the antipsychotic, but many would have. We had the luxury of time, after all; of twenty-four-hour observation, so that the risk of Mrs. Muller becoming psychotic as her medications were decreased was acceptable; we would notice if she started to get confused.

Many fewer doctors would have stopped her insulin, diabetes being a diagnosis that is hard to shake off once you have it. Still, with almost any physician at Laguna Honda, Mrs. Muller would have gone home. Because that was the nature of the place—with its open wards where patients could be monitored by observant if unsophisticated nurses; with staff physicians who could see the patient every day and notice changes; with an X-ray machine upstairs.

As I watched Mrs. Muller get into her car, I thought about the money that Laguna Honda's Slow Medicine had saved the health-care system. I was beginning to think of it as just that—as Slow Medicine, in the same way that there was Fast Food and there was Slow Food.

I was thinking about it especially because we were in the middle
of yet another budget crisis, and administration was sending us
memos about cost containment. We should pay attention to the costs
of what we did, administration advised. Perhaps we could avoid prescribing the newest medicine if an older, cheaper one would do; shelve
expensive tests if they had no clinical repercussions; order vans
instead of ambulances; or reconsider routine lab tests. Administration presented its suggestions as if doctors had to be convinced to
watch out for costs, and some doctors do take such suggestions as evidence for a capitalist invasion of the health-care enterprise. Yet the
real problem, Mrs. Muller showed me, was that administration's
thinking did not go far enough; it did not cast a wide enough net and
did not snare the real culprits.

In her case, what saved money were an accurate diagnosis and the
leisurely reevaluation of the patient. It wasn't much—a simple physical examination and an old-fashioned X-ray—but it did take time,
quite a bit of time, actually. A thorough exam takes me almost two
hours, and my daily visits, while not lengthy, were not rushed, but
they were what allowed me to see that Mrs. Muller was not demented,
psychotic, or diabetic.

Economists assume that this kind of care is expensive, but it is
still cheaper than an MRI or even a routine lab panel, not counting
the cost of keeping Mrs. Muller in the hospital for the rest of her life.
I worked it out. At $120,000 per year for the average six years a patient
lives at Laguna Honda, less the cost of Mrs. Muller's resurgery (and
not counting the cost for the care her retarded daughter would have
required), an accurate diagnosis of Mrs. Muller saved the health-care
system about $400,000.

The case of Mrs. Muller got me to thinking. If doctors were going to be held accountable for costs, why shouldn't we get some kind of credit for savings? To use for patients, for the kind of care that economists cut out as extravagances?

What was happening was the opposite: No expense was spared for medications, tests, and procedures, but to make up for that, staff, food, and accoutrements were cut to the bone. The calculus being that the medications, lab tests, and procedures were necessities, but that staff with enough time to do their jobs were an expendable luxury.

Doctors in particular. I was amazed at how expensive economists thought doctors were. They instituted many economic maneuvers—de-skilling medicine onto nurses and physician assistants; computerizing medical decision-making; substituting algorithms for thinking—because they assumed that doctors were such expensive commodities. And yet doctors were not expensive, at least, not the doctors I knew. We cost no more than the nurses, the middle managers, and the information technicians, alas. Adding up all the time I spent with Mrs. Muller, the cost of her accurate diagnosis was about the same as one MRI scan, wholesale.

Economists did the same thing with the other remedies of pre-modern medicine—good food, quiet surroundings, and the little things—treating them as expensive luxuries and cutting them out of their calculations. At Laguna Honda, for instance, while most patients were on fifteen or even twenty daily medications, many of which they didn't need, the budget for a patient's daily meals had been pared down to seven dollars, which could supply only the basics.

I began to wonder: Had economists ever applied their standard of evidence-based medicine to their own economic assumptions? Under what conditions, with which patients and which diseases was it cost-effective to trade good food, clean surroundings, and doctor time for medications, tests, and procedures? Especially ones that patients didn't need?

Although Mrs. Muller was an impressive example of Laguna Honda's Slow Medicine, she wasn't the only one. Almost every patient I admitted had incorrect or outmoded diagnoses and was taking medications for them, too. Medications that required regular blood tests; caused side effects that necessitated still more medications; and put the patient at risk for adverse reactions. Typically my patients came in taking fifteen to twenty-five medications, of which they ended up needing, usually, only six or seven.

And medications, even the cheapest, were expensive. Adding in the cost of side effects, lab tests, adverse reactions, and the time pharmacists, doctors, and nurses needed to prepare, order, and administer them, each medication cost something like six or seven dollars a day. So Laguna Honda's Slow Medicine, to the extent that it led to discontinuing ten or twelve unnecessary medications, was more efficient than efficient health care by at least seventy dollars per day.

I thought about what I could buy for my patients with seventy dollars a day. Good food. Not just tasty food, but excellent, organic, and varied food. Good wine. Hildegardian medicinal ales for the anorexic and digestives for the dyspeptic. Acupuncture. Massage. We'd be rich with seventy dollars per day to spend on each of our patients.

Over the next months, as I studied Hildegard's medicine, my thinking evolved. Suddenly it occurred to me: Why not have a ward at the hospital where Laguna Honda's Way of Slow Medicine could be tested for efficiency? Against the efficient health care of the economists? It would be easy to run a two-year experiment. All I would need would be a ward and an administrative dispensation from the forms and regulations raining down, along with a computer program to track the costs and savings incurred. I was pretty sure we'd end up in the black, and I knew just how I'd spend those savings.

I had a name for the ward, the ecomedicine unit, or ECU. Ecomedicine because it would be an *oikos*—a self-sufficient system at the level of the body, the ward, and the world. The patient's body would be an *oikos* because it would be envisioned not in isolation but as part of its environment. The ward would be an *oikos* because it would be in balance as a self-sufficient minihospital, with its own ecology within the larger ecology of the hospital and the world. The well-being of the staff would be taken into account as well as the well-being of whatever and whoever came into and left the ecomedicine unit: the plants and animals we ate, the stuff we used and threw away.

The ECU would be ecologic in a fractal sense, with ecosystems from smallest to biggest, lowest to highest.

I talked to Dr. Curtis about it. He would be the man to get the ecomedicine unit going.

It was a great idea, he told me, but he'd already planned his next move, which would be to New Zealand. The surfing there was terrific, and the medical system well run. He was looking forward to the change.

Then I told Larissa about my idea. Would she consider being the head nurse of the ecomedicine unit? Because a head nurse would be the first thing I would spend money on.

Of course she would. My ideas, after all, were not so radical; Russia had never lost touch with premodern medicine the way America had. In Russia, she'd often prescribed herbal medicines as tinctures and saunas. They were slower than synthetic medicines but worked pretty well, with fewer side effects. But did I really think that with everything happening at the hospital, with all the new demands of the DOJ and HCFA and Ellen Mary, I would be allowed to start something so, so . . . counterrevolutionary?

Dr. Major would help, I said. She would let me have an ecomedicine unit, I was certain.

Hadn't I heard? Dr. Major had resigned.

Larissa was, as usual, well informed. After twelve years Dr. Major was leaving. No one knew why, but she was as frustrated as the rest of us with the ever-increasing number of middle managers and the ever-decreasing clinical staff. Without Dr. Major, I would never be able to get the necessary dispensation to start my ECU.

It was just as well. It was time to write my PhD and a good time to take a break. I'd saved up enough money from Dr. Weitz's fellowship to take a year off. Why not go to Europe to write it, where premodern medicine had been born but did not die? I would escape the hospital during its painful metamorphosis; and I could visit Hildegard's monasteries and villages. I could study beautiful manuscripts in old libraries. And who knows? Perhaps I would never come back to the hospital or to medicine.

Over the next months I prepared my exit and then went one last time to Dr. Major's office. She was packing up. She was happy to hear about my plans for the future and happy to sign the form granting me a year's leave of absence. Then I went back to our doctors' office; said good-bye to Dr. Romero, Dr. Fintner, and Dr. Jeffers; took my white coat and stethoscope; and a short time later, got on a plane for Switzerland.

Six

DR. DIET, DR. QUIET, AND DR. MERRYMAN

I T WAS EVENING when the jet landed in Switzerland.

On the steps out of the plane it was foggy and cold, but inside the terminal it was bright, with posters touting the professionalism of a Swiss bank, the craftsmanship of a Swiss watch. How elegant everyone was! Slimmer than in the States, with shaped haircuts, gold around wrist and neck, and leather shoes. My train was just underneath the terminal, and in no time at all I was looking out a window at the dark lake and the lights across the lake, in France. It was all so different from the place I'd just left that it was as if I'd been dropped not simply onto a different continent with a different history but onto a different planet.

I arrived just a few days before an important conference about Hildegard, to be held in her town of Bingen, Germany, and I settled into my flat as quickly as I could. The conference was going to cover all of Hildegard's facets—her mysticism, her music, her art, and her medicine; and it was scheduled to take place exactly nine centuries after her birth in 1098, and to run through the anniversary of the day of her death on September 17.

Just knowing those birth and death dates is a lot to know about a medieval person. In the twelfth century there were no bureaus for the registering of birth, death, copyrights, or anything else. But Hildegard took care to mention dates in her writings and to preserve her work for the future. She kept copies of the hundreds of letters she wrote to popes and archbishops, kings and queens; and she made sure that her writings were preserved in a single volume, which has survived to this day. She even wrote a kind of autobiography. So that one of the most unusual things about Hildegard is how much we do know about her, given that she was not a king, a queen, or a pope.

She was born in Bermersheim, a tiny village in the southwest hills of Germany, and her family was well-to-do and devout. Two of her sisters also became nuns, and two brothers, monks. At eight, she was sent away to be schooled by a distant cousin, Jutta; four years later, she, Jutta, and Jutta's three other students were admitted to the formerly all-male monastery of Disibodenberg. This was remarkable because it meant that Hildegard would be exposed to the richer, more complex culture of monks.

After Jutta died, Hildegard took over as the head of the women's side of Disibodenberg. At forty-two, she began her first book, *Scivias,* which described and interpreted the spiritual visions she'd had since she was a girl. This was bold. Although the Church was the most powerful institution in Europe at the time, it was threatened by rising dissent. And authors who claimed independent insight into God's intentions, which was what Hildegard claimed with her visions, were not necessarily embraced. Sometimes they were brought to trial as heretics, imprisoned, and even executed. Hildegard, however, was able to convince first her abbot, then her archbishop, and finally the pope that her visions were from God and not the Devil, and they permitted and even encouraged her to keep writing.

Then, at fifty, she decided to leave the monastery of Disibodenberg and build her own monastery in Bingen. This was another bold move. Nuns and monks were expected to spend their lives in their original monastery, and her abbot forbade her to leave. Hildegard took to her bed with a serious, though undefined illness that lasted for months. Eventually her abbot gave in, and she made a miraculous recovery. She left for Bingen, taking most of the other nuns with her, along with their dowries of money and land. In Bingen she built a new monastery on the Rupertsberg hill.

There she spent the rest of her life. Over the next thirty years, she wrote two additional books of visions and composed more than seventy Gregorian chants. For the dedication of her monastery in 1152, she wrote the first musical drama of Europe, the *Ordo Virtutum*, which her nuns produced and sang, dressed in the scandalous costumes that Hildegard had designed for the occasion. In her seventies, she began to preach in towns across Germany, going out on four separate tours. She wrote many other works, including saints' lives, her interpretation of the Benedictine Rule, and medical and herbal texts, and she also built a second monastery for the many women who wanted to join her.

She lived through a fascinating time in Europe, the so-called Twelfth-Century Renaissance, when the West became intrigued by the Arabic culture it had discovered during the First Crusade and began importing, translating, and imitating Arabic music, medicine, astronomy, literature, and technology. In effect, Hildegard lived through a cultural revolution, and perhaps her biggest accomplishment was dying in her sleep at the age of eighty-one, in the monastery she had built, with her legacy and writings intact.

The conference was going to cover everything.

In addition to the conference, I wanted to see the village where she was born and what was left of her monasteries at Bingen and Disibodenberg. So as soon as I'd settled in my flat, I took the train to Bingen, and on the Sunday afternoon before the conference, I set off exploring.

There wasn't much left of the twelfth century in Bingen, I discovered pretty quickly. It was a forlorn little town on the edge of the Rhine, with a train running right through its center. There were a few structures that Hildegard would have known: Klopp Castle, which would have overlooked her monastery; Saint Martin's church, whose monks did not like her very much; a Roman bridge she would have used; but even they had all been destroyed and rebuilt many times. Her monastery was gone, destroyed during the Thirty Years' War, although I'd heard that there was one piece of it still standing, preserved inside a real-estate office.

It took me a while but I did find the office, which was closed, it being Sunday. I went around to the back anyway and climbed down through weeds to see if I could see inside. The blinds in the back were up and I put my head against the window. There was just enough light for me to make out polished cement floors, recessed halogen lighting, and sleek modern desks. After a while I got used to the darkness and then, suddenly, eerily, I saw it, coming out of the shadows— an immense arch, made of the huge white stone blocks they used in the twelfth century, curving from one end of the office to the other. That was all that was left of Hildegard's monastery: of the church, cloister, dormitory, refectory, scriptorium, hospice, and infirmary that she had, so radically, with such finesse, managed to build against all odds.

The conference was being held at the Hildegard Haus in the hills behind Bingen, and it wasn't fancy, just a few buildings with folding chairs. But planted all around were beds of the medicinal herbs that Hildegard had prescribed—sage and lavender, poppy, rosemary, borage, and many others—and there was a little Hildegard store selling Hildegard statues and calendars and books.

The talks were in the mornings and the afternoons, with lunch in between so the participants could mix and mingle. But they did not mix and mingle. They were too different. Because, as I gradually realized, there were two kinds of Hildegardians, and they did not see eye to eye. There were the scholars who gave the talks—serious, precise, and pale—and there were the enthusiasts who listened to them—Birkenstock-shod, amulet-wearing, and confident. While the scholars focused on the details of Hildegard's life, the enthusiasts were enthralled by the big picture, by the medieval woman who composed such grandiose music, painted such remarkable paintings, envisioned such marvelous visions, and brought a new kind of medicine to the modern West. Which was how they saw her medicine—not as an example of premodern medicine but as something new and brilliant. Thin and bright-eyed, the enthusiasts clustered together during lunch at the round dining tables, exchanging medicinal recipes and business cards for their Hildegard spas and Hildegard retreats.

It was no accident that there were two such different kinds of Hildegardians, because there were two Hildegards—the Hildegard who came out in her theology, letters, and autobiography, and the Hildegard who came out in her medicine. And the conference participants did not mix and mingle because these two Hildegards were seemingly irreconcilable. The Hildegard of the former was a nun who almost never left her monastery. Shy and devout, she lived a strict Benedictine life, with periods of prayer interspersed with rest and work.

The Hildegard who came out in her medicine was completely different. She knew about the body—all about the body—and gave prescriptions for everything that body was heir to: headache, toothache, earache; coughs, colds, and cancers; also for infertility, childbirth, and impotence—things no nun should know about. Even her tone was different: Unlike the mystical Hildegard, who was light-filled, abstract, and not of this world, the medical Hildegard was down-to-earth, forthright, and practical.

It was hard to reconcile the two of them. Most scholars left her medicine alone and concentrated on her theology, letters, music, and art. Other scholars questioned the authenticity of the medical writings ascribed to Hildegard, since all we know about her medicine came from two books, *Causae et Curae* and *Physica,* that surfaced only after her death. None of this, however, bothered the Hildegard enthusiasts. For them, her medicine was authentic, unique, and a gift from God to us moderns. It was the revelation of a spiritual medicine, and they took it at face value, planting her herbs, compounding her prescriptions, and drinking her potions.

I found myself somewhere in between. It was hard for me to imagine how the saintly Hildegard could have written—could have known and cared about!—all the symptoms and earthy problems of *Causae et Curae.* Yet there they were, and there seemed to be nearly as much evidence for the one Hildegard as for the other. During her life, Hildegard was known as much for being a healer as a mystic; the style of the Latin in *Causae et Curae* and *Physica* was the same as in her mystical writing; and in her theology, medicine was one of her main metaphors.

What finally would decide me was a puzzling but indisputable work by Hildegard, the *Lingua Ignota* (*Unknown Language*). It would reassure me that hard as it might be to accept that Hildegard was both a saintly mystic and a medical practitioner, that was our problem, not hers.

After the conference I went back to Lausanne in Switzerland, and I settled down in my flat that overlooked the lake. My study was white and quiet, especially when it was snowing, which it did a lot that year. All I had in it was a white trestle table, a blue chair, piles of books and papers, and a computer.

It was not a very exciting life. It was the opposite of the admitting ward. Instead of walking into the hospital not knowing what might happen, whether a patient would run off into the forest or even try to die, I was in charge of each day. My schedule was predictable: writing in the morning, research in the afternoon, walks in the evening. Now and then, I took a field trip to a Swiss library to examine some special medieval manuscript face-to-face.

There were other differences from my life in America. At Christmastime Lausanne decorated its streets with holly and candles; in the market there was a different holiday food every week. Advent meant *brunsli,* and Christmas meant *lebkuchen,* and if I didn't get *brunsli* at Advent, I wouldn't find it the next week. It was very medieval.

In fact, as the months went by, I began to understand that Switzerland, although modern, had not rejected premodernity as America had. Instead, the Swiss kept what they liked about the past and added the best of each period to their culture, consecutively. So when trains were invented, the Swiss took to them and put trains in everywhere, tunneling through mountains and laying tracks across peaks. But they kept their mountain paths and cobblestone streets for walking. When the automobile arrived, they took to it, too. They put in a bus system and highways, but still did not remove their trains, pave over the cobblestones, or put highways over their footpaths. They liked electric lights, installed them, and even improved on them. But they also liked darkness, and left their lakes and towns without much illumination, so that the stars were visible and the night sky not unfamiliar. Lausanne in particular liked its night watchman from the Middle Ages and still had one. At night, on the hour, I could hear his call that all was well.

The Swiss way seemed to be melding the medieval with the modern in a kind of additive fusion, like lacquering, perhaps. Or better, like evolution, where what works survives, and what doesn't work atrophies and disappears. This Swiss way was followed even in medicine, with the new ideas and medications of modern medicine integrated almost seamlessly into what had come before.

So in Swiss hospitals, I discovered, massage and brandy were prescribed at night for sleep, and herbal baths still used. When a physician found homeopathy useful or even convincing, he did not therefore resign his hospital position, but mixed the two practices, medieval and modern. In the pharmacy I found medieval potions on the shelves right next to modern pills. Old dicta that America had rejected long ago—that cold weather causes colds, that vinegar applied to the temples soothes headaches—were still believed and passed on. What I was discovering with such effort about health and the body from premodern medicine in general, and from Hildegard in specific, was, in Switzerland, nothing new.

The first thing I did in my quiet study was to take a second look at Hildegard's *Unknown Language*. I'd heard a talk about it at the conference and was once again intrigued by what it was and what it could tell me about Hildegard.

Of all her creations—her visions and illuminations, her Gregorian chants and letters—*Unknown Language* was the most mysterious. It was indubitably hers, because it was part of a manuscript that Hildegard put together while she was still alive. No one knew what it was supposed to be, however, because *Unknown Language* was simply five pages of words in some kind of language no one had ever heard of. Above each word was its translation in Latin or German. Hildegard never explained what it was for; a friend of hers had called it "the unknown language given to you by God," which is how it got its name.

A few scholars thought that *Unknown Language* preserved nonsense words that Hildegard uttered in a state of trance, like the talking in tongues of the Pythia or of certain Christian sects. But most scholars believed it was a glossary for a private language that Hildegard invented for her nuns to use when they were inside her monastery. Why, no one knew. The first time I looked at it, I wondered if it was a code masquerading as a glossary. The Middle Ages liked codes a lot, and a coded text would have been a way for Hildegard to write what she wouldn't have dared otherwise. I'd asked a computer specialist in codes to take a look at it, and he gave *Unknown Language* to his students to decipher. While I was in Switzerland, I received his summary of their research: Hildegard's *Unknown Language* was definitely not a code.

So now I was going to study it as what it seemed to be, a glossary for a Hildegardian language.

I started by counting. *Unknown Language* contained 1,011 words, and all of them, I noticed, were nouns. Which meant that if it was actually used as a language, it must have been with the grammar of another language—Latin or German, most likely. What nouns did Hildegard choose to translate? What order were they in?

The very first word in *Unknown Language*, I saw, was *aigonz*—God, according to the translation above it. Then came *aieganz*—angel; *zivienz*—saint; *livionz*—savior; and *divveliz*—devil. So, reassuringly, in her *Unknown Language* Hildegard placed spiritual beings above everything else.

Next came words for man, woman, and child, and words for the family—father, mother, brother, sister, son, daughter, and stepfather and stepmother, too.

In third place—and here I was pleasantly surprised—came medical words. There were words for the blind, the lame, the leper, the heart patient, and then for the parts of the body from head to toe. What was stunning was that Hildegard had words for all the parts of the body—not just lung, heart, and liver, but vagina (*fragilanz*), testicles (*virlaiz*), and penis. In fact, she had two words for penis—*creveniz* and *lizia*. Talk about hard to square with a modest, enclosed nun! Suddenly, reading that list of words in *Unknown Language* was like reading a mystery story. What would come next?

Next came words for bishop, priest, abbot, abbess—important positions in the Church. Then for building (Hildegard was building a monastery, after all). Then for workers and craftsmen: gardener, fisherman, weaver, goldsmith, silversmith. There were words for the tools of the scriptorium, where her manuscripts would have been copied—pen and parchment, ink and paints; and there were words for the days of the week, the months of the year, and the times of day.

It was fascinating. With its words and its ordering, Hildegard's

Unknown Language supplied an inventory of Hildegard's physical world as she saw it.

It also solved the problem of Hildegard's practice of medicine. Because not only were there words in *Unknown Language* for the humors, for the parts of the body, and for certain illnesses; there were also hundreds of words for the same medicinal plants that Hildegard recommended in her medical books. In fact, names for medicinal plants made up the largest section of the text. There was lavender (*liniz*), yarrow (*agonzia*), wormwood (*karischa*), marijuana (*aseruz*), and the opium poppy (*cuz*), to name just a few; and the only logical reason for Hildegard to have included so many medicinal plants in her glossary was that she did, in fact, use them.

Unknown Language was indeed a code, I concluded, but not a code to a secret text. It was a code to Hildegard's world. And in that world there was no contradiction between the mystical Hildegard, who needed words for God and angels, pen and parchment; and the medical Hildegard, who needed words for the humors, for the parts of the body, and for medicines. *Unknown Language* convinced me that it was one and the same Hildegard who wrote *Scivias* and *Causae et Curae,* who was stunned into silence by a vision of the universe, and who knew how to prepare a potion and touch a patient.

I f Hildegard did practice medicine, I asked myself next, then how did she learn what she knew? There was only one possible answer, which was that she had been the infirmarian for the women's side of Disibodenberg.

Now, every Benedictine monastery had a monk or nun infirmarian, whose special duty was to take care of the sick. The patients he or she took care of were more varied than I'd imagined at first because a monastery was not simply a place of worship but also a working farm. It employed many people, and the monk or nun infirmarian was responsible for all of them: for injured workers and their families when they took sick; for pilgrims and travelers; and for the monks and nuns of the monastery who became ill or old. Occasionally the infirmarian would be a physician who'd become a monk later in life, but most often he or she learned the healing arts as an apprentice to the senior infirmarian in the monastery.

This must have been how Hildegard learned her medicine. She would have had the perfect opportunity because Disibodenberg, with both a men's side and a women's side, would have needed a nun infirmarian for the women. She probably learned her medicine from the monk infirmarian for the men. Most likely, when she moved to Bingen, she wrote her *Causae et Curae* as a medical text for the nun infirmarian who replaced her when she herself became abbess.

So now I picked up *Causae et Curae* again, this time to study it as if I were Hildegard's twelfth-century student infirmarian. I decided to use only the information she provided in *Causae et Curae*, along with whatever would have been available to such a student. I would not use medical texts that came from before the twelfth century unless her twelfth-century student could have seen them, and no texts from after the twelfth century. I would try out what I learned, too, just as a student might. I would grow some of the plants she recommended, and I would prepare some of her prescriptions. I did boil up her sage cough lozenges; and I did prepare some of her medicinal potions.

Slowly I began to understand Hildegard's *methodus medendi*— her Way of Medicine. Not that she laid it out. Yet through her descriptions of diseases, her explanations of how medicines worked, and her teachings about diagnosis, I gradually put together an idea of what she must have done with her patients. Her method was very different from mine—and surprisingly similar.

Like me, her first and most important tool was observing her patient. She watched her patient as he walked in, sat down, and told his story. She noted how rich or poor he seemed, how clean or dirty. She looked at his color, his animation, and the brightness of his eyes; and she estimated the greenness of his *viriditas*.

Then, just as I do, she began her examination of the patient with the vital signs—the signs of life: temperature, respiratory rate, and pulse. Although not in the same way as I do. Hildegard didn't take a temperature with a thermometer, which wouldn't be invented for seven centuries; instead, she felt her patient's forehead, hands, and feet. I do that, too, nowadays, ever since the mercury thermometer disappeared from the hospital, to be replaced by the easy-to-use but unreliable electronic thermometer.

Next, she attended to her patient's respiration. But she was not getting a respiratory rate of so many breaths a minute the way I do; she was interested in something other than a number. Breath for her meant *spiritus*—the essence of life—and what she did was simply observe her patient breathing. Was his breath weak or strong? Fast or slow? Continuous? Or—most serious of all—discontinuous, with long spaces between each breath? Breath told her a lot about just how sick her patient was.

Last of the vital signs, Hildegard took her patient's pulse. But again, differently from the way I take a pulse. She was not counting the pulse for fifteen seconds and multiplying by four. That would have required a watch, also only invented seven centuries later. Rather, she was taking the pulse the way we speak of taking the pulse of a social group, by which we mean getting a sense of its emotional state—its enthusiasm, reluctance, energy. The pulse she took was the standard against which she measured the life force of her patient. It was not about heart, blood pressure, and circulation, but about the health and illness of her patient.

Sitting quietly, holding her patient's hand, she would first determine the temperament, since each temperament had a characteristic pulse. Her patient might be melancholic, sanguine, choleric, or phlegmatic, and was usually some combination, of the four. Because, just as DNA is made up of a combination of four basic nucleic acids, so every individual "temperament" was made up of a subtle combination of all four basic tempers, and the patient's pulse would reveal this unique temperament. Then she would decide whether that particular pulse was "normal," that is, "healthy," for that particular patient.

The rest of her exam was more focused and simpler than mine. She made sure to look at the part of the body that was bothering her patient, though not with flashlight, tongue blade, or stethoscope; instead with her eyes and her hands. Because her concept of the body was different from mine. She was not examining a body of fleshy organs linked by networks of vessels and nerves, but a body of liquid humors needing to flow freely and in the proper balance.

Last, she examined her patient's blood and urine. Again, not the way I examine blood and urine, sending them off to the laboratory for tests, although some of my tests are refinements of hers. What she did was, after drawing blood and getting a sample of urine, she waited for the blood and urine to layer out into their basic humors of blood, choler, phlegm, and melancholia. Then she "read" them, estimating their balance of the four humors and confirming her humoral diagnosis.

Finally she would come up with her prescription. It would have two parts: the first would be an individualized prescription for a "regime," and the second would be a prescription for some herbal mixture.

Regime—from *regula* (rule)—meant a set of rules for living. What you ate, how much you slept, how much you exercised, how often you had sex. Regime wasn't only for the sick; therefore, if you followed the right regime for your body, you had a good chance of staying healthy. Regime was personal, and it varied with your particular humoral makeup, the season, your age, and the climate in which you lived. Its principles were summarized by the proverb "Even without a doctor / You have three doctors at hand / Dr. Diet, Dr. Quiet, and Dr. Merryman."

Hildegard's prescription for regime would, consequently, include what her patient should and should not eat and drink (that was Dr. Diet); how much exercise, sleep, and rest he should take (Dr. Quiet); and how much sex and what kind of emotions he should allow himself (Dr. Merryman). Today all that we have left of regime is the monotonous injunctions to lose weight, lower our cholesterol, sleep eight hours a day, exercise, and be cheerful. Hildegard and premodern medicine were more subtle. Nothing was bad or good but as it suited the season, the climate, and the person. So she might recommend beer to fatten up the anorexic and forbid red wine to the choleric; in spring, fresh green shoots were good; in winter, stews. For the lovesick, distraction; for the scattered and anxious, focus.

The second part of Hildegard's prescription would be for a medicine, usually a mixture of those plants whose names she'd been so careful to put into her *Unknown Language*. She would prescribe just how the medicine should be made up and how it should be taken—eaten or drunk or applied to the skin so many times a day for so many days.

After I'd finished putting together my idea of Hildegard's

methodus medendi, what intrigued me most about it was how different it was from mine and yet how similar. The biggest difference was that her method did not use numbers. It was subjective. Almost everything I did had a number—blood pressure, pulse, and temperature; the width of the liver, the circumference of the calf, and all the measurements of blood and urine. Which made my method objective, to some extent, and reproducible by others. And yet, as different as they seemed, from a distance they wouldn't have looked all that different. Patients came to Hildegard with symptoms—pain, coughs, rashes— just as they do to me; and just as I do, she questioned and examined them, assessed their blood and urine, and gave them a prescription.

But did her method work?

Some of her prescriptions probably did. Her medicines were not as concentrated as the chemicals we have today; they took longer to act and were not so certain. Yet many of today's effective medications originated in the plants that she and other premodern practitioners prescribed. Opium, with its potent mix of morphine and codeine, was always grown in the infirmarian's garden, and it does work well for the pain, cough, and diarrhea for which Hildegard prescribed it. Ergot from rye fungus does control blood loss and instigate labor, as she used it; and we still use extracts of vinca and mistletoe for certain cancers. Doubtless there were active hormones and potent vitamins in the thyroid glands, bear's testicles, and liver she had her patients take.

There were even things to be learned from her method, I concluded, which we'd lost in our pursuit of the most reproducible tests and the strongest drugs: her patience, her skills at observation, her notions of the relationship between patient and environment—Dr. Diet, Dr. Quiet, and Dr. Merryman.

Nevertheless, as I closed *Causae et Curae* for the third time, I was

even more grateful for modern medicine than I'd been before, especially for its scientific method, which tests the past, rejects what is
ineffective, improves on what works, and passes to the future its powerful results. Taken all together, how jealous Hildegard would have
been of me and my technology! Of my amazing ways of examining the
blood, of peering into the body, of what I had to heal the sick.

The snow had started to melt in Lausanne; the days were getting
longer; and one day as I was out for a walk, I passed a woman
with a large thyroid. I could see it clearly, swelling at her throat, and
suddenly I found myself wanting to stop her and examine it. I didn't
stop her—it was Switzerland, after all—but I did begin to think about
medicine. I missed it. I wanted to see patients. And I still had a few
months to go before my leave of absence was up.

So that evening I contacted Dr. Hoefer, chief of community
medicine at the University Hospital in Geneva. I explained who I
was, what I was doing in Switzerland, and what I was missing. We
talked for quite a while. I wouldn't be able to practice medicine on
such short notice, Dr. Hoefer told me, but he could arrange a rotation
so that I could get a sense of how medicine was practiced in Switzerland. Why don't we meet next week at his hospital in Geneva? We
could have lunch, and in the meantime he would put together a schedule so that I could spend a day or two with each of his medical units.

The next week I took the train to Geneva for our meeting. The
train was one of those things that the Swiss made sure to save from
the nineteenth century, and I loved it. As an American I was supposed to have a love affair with the automobile, but in Switzerland
I'd learned it was more like a bad marriage, where you stay together
because there is no one else. In Switzerland there was someone else,

quiet and clean and safe, who arrived on time and took me exactly where I wanted to go. The train stopped in the center of town, and ten minutes later I was walking up the hill toward the Hôpitaux Universitaires de Genève (HUG). As I got nearer, I saw signs posted with increasing frequency; they showed a car horn with a red slash through it and the reminder QUIET: HOSPITAL ZONE.

I hadn't seen such signs in a long time, I suddenly realized as I was walking. When I first arrived at Laguna Honda, they'd been all around, and then, somehow, they weren't. What had happened to them? When did they disappear? Those signs had been a reminder not only not to honk your horn, but that the sick needed quiet, rest, and peace, and I missed them. Although it was just as well they were gone, I thought as I got nearer the HUG, because the one thing that Laguna Honda was not, was quiet, and car horns were the least of it. Televisions and radios; beepers and cell phones; overhead announcements, incoming faxes, IVs, oxygen equipment, EKG monitors— every new machine had its own signal and its own alarm. The only places at Laguna Honda that were quiet were the linen closets. And yet peace, rest, and noninterruption were healing, as everyone knew; they were Dr. Quiet; and the Swiss, apparently, hadn't forgotten him.

From the outside the HUG seemed like any hospital in the States—big, multistoried, an office building—but inside it was different. It was not crowded. Its floors were polished, and its light natural. Its patients looked different, too. They were dressed in slacks, shirts, and ties, or dresses, stockings, and heels, and they were waiting quietly in the lobby.

Dr. Hoefer met me at the elevator, and we went up together to his office, where he explained how his department worked. Community Medicine in Switzerland was where the Swiss put their public and social programs, he told me: their immigrant outreach programs, their alcohol and drug programs, their epidemiology and public health divisions, and their tropical medicine. He also had an acute medical division and an emergency room, as well. Then he passed me the schedule he'd made up for me; over the next few weeks I would get a chance to spend some time in each of those units. On my last day I would go with a team of his doctors to visit a rehabilitation hospital in France. And now, what about something to eat?

He took me down for lunch in the hospital cafeteria. I was impressed. It was a modern, spacious, and well-lit place, but what amazed me was the food. There were fresh salads and soups, and chefs in white hats slicing rack of lamb and preparing omelettes to order. Most remarkable, at the end of the line were little bottles of Swiss wine and three kinds of beer on tap.

Was this the doctors' cafeteria? I asked Dr. Hoefer.

No, it was for everyone, he said, doctors, staff, patients, visitors. The food that went up to the patients' rooms came from the same cafeteria, and, yes, patients were permitted wine and beer. As a matter of fact, doctors prescribed alcohol: red wine at meals, beer for the anorexic, sometimes schnapps at night, for sleep.

He ordered a small steak, a salad, a little bottle of red wine, and so did I. And as we ate, I thought about Dr. Diet.

At Laguna Honda, Dr. Diet had once had his day. There'd been a time when diet—good food and drink—was just about the most important thing the hospital had provided to its patients. I'd even seen menus from the century before, with their pint of wine or four ounces of whiskey every day, their beef stew for breakfast and dinner, their holiday meals of fresh game in plum sauce. Even when Dr. Jeffers had first arrived, he told me, the neighbors would still make a point of coming to the hospital for lunch and for dinner.

No longer. It wasn't that Dr. Diet wasn't considered, exactly.

There were almost as many dieticians as doctors at Laguna Honda, and each dietician made sure that each of her patients received the appropriate amount of vitamins, minerals, and fluids, and whatever special diet the doctor prescribed. But what with all the dieticians and special diets, there wasn't much left in the budget for chefs.

On the ecomedicine unit, I decided after I'd finished my steak and wine, once we discontinued all those unnecessary medications, we would use the savings to increase the food budget.

A lot.

For the sake of Dr. Merryman, as well as Dr. Diet.

spent two weeks at the HUG. I learned that public medicine in Switzerland dealt with the same problems we did in America and in many of the same ways, though with certain differences.

During my day on the medicine unit, one of the doctors called in sick, and I got the chance to see patients with the medical students. At the end of that afternoon, the chief of medicine, Dr. Mendes, showed me around. First we went to the acute medical unit, where patients were hospitalized when they needed an expeditious, thorough evaluation. Instead of having to spend weeks as an outpatient, getting tests and seeing different specialists, a patient could get all the tests, a diagnosis, and a plan in a few days, usually. It was much more efficient and sometimes safer, he pointed out.

We used to be able to do that, too, I told him, before the cost-effective, health-care efficiency movement took over. Now it was impossible to put someone in the hospital just for a workup, and sometimes it took us months to figure out what was going on. How was it that they could still do it in Switzerland?

No HMOs, he said. At least not yet. In Switzerland, medical care was still private; doctors had their own private offices; and patients had their own private doctors. The cost was manageable because of certain government policies. First, every Swiss citizen had to buy basic health insurance, which insurance companies were required to sell on a nonprofit basis. Under a certain level of income, the government subsidized those premiums. The insurance companies could still make a profit, though, because they were allowed to sell supplemental health insurance on a for-profit basis.

In addition, since there were always patients who fell through this net, the government subsidized public hospitals like the HUG, which incidentally provided places for medical research, and for medical and nursing training as well. The overall cost was also manageable because malpractice wasn't an issue in Switzerland. Doctors were never sued. He didn't know why. Maybe Switzerland didn't have enough lawyers.

Health care was still not cheap, of course—it made up 12.5 percent of the GDP—but that was still less than in the States, and almost everyone was happy with it. Doctors were not as well paid, it was true, but since medical education was free, they didn't have such huge loans to pay back and didn't have to make as much money.

"What about the emergency room?" I asked. "Your division runs that, too. Can I see it?"

"Of course."

He took me down a hall, to a large room whose door was open, though its lights were off. It had seven beds in it, each with plumped pillows and a down coverlet. But it was empty.

"Here's the emergency room," he said.

There must be a language problem, I thought. "The 'emergency' room?" I confirmed. "For emergencies? But it's empty. Where is everyone?"

Dr. Mendes shrugged. "It's usually empty. Trauma cases go to the surgical unit, obstetrics to obstetrics, and there aren't many medical emergencies because when patients get sick, they go to their own doctors."

We stood at the door for a minute while I looked at that non-emergency room. What kind of medical system had no emergencies? Even more remarkable, what kind of medical system fluffs up the pillows, starches the sheets, and lays down coverlets on top of its beds?

spent two days with the alcohol and drug rehabilitation unit, a day with the unit in charge of epidemiology and immigration, and one afternoon with Dr. Em, the tropical medicine specialist.

Dr. Em was short and round and energetic, with round glasses, and I sat with her all afternoon while patients from Africa and the Middle East came through her office. They spoke many languages and had diseases quite unfamiliar to me, but who I remember best is Miss Q. from Cameroon.

Miss Q. was tall, slim, and a very dark brown, and she wore her hair in woven rolls about her face. Her features were thin and delicate, and despite the pockmarks on her cheeks, she was pretty. Also, after her year in Switzerland, quite Swiss, wearing a dark gray skirt, close-fitting knit top, and stylish black-framed glasses. In French with an African cadence, she explained to Dr. Em that now that she'd finished her secretarial course, she was going back to her native Cameroon, and she wanted to find out if there was any new treatment for her disease.

What were her symptoms? Dr. Em asked.

Well, every few months she would get a fever, her muscles would ache, and her skin would start itching. A day or two later her vision would get blurry, and sometimes she would see a little worm shape crossing her line of sight. Then she would feel better until her next bout.

It was a bizarre set of symptoms, I thought, though I did remember something like it from medical school.

What did Miss Q. have? Dr. Em asked me.

I didn't know, but Miss Q. did because everyone in her village had the same thing. She had loiasis.

Then Dr. Em reminded me that loiasis was caused by the loa loa, a parasite spread by the tabanid fly of the African rain forest. It had a complicated life cycle, which depended almost entirely on human beings. People acquired the infection when they were bitten by a fly carrying the microscopic loa loa larvae in its proboscis. As the fly fed on the blood, those larvae entered the skin and migrated into the subcutaneous tissue, where they matured into the adult loa loa worm. Still under the skin they met each other and mated and reproduced the next stage of their life cycle, the microfilariae, which then entered the bloodstream by the thousands. When another tabanid fly bit, it picked up these microfilariae, which matured in the fly's gut into the infective larvae, and that was how the disease was spread.

The human body was allergic to the adult worm, Dr. Em went on, and so whenever the adult worm moved around, the body would react with the fever, joint pain, and itching that Miss Q. described. Sometimes the adult worms even migrated across the eye, causing the worm shapes that Miss Q. sometimes perceived. Loiasis caused much suffering and millions of dollars of lost productivity in Cameroon and other African countries, although it wasn't fatal. But the only sure way to get rid of loiasis would be to eradicate the tabanid fly, and that would mean eradicating the rain forest.

And—here Dr. Em turned to Miss Q.—there was a treatment for loiasis called diethylcarbamazine. But it wasn't perfect. It caused strokes and kidney damage in patients who were severely infected with loa loa, and treatment, therefore, had to be monitored closely. Also, it didn't reliably kill every adult worm, so the disease could recur even after treatment. And, of course, anyone living in Cameroon would likely get reinfected. Since Miss Q. was returning to Cameroon, where her treatment could not be supervised and where she would probably get bitten again, Dr. Em would not recommend a course of treatment.

As Miss Q. listened to Dr. Em, I watched her. She was quiet and composed. When she heard that there was a treatment for her painful, debilitating disease, but not for her, not if she wanted to go home, she didn't cry or get angry. She simply squared her thin and elegant shoulders, just a bit. Which meant that she would go back to her village, her family, and her country, and do the best she could with her fate.

I admired that. I didn't know whether I could do the same. I thought not. There was a whole tradition behind Miss Q.'s composure; it went way back; it was deep, mature, grown-up. Not American, with our youthfulness, our rebelliousness against fate, and our refusal of fate, too. Which rebelliousness was what led to the unraveling of the life cycle of loa loa, of course, to diethylcarbamazine, and would lead to other even more effective antifilarial medications.

I never forgot Miss Q. Partly because loiasis was an interesting, an unusual disease, one I had never seen before. There was something fascinating as well as horrible about living creatures for whom we are their homes and cities—where they are born, mature, grow old, and die, and where they travel, sightseeing in our blood, lungs, and even eyes. But mostly I remembered Miss Q. because it was the first time in many months that I'd been inside the special space that doctor and patient create together. Miss Q., with her quiet manner and her fortitude, had reminded me just how much there was to learn from patients, and not only about illness and disease.

M y last experience at the HUG was the next day. The rehabilitation unit was visiting a French alcohol and drug rehabilitation hospital in the Alps, and I went with them. Sitting in the backseat between two other physicians, I didn't see much during the drive, but when we arrived, I knew where I was. The Hospital of Saint Bruno, with its arched stone entrance and wings of high, arcaded windows, was a long-lost relative of Laguna Honda.

Dr. Lapin, its resident physician, met us at the entrance. He really was a resident, too—he lived in the Hospital of Saint Bruno just as the interns and nurses used to do at Laguna Honda, and just as the podiatry students still did, despite Dee and Tee. We would go on the tour first, he told us, and then we would have our lunch and our meeting.

The Hospital of Saint Bruno, he explained, had been built in the nineteenth century as a tuberculosis sanatorium, when the only treatment for tuberculosis was regime—a diet of eggs, milk, and meat; and the quiet, sunlight, and fresh air of the Alps. Although that treatment had worked surprisingly well, after antibiotics against tuberculosis were discovered, the hospital had been emptied and almost torn down. But then it was realized that its out-of-the-way location, fresh air, and good diet might make the hospital suitable as a rehabilitation facility for alcoholics and drug abusers, and it was reopened.

Dr. Lapin turned and walked through the arched stone entrance, and we followed him through a hall and out into a wide corridor. On our left were floor-to-ceiling windows; they faced south, he said, for the sunlight and vitamin D that did help cure tuberculosis. On our right were the rooms of the patients. The DOJ would have been pleased. Each one was private, with the narrow bed, small desk, and wooden closet that the French favor. But they were empty, the patients being at group therapy sessions that lasted all day.

We followed Dr. Lapin into the great room, which reminded me of Laguna Honda's hall for its smokers and poker players. Two patients were sitting in wooden chairs under the windows, and Dr. Lapin introduced them. Again I thought of Laguna Honda, because Madame Rouen was just as yellow, swollen, and spotted as Mrs. McCoy had been on the day she arrived; and Monsieur Noir, young, sallow, and shriveled, would have fit right in among our poker players, assuming he knew how to play poker. Then we went outside and saw the tennis courts for exericise, the green lawns for rest, and the wooded hills behind the hospital for meditative walking.

Finally Dr. Lapin led us to lunch in the doctors' dining room.

The dining room was entirely of polished wood—floors, walls, ceiling—and very quiet, without windows. Its long table was set for eight, with gold place plates, silver settings, three wineglasses, and one tiny glass for liqueur. And for the rest of the afternoon we ate and drank as course after course arrived, and wine after wine was poured.

Dr. Lapin and the HUG doctors discussed the treatment of alcohol and drug abuse, though I can't tell you what they said. I wasn't paying attention. Mostly I tasted and sipped, and looked around at the heavy, quiet walls. Especially after that third glass of wine, they seemed to exude stability and security, with their memory of many such meals, and their expectation of many more.

I thought about how, after tuberculosis was cured, the Hospital of Saint Bruno had not been torn down. Someone had recognized that there was still a need for such a place in modern France, this century for alcoholics and drug abusers. I thought about how, even after a cure for alcoholism and drug abuse was discovered, there would still be some such disease without a cure, some illness whose victims could profit from the prescriptions of those old-fashioned physicians—Dr. Diet, Dr. Quiet, and Dr. Merryman.

Sipping my cognac, it pleased me to think that the Hospital of Saint Bruno would have still another incarnation, another go at curing some illness in the old way. And I wondered for the first time in almost a year: What was happening at Laguna Honda? Was it going to be rebuilt as the Department of Justice had demanded? Or was it going to be closed and torn down?

So that night I called Dr. Fintner for news. I was scheduled to reappear on the first of July, and remembering the place as I left it, with Dr. Major packing up and the hospital's future uncertain, I telephoned with some anxiety.

Dr. Fintner answered, and she sounded just the same. Diffident and hard to bring out at first. Everything was fine, she said, and she was looking forward to my coming back.

But what was going on? I asked. Did Dr. Major leave? Who replaced her? What about Dr. Stein and the rebuild? What about the DOJ?

Oh yes, Dr. Major was gone. Dr. Romero was medical director now, and two part-time doctors had taken her place on the admitting ward. It had been kind of hectic. As for the future, well, Dr. Stein had just come out with his recommendation, which was to build a new and even bigger hospital, and the board of supervisors was looking into it.

It would cost hundreds of millions of dollars, though, and most people thought it would be better to just close the hospital down and use the money to take care of patients at home.

"But they don't have homes, Julie."

"I know. That's the problem."

"And even if we gave them homes, they don't have families to help out. And it would be expensive to provide everything they'd need at home—it would be like setting up a thousand minihospitals, with round-the-clock nursing care and daily doctor visits. Isolating, too."

"Well, it looks like the board of supervisors agrees with you, Victoria. Because it accepted Dr. Stein's report, and a bond measure is going on the ballot. But no one thinks it will pass."

"Anything else going on?"

"Well, Dr. Romero doesn't like being medical director much, and she's decided to come back to the admitting ward. But we're not. I guess it's been hard on her. It's been frantic here, actually. The DOJ came back thirteen times. So she's hired a new doctor, and just the two of them will be on the admitting ward."

"But what about us?"

"I don't know. I've heard we'll be taking over three of the long-term wards—a hundred patients between us. I don't know whether I can do that, Victoria. I'm thinking perhaps I'll retire."

That was sobering. Though interesting, I reflected, after I hung up. I would miss the admitting ward, for sure. And I did have an alternative. Dr. Hoefer had offered me a position as professor adjoint in the Department of Community Medicine. He was fine with my part-time practice and he liked my medieval research, and it would satisfy my ambition of living by that lake in Switzerland, writing in the morning and seeing patients in the afternoon.

But I missed my home, and I missed my hospital. I wanted to see what was going to happen; how it would all turn out.

S o right on schedule, I returned.

It was early in the morning when I parked in my usual space downstairs by the pigeons and the smokers who had, in my absence, been exiled outside. Laguna Honda was just as shabby-elegant as ever, I saw—peach-colored paint peeling from its walls and red-tiled roof. I went inside and up the stairs. But before I went into the medical director's office to get my new assignment, I took a stroll under the statue of Saint Francis and over to the admitting ward. Its double doors were, for the first time, closed, and a new sign was up on the wall next to them, in pink with a little pink heart: WELCOME TO THE ADMITTING WARD!

I walked over to the hall where the smokers used to congregate. It was empty, though the vending machines, tables, and floor-to-ceiling windows were still there. I stood for a while and just looked. Then I turned and started walking back to the medical director's office when I heard a voice.

"Is that you, Dr. S.?"

I looked around. I didn't see anyone. "Who said that?"

"Is that you?"

Then I noticed, in the corner of the hall, a wheelchair. And in the wheelchair, twisted and tiny, a patient I hardly remembered, a patient of Dr. Fintner's. I'd never paid him much attention. He was one of our developmentally disabled patients—blind from birth, twisted from birth, and, I'd always assumed, retarded from birth. How had he recognized me? How had he remembered me? After a year? Blind?

"Yes, it's Dr. S. How did you know it was me?" I asked.

"You've been gone a long time, haven't you, Dr. S.?"

"Yes. A whole year. But how did you know it was me?"

"Oh . . . I could tell it was you by your walk. You've been gone a long time."

"Yes. I have."

Then he smiled at me, and I smiled back and hoped he could hear my smile—who knows? But he was how I knew—I was back.

It was the first time I'd understood that I was not only in the audience at the hospital but on the stage, too. Of course, I'd always known I was an actor in the life of my patients, but I hadn't realized that my features, mannerisms, walk were scrutinized as much by my patients as theirs were by me; that as much as I examined them, they examined me and reached their own conclusions. Although why I hadn't realized what a stage it was—that spacious place with its wide windows, great hallways, and open wards—I don't know. It would be one of the big lessons in this next act of my time at Laguna Honda.

Then I walked down the hallway and went over to the medical director's office.

Seven

DANCING TO THE TUNE
OF GLENN MILLER

THERE WAS NO MEDICAL DIRECTOR in the medical director's office, not yet and not for many months, but it didn't matter much because there was Jerrie.

Jerrie was the secretary for the medical department, which consisted not only of doctors, psychiatrists, and psychologists, but also of the radiology department, the laboratory, social work, and rehabilitation. And Jerrie was the linchpin of the whole thing. She knew just about everyone in the hospital, and she always knew exactly what was going on. Her office was between Dr. Major's office and Miss Lester's, so she was even closer to the incoming and outgoing ambulance drivers than Miss Lester had been. Except at four PM, when the tide of nurses at change of shift surged past, her door was always open. Since Jerrie's desk faced the door, it was her smiling, amused face that met me on my first morning back.

"Well, well. Dr. S.... at last. Welcome back! And how was Switzerland?"

Hers was a small office, but it was gossip central, curbside-consult central, spontaneous-meeting central, and therapy central. Not just for the doctors but for everyone, even the patients. In fact, Jerrie had her own collection of patients—schizophrenic, brain-injured, demented, developmentally delayed, and often all four—who visited her daily.

For instance, Mr. Stuart Bayou was one of her patients. I'd admitted him years before. He was a grown man and virile, with a heavy five-o'clock shadow no matter how well the nurses shaved him, dark brown hair that the nurses combed over his balding pate, a strong jaw, straight nose, and full mouth. But because of a hip fracture that had knit poorly, he was confined to a wheelchair. He was confined also by a brain that had stopped maturing when he was five years old. So Mr. Bayou couldn't read or write, and, despite his athletic 180-pound frame and masculine habitus, he was still a five-year-old, with obsessions and even tantrums. But he did like the Beatles and could always be calmed by a positive response to his request: "Write me the Beatles. Write me the Beatles. Write me the Beatles."

He turned up almost every afternoon at Jerrie's office. She had paper and crayons ready, and every afternoon she wrote out THE BEATLES for Mr. Bayou over and over again on a piece of paper. She would hand it to him, and Mr. Bayou would scan it as if trying to figure out its magic meaning, then take it gratefully and put it away with his other papers and the magazines he'd lifted from the library. Then he would wheel off to visit someone else.

Jerrie was large though not fat, and a warm medium brown, with a lot of Native American and North African in her face. Her features were straight, her eyes golden brown, and her temperament cheerful but ironic, the sine qua non of her position. It was she who gave me my new schedule that day and explained the chess moves that had occurred in my absence. She confirmed Dr. Fintner's report: Dr. Romero and a new doctor, Dr. Dan Stanislaus, were now the admitting team for the admitting ward. Dr. Jeffers had moved to Clarendon Hall, and Dr. Fintner and I would share three wards, totaling 102 patients. I would have E4, a complex medical ward with rehabilitation patients; Dr. Fintner would have D5, also a complex medical ward, and we would share E6, a dementia ward.

I might want to get myself to my new wards and begin getting to know my new patients, Jerrie suggested, even though Dr. Fintner had not yet arrived.

I sighed. I loved the minihospital that the admitting ward was—the unpredictability of each day, the patients who came and so often went. It had suited me well. These new wards would be difficult, especially the dementia ward, the classic back ward of a state hospital. I thought about the HUG and the position I'd turned down, and then I started up the stairs for E6.

E6 looked almost exactly like the admitting ward except that it had been built during the Depression and had a narrower entrance and dimmer lighting. Otherwise its setup was the same. At the entrance, a few private rooms, a little kitchen, a cozy staff room, a linen room, a nursing station, and then the wide, open ward. Thirty-four beds lined the walls of the ward, each next to a window; at the far end, taking the place of the medieval chapel, was the solarium. Being one floor above the admitting ward, E6 had an even more beautiful, though more distant, view over the city to the ocean.

Dr. Kalma, the former doctor of E6, had left me with a good

ward, a straightened-out ward. He'd completed everything: the annual physical examinations, the monthly orders, the flu shots, the advance life directives. He didn't give me his set of index cards though—doctors didn't carry them anymore. Nor did he wait to walk me around the ward as Dr. Judd had done on my first day. But he didn't need to, because I would have plenty of time to learn about the patients all by myself.

Now E6 was part of the "dementia cluster," and this idea, of clustering patients with the same diagnosis together on one ward, was one of Ellen Mary's innovations. Before, patients had been assigned to a ward not on the basis of their medical diagnosis, but on some other basis, not always easy to guess—gender, nursing needs, and the mood, connections, and seniority of the head nurse. There were, after all, difficult patients and easy patients, satisfying patients and frustrating patients. And, since many patients stayed a long time and the head nurses even longer, over the years each ward evolved quite individually. Each had a reputation—of being good or bad, pleasant or not, for patients, staff, and head nurses.

Surprisingly, though, despite this individuality and the struggle of the head nurse for a manageable ward, each ward ended up with a near-identical mix of patients, as far as medical acuity and nursing needs went. Each ward had a few difficult patients, a few easy patients, some medically complex patients, some demented patients, and some little old ladies or little old men. This variety had had its advantages. It had been good for the nurses because it lent variability to their day and equalized the difficulty of their jobs across the hospital. It had been good for the doctors because it kept us on our toes medically. And it had been good for the patients because the disabilities in any particular ward were complementary—the physically disabled watching out for the demented; the lame leading the blind, in fact.

But that system was not the modern system, which was to cluster patients by their diagnosis. So as soon as Miss Lester retired, Ellen Mary Flanders reorganized the patients into new "diagnostic" clusters: the "complex medical cluster" for patients who were terribly but chronically ill; the "psychosocial cluster" for patients who were mentally as well as medically ill; the "chronic cluster" for the tiny ladies with nothing wrong with them except for Father Time. And there was the "dementia cluster." Each of the "dementia cluster" wards corresponded to a different stage of dementia: the stage when the patient forgets where he is and starts to wander; the next stage, when the patient forgets how to talk; and the last stage, when the patient forgets how to eat.

My new ward, E6, was one of the dementia wards.

Although it was a dementia ward, it was not an Alzheimer's ward, at least not according to the 1907 description of his disease by Dr. Alois Alzheimer. Today the diagnosis of Alzheimer's is practically synonymous with dementia, but that usage is often not accurate.

The word *dementia* comes from the Latin word *mens*, meaning *mind*; and to be "demented" signifies a kind of "de-minding," the gradual loss of intellectual functions—especially of memory, with its power for learning and planning. Premodern medicine usually called it *amentia*—that is, mind loss—and never could settle on whether aging alone caused it. For instance, the writer Cicero, who lived to be eighty-five, thought that dementia could be prevented by exercise, while Galen, the most famous physician of Rome, thought it was inevitable because of the cooling and drying of the body that naturally occurred over time. Which was how he understood old age: the warm, wet body of the infant gradually losing its warmth and moisture to end up as the dry, cold body of the elderly. This explained why the skin of the old was dry, the eyes dry, and the frame shrunken. The brain, according to Galen, also cooled and dried. And just as dried clay could no longer accept new impressions, so, too, the aged brain could no longer accept new impressions, which was why the elderly had trouble remembering. Galen did think that dementia could be delayed, however, by a regime that warmed and moistened the body, and Hildegard, who followed his teachings, did recommend just such warming and moistening herbs for dementia.

Our modern understanding of dementia is relatively new. It was first formulated in the early 1800s by Dr. Philippe Pinel of the Salpêtrière hospital in Paris. The Salpêtrière was an enormous chronic care hospital not unlike Laguna Honda, and over the years he practiced there, Dr. Pinel became fascinated by a group of patients for whom, as Henry Maudsley later put it, "the memory was impaired, the feelings quenched, and the intelligence enfeebled or extinct." Pinel named this condition *démence*—dementia. He made sure to autopsy the brains of his demented patients after they died and he was able to correlate their clinical course with what he found, generating a long list of causes for *démence*. His protégé, Jean-Étienne Dominique Esquirol, continued to study dementia and published his results in his 1838 *Des Maladies Mentales*. In it, he defined dementia as a "weakening of the sensibility, understanding, and will. . . . Incoherence of ideas, and a want of intellectual and moral spontaneity are the signs of this affection." He, too, correlated his patients' clinical courses with what he found at autopsy and concluded that dementia had many different causes, including: "strokes, head trauma, syphilis, mercury poisoning [for treating syphilis!], alcoholism, errors of regime, and trials, disappointments, and privation." What Esquirol did not describe, however, was what we know today as Alzheimer's. That would take another century and the formulation of new ways of staining brain cells.

In 1907 Dr. Alois Alzheimer published his case of Auguste D, a fifty-one-year-old woman who had had an unusual, rapidly progressive dementia. After she died, he did an autopsy, and he prepared her brain with silver stain. Then when he examined the brain cells under his microscope, he saw that they were filled with thick black tangles, which he called "neurofibrillary tangles." Outside the cells he saw thick white plaques—"extracellular plaques." These tangles and plaques, he proposed, must have been the cause of her unusual dementia, and a few years later, his discovery was named after him.

For many decades after its description, Alzheimer's disease was a very rare cause of dementia because of the way Dr. Alzheimer had defined it. Alzheimer's dementia had to be a "presenile" dementia—that is, it had to have started in middle age, and this was rare. The patient's brain had to show neurofibrillary tangles and extracellular plaques, and this meant that a biopsy or autopsy had to have been done, which was also rare.

But then, in the 1970s, there was a research push to understand the dementia of old age, and when silver stains were applied to elderly demented brains, many showed neurofibrillary tangles and extracellular plaques. Scientists, therefore, concluded that Alzheimer's disease was not a rare but a common cause of dementia in the elderly, and money began to flow into researching the reason for these tangles and plaques.

There was a problem, however. In order for scientists to do research on Alzheimer's disease, there had to be a way of identifying which demented patients had those tangles and plaques. Yet, except for a brain biopsy or an autopsy, there was no way of determining that—no blood test or X-ray. So in the 1980s a crucial redefinition was made. Instead of continuing to use Alzheimer's original definition of a presenile dementia with neurofibrillary tangles and extracellular plaques, a new definition of Alzheimer's was put in place: it was any dementia without another known cause. This was a huge change since it meant that the diagnosis of Alzheimer's depended, not on a brain biopsy or on an autopsy, but on doctors excluding all other causes of dementia—in theory, the whole list that Esquirol and others had developed over the preceding hundred years.

At first doctors were careful to look for other causes of dementia before they made the diagnosis of Alzheimer's. But as time went on, and the management of health care became tighter, demented patients stopped getting this full dementia workup. It was easier, faster, and cheaper to just assume that a demented elderly patient had Alzheimer's, which was so common anyway.

And what was wrong with that? What was wrong with changing the definition but keeping the old name if we all agreed on the new definition?

What was wrong was that in the past Alzheimer's had been defined as a rapidly progressive, presenile dementia with neurofibrillary tangles and extracellular plaques. And that meant that the diagnosis of Alzheimer's implied a course and a prognosis: It was rapidly progressive and relentless. But if, instead, Alzheimer's meant any dementia for which we can't find a cause, then this prognosis might be inaccurate, and patients and families would make incorrect decisions about future care, inheritances, and wills.

Even worse, all the past research on Alzheimer's had concentrated on those neurofibrillary tangles and extracellular plaques, and Alzheimer medications had been developed for them specifically. If they were given instead to a patient whose dementia had nothing to do with neurofibrillary tangles and extracellular plaques, then they wouldn't be effective. A patient would get all the side effects but no improvement. That is what was wrong with redefining Alzheimer's

dementia as any dementia with no other known cause. On the admitting ward, I'd already seen many patients who had the diagnosis of
Alzheimer's but, in fact, turned out to have a different cause for their
dementia—and sometimes a treatable cause, such as B_{12} deficiency,
AIDS, depression, or a thyroid disorder. With the correct diagnosis
and the corresponding treatment, many of these "Alzheimer" patients
improved, sometimes enough to go home.

On E6, too, none of its thirty-four patients had Alzheimer's, as I
would gradually realize when I got to know them, although many had
that diagnosis in their charts. Instead, each one had some other cause
for their dementia—and usually many causes.

There was Mr. Essem, for instance. He was my youngest patient
on E6.

When Mr. Essem was twenty-eight years old, a blood vessel burst
in his brain. He collapsed and went into a coma, but then through the
miracles of modern medicine, he was saved. He was rushed to surgery; the bleeding blood vessel was clipped; and the blood in his brain
was removed. He was sent to the intensive care unit, where he
remained in a coma for weeks. Then he woke up. He was bright and
alert, and could move all his limbs, but he didn't speak, and no one
could tell how much he understood. So he was sent for rehabilitation,
but didn't improve. He was pleasant and cheerful, but if left alone,
Mr. Essem simply sat. Finally he came to us, and by the time I met
him, he'd been on E6 for more years than I'd been at the hospital.
Each morning the nurses got him out of bed, shaved him, dressed
him, fed him, and put him in his chair. And there he sat all day long,
with his round young face, his round ears, and his round, attentive
brown eyes. He never spoke, but he did smile, a tiny, pleasant smile, as

he watched the ever-changing, mysterious scenes on his ward. He was demented, but he didn't have Alzheimer's. He had a traumatic brain injury.

The oldest patient on E6 was Mr. Hernandez, who, when I met him, was ninety-eight years old. He was short, stocky, and well muscled, with thick, slightly graying hair, all his teeth, and a raspy voice. Whenever I pointed out to him that he was my oldest patient, he would reply defiantly, "No, I'm not!"

"Yes, Mr. Hernandez, you are."

"No, I'm not," he would repeat. "Bring me a woman, and I'll show you how old I am!"

Although we never did bring him a woman, on his 104th birthday the nurses arranged for a stripper—mostly dressed—to come to E6 and present Mr. Hernandez with a bouquet of balloons. He was very pleased. Mr. Hernandez was old enough to have real Alzheimer's as a cause for his dementia, but I was skeptical of that diagnosis because in the years I knew him, he never deteriorated. He didn't get better, but he didn't get worse. His son told me that his father wasn't much different from how he'd ever been, so perhaps Mr. Hernandez was just being Mr. Hernandez, only older.

Between Mr. Essem and Mr. Hernandez, there were examples of just about every other cause of dementia on E6—except Alzheimer's. There was Mr. Richard Temkin, for example. Mr. Temkin was a depressed alcoholic who, one evening when he was fifty-four years old, left his usual bar, went back to his single room above the bar, took a loaded gun out of his bedside drawer, opened his mouth, and put a bullet through his head. Right through it—through his hard palate, and then through those frontal lobes that neurologists say we need in order to have "executive power"—to think and to plan.

Apparently we don't need them; at least Mr. Temkin didn't, although it did take him quite a while to get used to life without them.

When he first arrived at Laguna Honda, he was just waking up from his coma. It took a few months, but he did wake up, and eventually his Self—morose, insulting, and irritable—came right back to him uninjured, despite those missing frontal lobes, along with enough executive power to insult the other patients and order his own meals from the cafeteria. He continued to improve, and a year later was able to go back to his room above the bar, the only apparent difference in his mental state being that after his attempted suicide, he was no longer suicidal. He, too, had a traumatic brain injury and not Alzheimer's.

There was Mr. Bailey, a diabetic who had been obsessive about treating his blood sugars. He'd kept them so low that he'd had many episodes of hypoglycemia—when the blood level of sugar is too low for the brain to function. Which was how, over time, he, too, had become demented—from recurrent episodes of hypoglycemia.

Then there was Mr. Powell, whose dementia had been caused by a series of small strokes. He was also a diabetic, and his right leg had been amputated in consequence. He was none too bright to begin with, and now demented, too. I was all the more impressed, therefore, when he showed me how, lacking any locking drawers in his bureau, he used the space inside his artificial leg to keep his money, cigarettes, and contraband matches.

Of all the patients on E6, only Mr. Stembel seemed a candidate for real Alzheimer's. His dementia had started when he was only thirty-eight and had progressed so rapidly that by the time I met him he was mute, unable to sit up in a chair or swallow his own spittle. So he did have a rapidly progressive, presenile dementia. I decided to try

Aricept, therefore, one of the few medications we have for Alzheimer's. Aricept interferes with the body's ability to break down acetylcholine (ACH), an important neurotransmitter in the brain. This lack of acetylcholine was, at one time, thought to be the cause of Alzheimer's dementia, although the fact is that Aricept works well in only a few patients, perhaps because of our redefinition of the disease. I started Mr. Stembel with the very tiniest dose, and I was shocked the next morning to find him sitting up in his chair, smiling, no longer drooling, and trying to walk. So perhaps he did have Alzheimer's. Although our neurologist thought not. Mr. Stembel's reaction to Aricept was so exaggerated that it was more likely he'd stroked out the part of the brain that modulates the response to ACH, he hypothesized. In any case, there was no long-term effective medication for Mr. Stembel. Just those few minutes every day when he suddenly sat straight up, swallowed his own spittle, raised his eyebrows, and opened his eyes wide, with a broad, delighted smile.

These six, and the other twenty-eight patients on E6, had just about every cause for their dementia except Alzheimer's—and usually a mix of many causes: stroke and alcohol and head trauma, drugs, deprivation, disappointment, and want—all the causes that Dr. Esquirol had described almost two hundred years before.

Although the patients on the dementia ward did not have the feared diagnosis of Alzheimer's, they were certainly "de-mented"— deprived of parts of their brain and mind. Now, I'm an optimist; I believe that there is meaning to life and that this meaning has something to do with soul or spirit; and the men of E6 worried me. Death is one thing. When a vibrant, intelligent being dies, it is devastating, but it is not difficult to believe that his *anima,* his spirit, survives that sudden loss of body, the difference between the living and the dead being so bright, so clear, so distinct.

But the demented men of E6 gave me pause. They weren't all there, and they weren't all not there either. They were demented, but not de-souled or de-spirited. They certainly had the "impairment of memory" and "enfeebling of intelligence" that Maudsley used to define dementia. I'll grant, too, that many had Dr. Esquirol's "weakening of the understanding." But they did not have "a quenching of feelings" or "weakening of the will." Indeed, I learned a lot about sensibility, feeling, and will from those demented men of E6.

Still, Alzheimer's or not, dementia is challenging. It challenges what we think of soul, spirit, and personality. Which was why, when I saw Mr. Bramwell dancing to the tune of Glenn Miller, I never forgot it.

met Mr. Bramwell for the first time on the day he was transferred up to E6 from the admitting ward.

He was sitting in the chair by his bed, dressed in dark blue pressed chinos and a green plaid shirt with the collar buttoned all the way up. He was African-American and dark brown, with a wide face, slack jaw, and incurious eyes, which stared at his own hands tapping softly on the table in front of him. Mrs. Bramwell was standing next to him. She was beautiful. Tall and statuesque, she was calm and confident in high heels and nylon stockings, a maroon skirt-suit, and an elegant green wool coat. Which sounds like it would clash, but against her dark, clear skin, did not. She was probably the same age as Mr. Bramwell, which was seventy, although she could have been ten years younger.

She just couldn't manage Mr. Bramwell any longer, she told me. The Alzheimer's was just too hard. Her husband had been a family man, and they had six children, three boys and three girls; he'd worked in construction and had a business with his son and son-in-law. He drank too much, yes, but they hadn't noticed much wrong with him until the time he got in an argument with his son-in-law and took an ax to him. That was six years ago. After that, he stopped drinking, but gradually, maybe four years ago, they started to notice he wasn't quite right. Didn't talk as much. Seemed slowed down. Then a year ago he began to act really crazy. He got lost in places he knew, and then he started to soil himself.

So she took him over to the County Hospital, where they told her he had Alzheimer's and sent him to Laguna Honda. He stayed for several months, and he got better, and she took him home. But now she just couldn't manage him anymore, even with their children's help— the wandering, the sleeplessness. If he got better again, she would take him home. She wanted to take him home; they'd been married fifty years, and he'd been a good husband, a good father, a good provider.

While Mrs. Bramwell was speaking, Mr. Bramwell sat quietly, with a faint smile on his face, his eyes not blinking much, and his fingers tapping on the table. When I introduced myself and asked him how he was, his eyes turned to me, but he didn't answer, and then they went right back to the spot he'd been looking at before I spoke.

He'd already been examined and worked up by Dr. Dan, the new doctor on the admitting ward, so I went back to the nursing station to sit down with his chart, his old tests, Dr. Dan's examination, and his previous admissions to us and to the County Hospital. I would examine him myself later on.

Mrs. Bramwell had the story exactly right, although when I went through the records, they provided more detail and a different emphasis on the facts. Mr. Bramwell had been a very heavy drinker, although he had stopped three years before. He'd had some kind of head trauma, too, in a car accident many years before. Also, he had a psychiatric diagnosis; he was "schizoaffective," a handy diagnosis that meant whatever we wanted it to mean—a mixture of schizophrenia and manic depression or just depression. What made that diagnosis interesting was that untreated schizoaffectives sometimes use alcohol to self-treat their mental illness. Though I doubted that Mr. Bramwell was schizoaffective. Not many schizoaffectives have construction businesses, houses, six children, a fifty-year marriage, or Mrs. Bramwell, for that matter, and it was more likely that the diagnosis crept into his chart thanks to some overenthusiastic intern who had just heard a lecture on it.

As I went through his records, I was trying to determine the basis for Mr. Bramwell's profound but rather static dementia. He did have the diagnosis of Alzheimer's, of course, passed along from doctor to doctor, but real Alzheimer's didn't seem likely. Not the Alzheimer's defined by Dr. Alzheimer, with its neurofibrillary tangles, extracellular plaques, and rapid progression, nor even the new Alzheimer's, which required only that no other causes for dementia be present. Mr. Bramwell had many causes for his dementia. There was his heavy drinking, which pickles the brain and causes a specific dementia called Korsakoff's dementia. He had head trauma from his car accident, which can cause the traumatized part of the brain to deteriorate into the encephalomalacia of post-traumatic dementia. If he really was schizoaffective, then he might have the "pseudo dementia" of a psychotic depression, which can look like dementia. Almost certainly, he had some component of multi-infarct dementia, where patients with high blood pressure suffer small, silent strokes that gradually damage their brains. Given his rigidity, lack of blinking, and slow movements, he might even have Parkinson's disease or its relative, Lewy body disease, both of which can also cause dementia.

But what was most likely, I thought, after I finished going through his records, was that Mr. Bramwell had what so many of our patients had—a mixed dementia from a combination of causes. Indeed, I was beginning to think of dementia as a kind of polynomial equation, or as some kind of weird recipe: three parts multi-infarct plus two parts alcohol, and one part each head trauma, depression, and the side effects of medication.

What was important about this recipe was finding the ingredients in it that were treatable. A medication the patient was taking that caused confusion; an underactive or overactive thyroid; a vitamin deficiency, an imbalance in the blood, or a depression; all these can be treated, and doing so often improves the dementia enough to make a difference—to send the patient home, for instance.

Mr. Bramwell did not have any of the unusual but correctable causes of dementia, though he did seem depressed, and he was on quite a few medications. We could try decreasing or even discontinuing some or all of them, and we could try treating depression. We would see, I told Mrs. Bramwell, how well he would do.

It took more than a year to get Mr. Bramwell off his medications and to treat his depression. And I wish I could say that he had a remarkable improvement. But he did not. He continued to be kempt and shaved, with his little smile and his tapping hands; and Mrs. Bramwell continued to visit him every day, bringing in home-cooked food. She did take him home now and then, but only for a few days; and every time she had to bring him back. Partly because she had kidney failure herself and went to dialysis three times a week, and partly because, well, he just didn't get better. He didn't get worse either, which made Alzheimer's all the less likely. He simply stayed the same, a sad shadow of his former self, a warning that time is short, that we must live our lives to their fullest while we can.

Then one day Mr. Bramwell demonstrated one of the oldest

observations about dementia: that even when a patient is de-mented—deprived of mind—his soul, his *anima*, is still . . . somewhere.

Now, every ward at the hospital had an activity therapist (AT), and so did E6. The ATs had a hard job—to come up every day with an activity that would engage the demented and the disabled, who were also mostly very sick; an activity, too, that would work the joints and muscles, stimulate the mind, and encourage social interaction. I don't know what their training was, but, as with all of the new health-care professionals, it was, doubtless, long and rigorous.

The ATs were mostly women; kind and intelligent, they loved their patients; it was easy to see by the passion they put into their wheelchair dodgeball, their bingo games, newspaper readings, poker, blackjack, and baking in the portable ovens. I didn't like their title though. It was too bland, too nondescript for what they were trying to do. The French is better: Activity therapy is called *animation* and the activity therapist an *animatrice*, as in *anima*—that which animates the body, which makes it come alive and stay alive, and which leaves the body after death.

Activity therapy had replaced the previous activities at the hospital that had been called "work." Along with giving us the word *dementia,* Dr. Pinel had also observed that work was therapeutic for the demented, and he had assigned his patients chores—gardening, sewing. At the early Laguna Honda, too, patients had been expected to work if they could. And they did work, farming its sixty-two acres, weaving the cane chairs they sat in, sewing the bandages they used. As late as Miss Lester, the head nurses still assigned patients to feed other patients, read to other patients, and push the wheelchairs of other patients, if they could.

But by the time I arrived, that system of work had been discontinued. It was too complicated; it had too much liability; it took away union jobs. All that was left of it were two patients who worked in the little store, selling candy and shaving supplies, and Mr. Sanchez. Mr. Sanchez was a diabetic who'd lost a leg from his diabetes. Nevertheless, leaning on his wooden cart, he still delivered newspapers to all of our 1,178 patients. He didn't get paid, but he loved his job, and smiled his way into many an illicit Coke on the wards he visited every day.

Except for those three patients, however, paid workers had replaced the rest of the worker patients, and activity therapists had been hired to provide activity therapy instead.

One of their most popular activities was dancing. There was the Valentine's Day Dance, a formal affair for the whole hospital; and there were the weekly dances on each floor. Three wards would participate in a weekly dance—ninety patients sitting in rows of folding chairs or in their wheelchairs. There would be music, and the nurses would dance and try to cajole the patients who could to dance with them.

And so it was on this day, when I came around the corner on my way to E6. A volunteer was playing the piano, boogie-woogie and jitterbug, and three of the pudgy, youngish Filipino nurses were dancing by themselves.

They were not very good dancers, kind of stiff and slow, but they were enthusiastic, and I stopped to watch. The patients sat in various attitudes of attention and slumber, and none was brave enough to join them. Suddenly one nurse threw out both arms and pulled up a patient to dance with her. It was Mr. Bramwell.

He stood for a moment in front of her, confused and uncertain. He swayed a little, and I was afraid he might fall. With his slack jaw and open mouth, he stared at the nurse, puzzled. Then, slowly, he lifted his right hand and took her left hand, and her right hand in his left, and he began to dance. And though he no longer remembered how to talk, how to clean himself, and barely how to eat, he wasn't a bad dancer.

Actually, he was a very good dancer. After a few turns with the first nurse, he held out his hand in a gentlemanly way to another nurse, and she obliged him and stepped up. And then he was spinning her under his arm, twirling her in and out and smiling—just a bit, not too much. He was manly, in control, and suddenly young. Though he'd forgotten everything else, he still did know how to dance, and with the dancing, he remembered not only his steps but his style, his manners, and his charm.

The music stopped eventually, and Mr. Bramwell stopped, too. He slumped, he stooped, he came to a halt; he forgot the dancing and shuffled with the nurse back to his ward.

But I didn't forget. And ever after on my morning rounds, when I came to Mr. Bramwell sitting so stiffly in his chair, with his left foot tap-tapping on the floor, and his hands drumming out a little tune on the table in front of him, I read him differently. With that slight smile as he stared at his hands, he was waiting, I thought, for those first strains of Glenn Miller to sound in the hall.

Ever after, too, when I passed the other patients on the dementia ward, I wondered: What tunes would get them dancing? What did their blank faces hide? What worlds of talent did their eyes shutter?

Long ago Saint Isidore wrote that dementia showed that life could go on even without the spirit. I knew what he meant. Those were the patients on the feeding-tube ward, mute and still. But, he continued, sometimes in dementia, the soul—the *anima*—remains in spite of the loss of mind. I learned that from Mr. Bramwell. No matter how demented a patient seemed, it just might be that deep within he still had his *anima*, his soul. If we could just get to it!

That wasn't all I learned from Mr. Bramwell. There was his sister-in-law, Lorna Mae.

Lorna Mae was Mrs. Bramwell's sister. While not as beautiful or as statuesque as her sister, she was just as tall and just as dark and rich a color, and a year into my rather ineffectual treatment of Mr. Bramwell, she turned up one day at his bedside. At once, as soon as she saw me, she burst out, with a big, embracing smile and a lit-up face, "Is that you . . . Miz Altman's great-niece?"

I looked at her. It took me a while to remember.

"How is your dear mother? And your sisters? And how are you?" she went on.

Suddenly it all came back. Lorna Mae had taken care of my great-aunt Bess years before. I remembered her walking out of the kitchen, as I was sitting with my aged, feeble great-aunt, to bring her soup; and I remembered her at my great-aunt's funeral, too.

She'd come to the funeral with two other friends, and they sat in the back. It was a formal funeral, attended mostly by white-haired little white people in black suits and ties, black dresses and pearls. Since my great-aunt was not religious, in lieu of a service there were a violinist and a cellist, playing Bach. I sat on the side of the chapel, and the mood was somber, staid, and philosophic. The little white-haired white people sat in front, listening in silence to the cello and violin, and dealing as best they could with the meaning of life in the face of death.

But I could see Lorna Mae in the back row. I didn't know why she came, whether to mourn my great-aunt, to honor her, or, perhaps, from a sense of accomplishment—a job done well, now over. She was not dressed in black, but wore a heavy dark purple silk dress and a huge purple felt hat with a swooping green feather. She did not seem sad or dismayed; she sat confidently, with satisfaction, I thought, in the sure and certain hope of resurrection and faith in a life to come. Her confidence and her purple hat with its green feather became the focal points in the first piece of writing I'd ever published.

And here she was, fifteen years later.

Sitting by the side of her brother-in-law's bed, she looked at me expectantly. What would I do for him? And what hit me at that moment was the reversal of our positions. Once I'd been sitting by my relative's bed, and she'd been the giver; now she was sitting by her relative's bed, and I was the giver. It was the reversal of our positions that struck me. It illuminated something I'd been puzzling over, which was that the root of *hospital* is *hospitality*, and the root of *hospitality* is *hospes,* which can mean either "guest" or "host."

In Rome *hospitalitas*—hospitality—meant caring for the traveler, the stranger, and the pilgrim, but only when he was of the same class as oneself, because then one could expect an equivalent return. So Roman hospitality was a kind of fair exchange. It was based on the idea that every host (*hospes*) was also a guest (*hospes*) somewhere else; that one's identity as either host or guest was interchangeable.

After Rome collapsed, the monasteries grew out of their old villas, and took over many of the social contracts left in Rome's dust, especially that of hospitality. But the hospitality of the monasteries was radically different from Rome's, because the monks and nuns opened the door of their hospices to everyone, regardless of their social standing. To rich and to poor, to travelers, pilgrims, and the sick, to Muslim and to Jew. The reason for that was Matthew in the

New Testament, who had quoted Jesus as saying: Whatever you do for the least of these, you do for me. Which was interpreted by the monks to mean that any guest was welcome in the monastery because any guest could be—and therefore was—Christ. That was how the Roman *hospitalitas* turned into the medieval hospitality of the monastery's hospice.

What I'd been puzzling over when Lorna Mae and I recognized each other was why, in Latin, French, and even, originally, in English, the concepts of guest and host were not differentiated; there was no word for telling them apart. They were the same. And at the moment when I recognized Lorna Mae, I suddenly understood why: It was because our parts are, in fact, interchangeable. The essence of hospitality—*hospes*—is that guest and host are identical, if not in the moment, then at some moment. Whatever our current role, it was temporary. With time and the seasons, a host goes traveling and becomes a guest; a guest returns home and becomes a host. That is what the word *hospitality* encodes. And in a hospital, the meaning of that interchangeability is even more profound, because in the hospital, every host will for sure become a guest; every doctor, a patient.

That is what I realized in that moment with Lorna Mae. I, too, would go from being a host in the hospital to being its guest; I, too, would become a patient. Although sobering, that was the essence of the matter.

Mrs. Bramwell's sister takes care of my great-aunt; I take care of her brother-in-law. I teach my medical students to be good doctors, and it is not entirely unselfish, because sooner or later, they will be taking care of me. It was the measure of the Golden Rule and a good, selfish Golden Rule: Do unto others as you want them to do to you because pretty soon they will be doing unto you, directly or indirectly.

It was in this sense—*hospes*, the non-distinction between guest and host—that hospitality was, and should be, the essence of the hospital. That is what I learned from Lorna Mae.

And although I never heard it talked about, the longer I was at Laguna Honda, the more sure I was that its first principle was not medicine, nursing, or a balanced budget, but hospitality in the sense of taking care of anyone who knocked at the door because—it could be me. It was me.

As I was getting to know the Bramwells, the politics of the hospital were complexifying. The Department of Justice was adamant: If the city did not correct Laguna Honda's violation of the patient's right to privacy, it would be closed.

Dr. Stein spent almost a year working up every one of his options. He looked at shutting us down and using the money saved to take care of our former patients at home. He looked at building several mini-hospitals scattered around the city. He looked at renovating the old buildings. Last he looked at the most expensive option: tearing down the old Laguna Honda and rebuilding a new Laguna Honda as a modern, state-of-the-art health-care facility with two thousand beds.

Each option was costly—many hundreds of millions of dollars costly. There seemed to be no way around it. And I sometimes wondered whether Dr. Stein ever thought, as I sometimes did: Why not just let the place close down? Almost every other county had closed its almshouse, and their citizens seemed to manage. True, their private hospitals were even more jammed up than our city's, and their streets were filled with even more of the sick poor. Or perhaps not. Our city was a magnet for every loose iron filing in the country, and no matter how large Dr. Stein made the new Laguna Honda, it would never be big enough to take care of them all.

If he did think it, Dr. Stein never said so. His final recommendation was to rebuild a huge new health-care facility, one big enough to accommodate the wave of frail elderly, destitute disabled, and mentally ill expected to deluge the city as the Boomers aged.

He presented his recommendation to the board of supervisors. The supervisors were aghast. Five hundred million dollars. Not all of the money would have to come from the citizens, fortunately; half would come from what the tobacco companies were going to pay the city for tobacco's role in lung disease. But the other half would have to come from a bond, and the bond would have to be approved by a two-thirds vote of the citizens. Times were not good, and the mayor did not want to put the bond on the ballot. He did not want to support something he knew would fail. But he succumbed to pressure, and the bond for a new Laguna Honda did go on the ballot.

The bond had many enemies but, since no one imagined it would pass, the forces against it were lackadaisical. The Republican Party was against it, arguing that the rebuild was unnecessary because Laguna Honda's patients could be cared for more cheaply elsewhere. The mayor's opponents were against it: the rebuild was simply a boondoggle for the unions that supported the mayor. Disability activists were against it: The disabled had a right to live at home, and the city should spend its money providing homes or homelike places so every patient could live in the community.

Still, all considering, there was only lukewarm opposition.

By contrast, the pro–Laguna Honda forces were passionate, organized, and active; and the arguments in favor of the rebuild ran to thirty-five pages. The Society of Architects argued that no matter how expensive a new hospital would be, it would still be less expensive than any alternative. The unions argued that a new hospital would provide jobs and maintain a safety net for disabled workers. Nurses, doctors, and patients argued that a new hospital was simply the right thing to do, no matter how much it cost. AIDS groups, Hispanic groups, African-American, Asian, and Catholic groups all spoke up for a new Laguna Honda, too.

And there was Miss Lester, who though retired was still active in the hospital's politics. Of course, except for Miss Lester, it could be said that everyone in favor of the bond was arguing from self-interest. Miss Lester did not even argue. She wrote: "After forty-four years of caring for thousands of our brothers and sisters who were restored and returned to their homes, and for thousands who were cared for in love and respect until their final hour, I am convinced that Laguna Honda must forever be part of our city. Vote Yes on Proposition A."

And the citizens obeyed her. They did vote Yes. It was stunning. It was unexpected. In the middle of a recession, with job losses, deflation, and a frightening future, the bond passed by nearly three to one. Although given the times—times when anybody might need the almshouse—it was less surprising than it might have seemed. Still, Dr. Stein, the mayor, and the board of supervisors were astonished. They scratched their heads, smiled and frowned, and began to put the structures in place to collect the five hundred million dollars they would need.

Believing for quite a while that our hospital would close, and then finding out instead that there would be a new, enormous, and expensive health-care facility built next door was stressful to us all, and I cherished even more those Tuesdays, Thursdays, and Saturdays, when I could hide out in the library with Hildegard and premodern medicine. Having studied her context and her medical practice in Switzerland, I now turned to understanding her medical theory: that is, how she conceptualized what she did with her patients—her framework.

For us, for modern medicine, our basic framework is the cell. We begin life as a single cell, the fertilized egg, which then multiplies and divides and differentiates into all the different cells of our body. Inside each cell, we believe, is a kind of chemical factory, with production machinery, communication devices, and energy machines; and their programs are contained in the code called DNA. Each cell follows its DNA instructions and so produces the chemicals necessary for its life. To communicate with other cells, each cell secretes certain of these chemicals into the blood. There they circulate and interact with other cells, modifying these other cells' DNA orders, and so unite the individuality of each cell into a corporate whole.

Modern medicine's framework for the body, then, is industrial, mechanical, and democratic: The body is a factory with workers; a machine with parts; a democratic republic of cells, each obedient, hardworking, and united for the common good. Though complex, our cell model of the body obeys clear laws; it is orderly, rational, and predictable, up to a point. Once the cell is understood, it is easy to understand how each organ functions, how diseases injure, and how medications work.

And so I asked myself: What was Hildegard's framework for understanding the body? What was her intuitive, internal model of the body, which worked for her the way the cellular model worked for me?

It took me a long time to grasp Hildegard's framework. Even now I'm not sure I understand it fully, but I do understand it enough to put myself inside it and even use it sometimes, as a way of thinking about a patient, a disease, or a medication, as a way of thinking outside my box. Because, although Hildegard's framework could not be more different from cell theory, it is not unfamiliar. It is our oldest way of thinking about the body, preserved in the etymology of our words and in our proverbs. Alternative medicine, homeopathy, naturopathy, and even astrology use this premodern model, which is, doubtless, one of their attractions for the modern temperament.

Hildegard's framework was based on the classic system of premodern medicine—humoral medicine—which was also known as the System of the Fours. What were the fours of the System of the Fours? They were many, and they were all related: four elements, four qualities, four humors, four directions, four colors, four temperaments, four ages, four times of day, four seasons.

It is best understood with a diagram (see page 203).

The way the diagram works is this. The world is made out of four basic elements—Earth, Air, Water, Fire, each of which occupies one of the four corners of the diagram. Each element is made up of two of the four qualities—hot and cold, and wet and dry. Earth is cold and dry; Water is cold and wet; Air is hot and wet; and Fire is hot and dry.

Like the world, the body is also made up of a "four": the four humors—blood, phlegm, bile, and melancholia. And just like the elements, so, too, are these humors made up of two qualities, each humor corresponding to an element. The humor blood is hot and wet, and corresponds to Air; phlegm is cold and wet, and corresponds to Water; bile is hot and dry, and corresponds to Fire; and melancholia is cold and dry, and corresponds to Earth. In the diagram, they are placed with their respective element at each of the four corners.

Since the qualities of hot and cold and wet and dry are also the qualities of weather and climate—that is, of temperature and humidity—each of the four elements and each of the four humors is related to one of the four seasons and increases during that season. For instance, in spring, which is hot and wet, the element of Air increases outside the body, and inside the body, the humor of blood increases. In summer, which is hot and dry, outside the body the element of Fire increases, and inside the body, the humor of bile increases. In autumn, the dry, cold element of Earth and the dry, cold humor of melancholia increase; and in winter, the moist, cold element Water and the moist, cold humor phlegm increase. This is true not only for human bodies, but also for animals and plants.

As the year passes, and the Sun moves around the Earth—clockwise during the day; counterclockwise during the year, and from south to north and back again—what is wet, dries; what is hot becomes cold. The seasons give way to one another, and the four elements rise and fall. For instance, as spring turns into summer, *Air* decreases and *Fire* increases. There is a corresponding change in one's lifetime: The hot, wet youth becomes the cold, dry elderly. Since health results from the right balance of the four humors inside the body, the way to ensure it is to compensate for the seasonal changes outside the body by modifying the humors inside the body.

This was where Hildegard's prescription for "regime" came in. Regime was made up of all those things that could be changed as the seasons changed—the kinds of food we eat, the kinds of drink; the amount of rest and exercise, sex and emotion. For example, since summer was by its nature hot and dry, Hildegard typically prescribed a regime that was cold and wet: so beer instead of wine; tepid bathing instead of hot baths; less sex, less stress, and more relaxation.

It wasn't just the human body that had a temperament affected by the seasons. So did animals and plants. In fact, every plant had its own balance of the four qualities, being more or less hot or cold and wet or dry; its qualities being determined by its taste. (We still do this today, but only for wine.) It was by their qualities that plants could counteract the effects of the seasons, and many of Hildegard's

THE SYSTEM OF THE FOURS

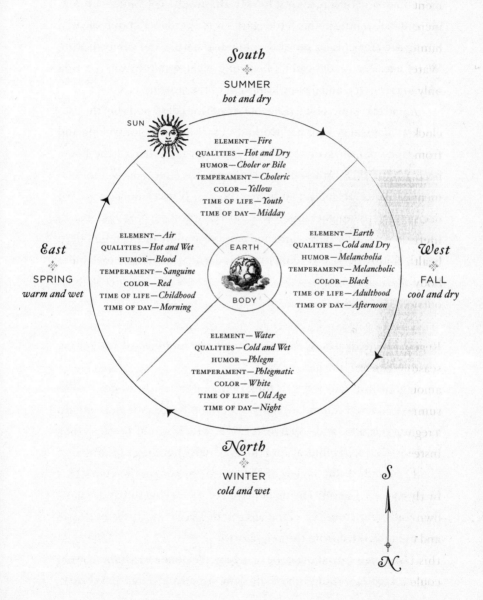

South

SUMMER
hot and dry

SUN

ELEMENT—*Fire*
QUALITIES—*Hot and Dry*
HUMOR—*Choler or Bile*
TEMPERAMENT—*Choleric*
COLOR—*Yellow*
TIME OF LIFE—*Youth*
TIME OF DAY—*Midday*

ELEMENT—*Air*
QUALITIES—*Hot and Wet*
HUMOR—*Blood*
TEMPERAMENT—*Sanguine*
COLOR—*Red*
TIME OF LIFE—*Childhood*
TIME OF DAY—*Morning*

EARTH

BODY

ELEMENT—*Earth*
QUALITIES—*Cold and Dry*
HUMOR—*Melancholia*
TEMPERAMENT—*Melancholic*
COLOR—*Black*
TIME OF LIFE—*Adulthood*
TIME OF DAY—*Afternoon*

ELEMENT—*Water*
QUALITIES—*Cold and Wet*
HUMOR—*Phlegm*
TEMPERAMENT—*Phlegmatic*
COLOR—*White*
TIME OF LIFE—*Old Age*
TIME OF DAY—*Night*

East

SPRING
warm and wet

West

FALL
cool and dry

North

WINTER
cold and wet

S

N

prescriptions rely on those qualities for their medicinal effect. For instance, for Mrs. McCoy's cold, wet edema, Hildegard would have chosen hot and drying plants; for Mr. Bramwell's cold and dry brain, hot and moistening plants. Hildegard's was a gardener's point of view, taking account of each patient's individual nature and compensating for its excesses or deficiencies—drying what was too wet, wetting what was too dry, and paying attention to the seasons.

It had taken me a long time, but I finally understood why the premodern medical system had worked so satisfactorily for so long and then fallen out of favor so quickly. Hildegard's System of the Fours was based on the simplest of observations—the effects of the four seasons on plants, animals, and human bodies. It was a holistic system whose underlying metaphor was horticultural, and it had corresponded perfectly to the rural and agricultural life of the premodern world. With the rise of industrial modernity, it disappeared quite naturally, if abruptly.

It took Dr. Stein almost as long to begin the rebuild as it had for me to understand Hildegard's Way.

It took him four years. It took that long to sell the bonds for the new hospital, to accumulate the first of the tobacco money, to obtain building permits, and to choose a site, which would be the valley between the main building and the even older building of Clarendon Hall. From the point of view of Hildegard's System of the Fours, this valley was insalubrious, being deprived of the drying sun and cleansing winds, but from the point of view of Dr. Stein, it was perfect—vacant and hidden from the neighbors.

The plan was that once the new Laguna Honda was built, the old Laguna Honda would be partially demolished and a multilevel parking lot constructed in its place. It could not be completely demolished, though, because the front part of the main building was on the Register of Historic Places and would, therefore, be saved from the Grim Reaper—saved and renovated and turned into offices for the city's administrators. It was, after all, a beautiful if decrepit building, with spectacular views of the city and the ocean.

Finally, Dr. Stein had everything ready, and the archeological excavations commenced with bated breath. Because if any human bones were discovered—Native American burials, for instance—construction would come to a halt. Amazingly, fortunately, suspiciously, not a single bone was uncovered by the archeologists. Only whiskey bottles turned up—a veritable museum of whiskey bottles, some of them one hundred years old, thrown into the valley by rapscallion patients long since dead.

So then it was time for a party, a groundbreaking ceremony. The day was chosen and invitations sent out to the outgoing mayor, the incoming mayor, the Board of Supervisors, Dr. Stein, the press, the staff, and the patients.

I made sure to attend.

It was not only gray and foggy that day, to be expected in our city, but drizzly and even rainy; still, the volunteers and nurses managed to find umbrellas for the patients, and even some waterproof orange jumpsuits. The dignitaries gradually arrived, and after posing with hard hats and shovels, made their way to the dais. There was the outgoing mayor in his black fedora and long cashmere overcoat; there was the new mayor-elect, baby-faced, with his hair slicked back and his white smile. There was the city attorney in her gold pompadour, high heels, and skirt; the head of the hospital in his stiff black suit, grown a little pudgy and a lot older since he took over; and, in a wheelchair, a patient.

From where I stood in the valley I could see the old hospital high above our heads, with its square bell tower and red-tiled roof, and the trees sloping down the hill toward us. Dressed in black with gold buttons, and carrying polished brass instruments, was a band, playing Big Band music from the 1920s, 1930s, and 1940s. There was food—plates of smoked salmon, hot black coffee, even French champagne—and the able-bodied and mobile helped themselves. Wandering through the crowd were a few orange jumpsuited patients, including one I couldn't help noticing because he seemed so out of place, a tall, white-haired, blank-faced man with a gap in his teeth and the halting Parkinsonian gait.

Light rain came and went. Everyone had something to say. The old mayor, the city attorney, the head of the hospital, all talked about how difficult it had been to persuade the city to rebuild. Ironically, it was thanks to Demon Tobacco that the city had been able to afford the five hundred million dollars the new hospital was going to cost—fifty times what the present hospital had cost and five thousand times what it had cost to build the original four-story building.

Last to speak was the patient in his wheelchair. He took the microphone and looked out over the crowd. It was great that the city was going to build a new hospital, he said, great and laudable and charitable. And yet, somehow, he was concerned. The old hospital—we all looked up to see it in the drizzly rain, high on the hill behind him—with its warrens of rooms and wards, was a kind of storehouse, he said, or a sponge, or, perhaps, an old body, which had absorbed all the things that had ever happened within it and been subtly changed by them. Small and big kindnesses; suffering quietly or not so quietly but courageously borne, or at least borne. Or perhaps the old hospital was like the air in an old church, redolent of once-burned incense and living mold. Best, perhaps, the old hospital was most like what it actually was—an old, old house, and it had its ghosts.

He was right about that. Walking through the wards, turning down hidden corridors, I did feel ghosts sometimes, just like in an old house—ghosts of patients past, suffering past, death past, Christmases past.

Mainly, he went on, he thought the move would be a good thing, but now that we would be starting with a fresh building, with new walls and windows, what would happen to the spirit of the old? Since everything old—the beds, bureaus, curtains, tables, the oak chairs in the library, the wooden desks in the nursing stations—was going to be discarded, the old spirit would have to be carried to the new hospital, he said, ending his speech, transported somehow by all of its people—by all of us—patients, visitors, staff.

We all knew what he was trying to get at, but I wasn't sure it would work. Moving from an old, old house, leaving all the old possessions behind, to a new, new house, what can be transported? Within those new, spiffy walls of the new hospital with its fresh carpet, clean and shiny doorknobs, sharp edges, how would we remember, what would remind us, of the old patients and the old ways?

I couldn't imagine that they, the ghosts, would move with us, without their beat-up furniture, the easy chairs with the torn Naugahyde, the cracked and peeling many-times-repainted walls. I doubted that the ghosts would feel all that comfortable in the new climate-controlled, computer-designed building anyway. Instead of moving with us, they would stay on in the old building, I thought, lurking in their accustomed places like ghosts always do. And, since the city's administration was going to move into the old building—renovated, to be sure—in the end, the ghosts might do more good by staying put.

Because even after the renovation, the old walls, the jail cells, the breezeways—all those haunts of the old ghosts—would survive. And there would sit the city's strategists and implementers, suddenly taken by a momentary lapse of focus—by a breeze of boozy breath, of long-banished cigarette smoke; by the phantom squeak of a wheel-chair, music from an invisible piano, or the whisper of a ghostly deck of cards being shuffled somewhere in the hall.

Though that was a long time off, I reflected as I walked back up the hill.

We didn't even have blueprints yet. Still, the new health-care facility would look nothing like the old. It would have private rooms and flat-screen TVs—all the accoutrements of modernity. It would reference the hotel branch of its etymological family tree, not the monastic hospice branch. There would be no open wards to encourage community; no wide hallways for fortuitous meetings; no Romanesque arches to remind us of the religious and spiritual roots of *hospital*. No solarium standing in for the chapel, no turret for a live-in priest. I wasn't sure how much these architectural reminders influenced the hospitality of the old hospital, but I did wonder whether we could transport the spirit of the old to the new.

Perhaps the patient on the podium was right; perhaps the spirit was not mainly in the building itself, with its memories, its ghosts, and its references to medieval hospitality. Perhaps its spirit was in the people, in the nurses, the doctors, and especially the patients; and perhaps the new Laguna Honda would be as tender, as intense, as the old.

Well, I would find out, eventually—later rather than sooner, as it turned out. In the meantime, I still had a lot to learn from my patients, especially from my new patient, Mr. Thomas Teal, and his bride, Mrs. Thomas Teal.

Eight

WEDDING AT CANA

I T WAS UNUSUAL for E6 to get a new patient.

Its demented patients didn't come or go, and by and large, if I
didn't bother them, they didn't bother me. In fact, it was amazing to
see how little medical care they required. They hardly ever needed
the blood-pressure medications they'd been taking; on E6 their cho-
lesterols mysteriously normalized; their diabetes improved; and their
cancers stopped growing. Diseases that would have killed an intelligent and thoughtful person didn't phase E6's demented patients one
bit. They danced to the tune of Glenn Miller; they tapped on their
tables; they read their newspapers every morning, though sometimes
upside down. They rarely got sick, and none of them died.

But after we discharged Mr. Temkin back to his single room
above the bar, we did have an open bed, and I did get a new patient.
And if Lorna Mae, Mr. Bramwell's sister-in-law, taught me the
first principle of Laguna Honda—which was hospitality—then Mr.
Thomas Teal taught me its second principle, which was community.

Among the other things he taught me, such as unselfish love and a certain kind of resurrection.

Mr. Teal was admitted because he was, as the law put it, "gravely disabled" from dementia. On the admitting ward, Dr. Romero did her usual thorough workup and concluded that he was demented, and that there was nothing more to be done for him. So she sent him up to E6, where he inherited Mr. Temkin's bed in one of the semiprivate rooms. This turned out to be a good thing because Mr. Teal was a bit of a loner, and I doubt he would have tolerated the open ward long enough to undergo the various miraculous transformations that awaited him.

When I met him for the first time, he was alone in his room, a lanky figure curled up on his right side, with the covers pulled up over his head. He did pull them down when I came in, however, and greeted me in a slow drawl. His face was leathery and weather-beaten; his hair, white, thin, and scraggly; and his nose was crooked, broken at some time and never set.

He did not do well on the mental status exam.

He was demented; yes, so it seemed. He thought he was in Jefferson Memorial Hospital in Florida, which was not good, and that it was 1983, which was particularly bad, because I'd noticed that the depth of dementia could be measured by the difference between the actual date, the actual place, and the actual president, and the date, place, and president that the patient answered when asked. So "Obama and 2012" was great; it signaled a quick recovery and probable discharge. "Roosevelt and 1936" was bad; it meant a severe and irreversible dementia. Mr. Teal's "Florida and 1983" was not hopeless, but it wasn't good either.

Then I began my physical exam. I looked at Mr. Teal's hands, with their fingertips stained with nicotine, the slight curve of the nails, and the calluses of the once-working man. His eyes were blue, dull, and a little puffy; his teeth poor. His lungs were fair, with some evidence of his fifty years of smoking. His heart was better than I'd expected, given his three heart attacks; it beat sluggishly, but, all considered, it was a pretty good heart. The rest of him, too, was serviceable, I found, except for his right hip, that, after a fracture he must have ignored, had twisted and contracted into an unusable position. My exam concluded, I went back to the nursing station to read about the life that Mr. Teal could not or would not recount.

He grew up in Alabama, I learned, and dropped out of school in the twelfth grade. He made a living painting houses and had also studied religion, he told Dr. Romero, through correspondence courses. Eventually, like so many others, he decided to leave Alabama and come to California. To make his fortune? To escape bad debts, enemies, a prison sentence? To become a hippie or, given his correspondence courses, to find God through LSD? In any case, he ended up an alcoholic, living in shelters or on stoops or under bridges, with frequent visits to the County Hospital.

Then a few months before, he was picked up by the paramedics because they'd seen him "down"—that is, collapsed and unarousable— on the street. They stopped, examined him, and found that he had a bad cough and swollen legs, and they took him to the emergency room. This was the first miracle. If the paramedics hadn't stopped, examined him, and taken him to the emergency room at that very moment, Mr. Teal would have soon been dead.

Because, just as they got to the emergency room, Mr. Teal's heart stopped beating. The emergency room called for the Code Blue resuscitation team, which came running; and they were able to resuscitate Mr. Teal, with the shocks and tubes and magic medications of modern medicine. This was the second miracle, since, in spite of what we see in the movies, only one in twenty-five cardiac arrest victims are successfully resuscitated; of those who are, only one in a hundred survives to discharge. But Mr. Teal was successfully resuscitated and then sent to the intensive care unit, where, a few hours later, the blocked blood vessel that had caused his heart to stop was opened with a stent. His heart attack was massive, however, and he needed a heart pump to keep him alive. Eventually he recovered, though not enough to go back to his stoop and his vodka. The County psychiatrist found him so demented from the cardiac arrest and his vodka that he could no longer manage for himself and determined he would need care for the rest of his life.

For the next many months, Mr. Teal did not move from his room on E6. Withdrawn and reclusive, he stayed in bed, curled up on his right side twenty-four hours a day. Whenever I came in to ask him how he was, and urge him to get up, to use his wheelchair, to go to physical therapy, he was pleasant enough. His weathered face would crease into an apologetic smile and with a drawl he would respond, "No, ma'am, Ah don' feel bad; Ah jest don' want to git up." Eventually, though, he did agree to see the physical therapist, who fitted him with a wheelchair and tried to get him to exercise his stiff and contracted hip. But he wouldn't. He just would not. Nor would he take the heart medications I prescribed to prevent another cardiac arrest. He understood that I meant for the best, and often he told me he would take them, but he never did.

He did, however, uncurl himself eventually and take to his new wheelchair, and soon he was gone from the ward all day long, coming back only at the end of the day, reeking of alcohol and cigarettes. He'd discovered the coterie of miracles like himself—the group of resuscitated or grafted or operated-on drinkers, smokers, and drug addicts who congregated outside in the smokers' ghetto named "Harmony Park," to smoke, drink, and sometimes talk.

The nurses didn't like this new behavior at all because, looped and high on whatever he was drinking, though pleasant as always and turning ever more brown and leathery outside in the wind and sun all day, Mr. Teal began to refuse not only his medications but also his daily, then biweekly, and, finally, weekly baths. He started to look and—worse—smell, like the homeless wino he was. He was unshaven and dirty in the way that the movies can never portray, with a dirt deep in the creases and the pores and the cuticles and the hair and the hair follicles, back of the neck, ears, clothes—layer upon layer upon layer. And smelling of a really dirty dirt, mixed with old cigarette smoke, old nicotine on fingers, yesterday's alcohol, and today's and the day before yesterday's.

Then Mr. Teal began to insist that we discharge him, preferably to Reno, Nevada, but, if necessary, back to the streets of our city. Our kindly psychiatrist objected; she was sure that Mr. Teal was still gravely disabled from the many insults his brain had suffered over the years. So we tested him, and Mr. Teal was able to demonstrate that he still knew enough to meet the minimum criterion of the law: He was able to provide for himself as well as he had provided before his miraculous resuscitation—that is, sleeping on stoops, begging for money, and drinking on the streets. So the law decreed that Mr. Teal could leave whenever he wanted, and the social worker began looking around for a room. This was more difficult than we'd imagined, because Mr. Teal turned out to be well known for setting fires in his rooms, and no one would take him even when a room was vacant and even if the state paid for his discharge.

So Mr. Teal stayed on.

He spent less and less time in his room, however, showing up late at night, unkempt and rowdy and, sometimes, angry. Still, we couldn't quite bring ourselves to discharge him in his wheelchair onto the streets of the city. But the nurses were beginning to find half-pint bottles of vodka in his bureau, and administration was starting to crank up the pressure for just that kind of discharge when suddenly . . .

Well—nothing. It took me a while to realize that Mr. Teal had stopped being an issue. True, he was never in his room during the day, so I never saw him, but the nurses no longer told me about liquor bottles, and his room, when I passed it, seemed less like a flophouse and more like a boarding house room—plain and simple, but neat and clean, and not aromatic of alcohol and dirt. Finally I asked the nurses about him.

"Mr. Teal? Oh, he's not a problem anymore. He stopped drinking. Because he has a girlfriend. In fact, Dr. S., they're going to get married in the chapel next month; do you think you can be there?"

"Married? A girlfriend? Who is it?"

"Oh, it's Jessie, one of Dr. Bart's patients on the women's ward downstairs. He's been seeing her for quite a while. Since he met her, he takes his bath and lets us shave him every day. They're getting married in June on the fifteenth; it's a Wednesday; don't forget."

t was very busy at the hospital, though, and I did forget. Fortunately, I ran into Mr. Teal on the morning of his wedding.

It was one of those beautiful spring days we sometimes have in our city, when the fog is blown off by a crisp wind coming in from the ocean, up our hill, and through the hospital. Mr. Teal was sitting in his wheelchair in the breezeway, smoking, but I didn't recognize him at first. He was spotless, kempt, immaculately groomed—his silver hair pomaded, wavy, and parted on the left; his face meticulously shaved; and the pungent, attractive, and masculine smell of after-shave lotion was the only smell coming from him. He was dressed in a gray-green silk Armani suit, a starched and very white shirt, and a white silk tie. There was a white carnation in his buttonhole, his slacks were creased, and I could see gray silk socks in polished brown leather shoes on the footrests of his wheelchair.

As I came up, though, he smiled at me, and I recognized him—his cornflower blue eyes in that brown leathery face gave him away. Then I saw that his hands were shaking as he held his cigarette, and he told me that today was the day he was going to the chapel to get married. At eleven AM. Would I be there?

I would be there, I told him.

I kept track of the time, and a few minutes before the ceremony, I started for the chapel, which was downstairs at the front of the hospital.

I wasn't the only one. As I made my way, I was amazed to see how many people were walking in the same direction. There was my friend Dr. Bart, who was the bride-to-be's doctor; there were the physical therapists, the speech therapists, and the activity therapists; there were nurses, social workers, volunteers, and many others, all heading to the chapel. There were patients, too, limping or wheeling themselves down the corridor. I could barely find a seat in our chapel, which was not really a chapel but a small church, with stained-glass windows and rows of polished wooden pews.

The nurses of E6 and the nurses of L5, the bride's ward, were in the back, dressed in mothers-of-the-bride-and-groom dresses. They had on pearl earrings; their hair was done; and they were fussing with the reception table, which had on it presents, a cake, and two bowls of punch. Mr. Teal was already there in his wheelchair, nervous, and smiling shyly. The chapel was full.

I looked at my watch. It was 11:02 AM. Where was the bride? There was a bustle and a whisper. 11:05 AM. She was still on her ward, someone said, getting the finishing touches put on her coiffure. 11:10 AM. We heard she was coming, being wheeled off the elevator and down the corridor that leads to the chapel. 11:15 AM.

Here she was. And she was beautiful. "Bright as the sun and beautiful as an army with banners" as the Song of Songs has it. She was a warm mahogany brown, and she was wearing a diaphanous silk dress with light golds, yellows, browns, and reds in an African pattern. The dress was long and flowing; it covered her body and her wheelchair, and made her look, not like the stroke patient she was, but like a queen on a wheeled throne. Her black hair had been straightened and curled and woven with tiny rhinestones. Her earrings were gold; she wore a heavy gold necklace; and she was beaming, smiling so widely that even the paralyzed side of her face was lifted. Everyone turned their heads to see; several went over to her, to touch her and exclaim.

Mr. Teal, sitting in his wheelchair, was also smiling, a kind and grave and gentle smile. The organ began Mendelssohn's "Wedding March," and people hurried back to their places as the rest of us stood up, turned around, and looked at the bride and groom in the back.

Dr. Bart, the bride's doctor, and I looked at each other from our pews. It just didn't seem the moment to let our patients struggle by themselves down the aisle, rolling their wheelchairs as best they could. So Dr. Bart walked to the back and went over to the bride, and I went to the back and over to Mr. Teal, and we grasped the handles of their wheelchairs. Then Dr. Bart and I, with our charges, paced slowly in time to the music down the aisle, side by side. We left the bride and groom at the altar.

Meanwhile the minister had appeared. He was in front and dressed in black with a clerical collar. The organ music stopped, and there was a minute of silence while he looked at the couple in front of him. He cleared his throat and took a piece of paper from his inside pocket. Then he looked out at us, sitting in our seats, not knowing what to expect.

"Thomas and Jessie came to me several weeks ago," he began. "They told me they wanted to compose their own wedding vows. They worked very hard on them." He cleared his throat again, unfolded the sheet of paper, and began to read from it.

"Will you, Thomas Teal, take Jessie to be your wife, to love her as best you can for your whole life that remains to you?"

"I will," said Mr. Teal, blushing as we looked at him and turning to his bride with an indescribable smile.

"Will you, Jessie, take Thomas as your husband, to love and to hold, to cherish and take care of, as best you can, as long as you shall live?"

"Yes, I will." She was beaming so brightly when she said this and looking right into Mr. Teal's eyes, returning his glance as we seldom return a glance.

"Then I declare you husband and wife," said the minister. "You may kiss the bride."

We all held our breath. They were sitting next to each other in their wheelchairs, and Mrs. Teal couldn't move her left side, and Mr. Teal couldn't walk, but he could turn to her and throw himself slightly out of the wheelchair and grab her in his arms and give her a real, passionate kiss. Which he did.

never forgot that moment. The wedding of the Teals crystallized something for me that had been hard for me to conceptualize, but it had something to do with miracles and transformations and community. I thought of it as the "Wedding at Cana."

The Wedding at Cana was where Jesus performed his first miracle—the transformation of water into wine. And Mr. Teal's survival and transformation had certainly been miraculous. There was the first miracle that the paramedics had bothered to pick him up at all; and the second miracle, that he arrived at the County Hospital just in time for his resuscitation. There was the third miracle of his reconstitution in his bed on E6; and there was the miracle of his transformation—falling in love with Jessie.

But it was not only miracle and transformation that made the wedding of the Teals stand out in my mind as the Wedding at Cana. It was also, and even more—Cana.

Cana was just a little village in Palestine, and the wedding was nothing special. Yet everyone in the village attended—Jesus' mother and cousins, his aunts, his friends and relations, the rich and poor, the children, the elderly, the beautiful unmarried women, and the men looking for wives.

And at the Teals' wedding, when I saw the nurses in their mothers-of-the-bride-and-groom outfits; the other patients, dressed up and streaming into the chapel; Dr. Bart; and many others I didn't even know, what hit me was that the hospital was Cana—a little village and a true community. And that a great part of Mr. Teal's transformation had to do with this community—with its patients, its staff, its priest and nun, its open breezeways, its groups of smokers and scalawags, its doctors, nurses, and administrators.

After hospitality, I decided, community was the second principle of Laguna Honda.

What do I mean by community?

Community comes from the Latin *communio*, for which the *Oxford Latin Dictionary* gives two derivations. *Communio* as a verb comes from *munio*—wall—and means "to build a wall around." So a community is defined by the wall—symbolic or otherwise—around it. Everything inside the wall is the community, and everything outside the wall isn't.

That was a good definition of the community of Laguna Honda: You were a member of it just by being inside its wall. Because the hospital did have a wall, a real wall of polished rocks, piled up and shellacked by patients long ago. And we were a community simply because we were behind that wall and stuck with one another—doctor, patient, nurse, administrator, and budget. We had to do the best we could with what we had.

But *communio* as a noun derives from *munis*—gift; so *communio* also means "those who share a gift in common." That was true of the hospital's community, too, though it was not as obvious as the wall. At the Teals' wedding, when I saw almost all of Laguna Honda pouring into that church, sitting rapt during their vows, and, yes, even crying, I understood that it wasn't only me who was interested in the Teals, who made time, who was touched by them. Almost everyone was there; the wedding was a gift we shared in common, and that sharing made us a community.

For all the years I knew him after his wedding, Mr. Teal remained transformed.

He never went back to drinking and, although he was never as clean and handsome as he was on the day of his wedding, he stayed married. By that I mean, when Mrs. Teal had another stroke, he sat by her in his wheelchair and held her hand and worried; and when she recovered, he waited for her to appear in her wheelchair, with his sad and patient face, his bright blue eyes, and his farmer smile.

I saw them often sitting together on the nice days in the breeze-way, on the cold days just inside, sharing their smokes and, I believe, even getting into marital tiffs. Possibly about Mrs. Teal's flirtatious-ness and Mr. Teal's jealousy. Because there were days when Mr. Teal sat alone, and Mrs. Teal was nowhere to be seen. But then a few days later, there they would be again, together; and Mr. Teal would be, well, joyous; there is no other word for it.

Not too long ago, I asked him about his wedding. Wasn't his anniversary coming up?

He couldn't remember; I should ask the missus about that; she knew, she would remember.

Now, we had e-mail at the hospital, and I did use it, but when I wanted to meet someone, I didn't bother with it; it was too inefficient. Instead, I thought about whoever it was, his or her face fluttering across my mental screen, and in spite of our sixty-two acres and 534,000 square feet of building, I would run into him or her within a few hours.

So it was with Mrs. Teal. After I talked to Mr. Teal that day, an hour later there she was in her wheelchair, wearing a new wig, straight and reddish, and smiling gap-toothed at me.

"Well, well, Mrs. Teal! How perfect. We meet again. How are you?"

"Oh, fine! I'm fine, Dr. S.! But I'm going for a smoke. I started smoking again."

"Oh, well. You'll stop again, I'm sure.... I've got a question for you. When is your anniversary?"

She smiled more broadly. "I can't quite remember. It's in the book, though."

"The book?"

"The book the nurses made me—the wedding book. It's by my bed. Do you want to see it? It's got the date in it."

Of course I did. So we went over together to Mrs. Teal's ward, to her bedside.

"It's in the third drawer," she instructed me. "In a maroon pouch."

She was right; there it was. I took it out, sat down on her bed; and we turned the pages together. There was Mr. Teal in his gray-green Armani suit and white silk tie; there was Mrs. Teal in her gown; there were Dr. Bart and me in our white coats, giving the bride and groom away. There was the minister, and there was the kiss. On the reception table I saw the wedding cake; and there was Mr. Teal, feeding Mrs. Teal cake.

"They call us Mr. and Mrs. Laguna Honda," Jessie told me, "'cause we were the first to get married in the church. I'll never forget the day we met."

"How did you meet?"

"Didn't I ever tell you? We were in the smoking area. I asked Thomas for a smoke and he smiled and gave me one. He was so nice! Then I thought to myself, I've never kissed a white man before! And we kissed! It was so nice! That's how we met, and we've been together ever since."

And they did stay together. Mr. Teal's pyromaniac reputation continued to prevent him from being discharged, although his social worker did keep trying. He wouldn't have gone anyway without his missus, he told me, who could not be discharged because she was just too disabled to live outside the hospital.

I worried a little that once the new hospital was built, there might be efforts to move Mr. and Mrs. Teal together into one of the semiprivate rooms. That, I thought, would be a mistake. Because theirs was not a modern marriage, privileging intimacy over privacy; theirs was an old-fashioned, a Victorian marriage, where you sleep in separate bedrooms, keep your separate friends, and live your separate lives, meeting coifed and shaved at dinner.

The Teals' future—and the future of my other patients—was on my mind especially at this time because the city had just received a second letter from the Department of Justice. This one accused the city of discriminating against the disabled by keeping them at Laguna Honda, and it demanded immediate remedial measures. The DOJ's first letter had accomplished its main goal; a modern hospital was in the works. Despite, or perhaps because of, this success, the DOJ continued to investigate us, arriving several times a year, though never stating its objectives.

Finally, its second letter arrived, long and detailed, and summarized the investigation so far. Its main complaint, now, was that the city was violating the 1999 *Olmstead* decision, which ruled that disabled persons had a right to live in the community. Since our city did not provide alternatives to Laguna Honda for all its disabled citizens to live in the community, it was violating this civil right. So the letter stated.

The DOJ this time demanded that the city remedy the situation immediately, and the letter provided thirty-two minimal remedial measures for that purpose. Most of them had to do with discharging as many patients as possible and preventing any new admissions.

For instance, Laguna Honda was ordered to revise its admission assessments and utilization review procedures; institute new policies regarding admission and discharge; and create a complete database of its patients. Most important, it was to reassess, once again, all 1,178 patients and discharge the eight hundred patients that the DOJ believed did not have to be in the hospital.

It was a tough letter, and administration threw itself into the DOJ's demands with a flurry, nay, a snowstorm of activity. It was impressive.

To prevent future admissions, a team of doctors and nurses was put together to screen any potential Laguna Honda patient. The team would review the potential patient's chart and sometimes even go over to the acute hospital and examine the patient there. Did the patient need our care? Was there a community alternative? It was a thankless task, and I was glad it wasn't mine, because trying to figure out how sick a patient really was when an entire acute hospital was determined to stack the deck in favor of Laguna Honda must have been stressful.

For the patient database, administration installed the minimum data set (MDS) on our computers. This was a form to be filled out for each patient. It was twenty pages long and had hundreds of questions, the idea being to have a computerized measure of how sick every patient was. On a scale of one to four, how demented was the patient? On a scale of one to ten, how dependent? In how much pain? The MDS form was so complicated that a full-time MDS coordinator had to be hired for each ward in order to fill them out. Ellen Mary found the best nurse on each ward, had her trained, and then installed her in

one of the few private rooms on the ward, where she henceforth spent
all day entering data into the MDS.

To accelerate discharges from the hospital, administration
decreed that every patient was to be reevaluated quarterly as to his or
her potential for discharge, even if he or she had been comatose for
years.

Last, a second team of doctors, nurses, and social workers
reviewed every patient for discharge. Once again, this took weeks.
The team did find eight patients to discharge, which wasn't the eight
hundred patients the DOJ estimated could be discharged, but it was
something.

I n addition to the DOJ investigation, the city was facing a lawsuit,
called the *Davis* lawsuit, put together by disability-rights lawyers
in order to stop the city from building a new Laguna Honda. These
were the same lawyers who, in the 1970s and 1980s, constituted
the "Mental Health Bar," which had successfully closed the state
mental hospitals. Now they had set their sights on closing the country's long-term-care institutions, and Laguna Honda was one of their
test cases.

Initially they had opposed the bond for the rebuild on the
grounds that it would be cheaper, as well as more just, for the city to
close Laguna Honda and care for patients in the community. When
the bond passed anyway, the lawyers strolled around the wards and
finally found Mr. Davis and seven other patients willing to join him in
alleging that by keeping patients at Laguna Honda, the city was deny-
ing them their civil rights. This was *Davis*.

Davis had many demands, but its main one was that the city fund
a new program to assess—yet again—each Laguna Honda patient for

discharge and every potential new admission. This multimillion-dollar program, Targeted Case Management (TCM), would have its own director, nurses, and social workers (though not its own doctors) and would be independent of Laguna Honda, since the disability-rights lawyers did not trust Laguna Honda's own staff to evaluate its own patients. *Davis* also demanded that the city decrease the size of the new hospital by one-third.

The city did not fight *Davis* but settled. It refused to reconsider the size of the new Laguna Honda but it did fund TCM, whose staff began appearing on the wards soon after. I was surprised that they never examined or even met the patients they took on, and that they never talked to the patients' doctors. They read the charts we wrote and studied the MDS forms. And almost invariably they picked the patients for discharge who were the least likely to be discharged—the comatose, the terminally demented, the severely developmentally disabled. It was a little strange.

During TCM's first year it discharged two patients from Laguna Honda. After three years, it had discharged 139, many of whom were scheduled for discharge anyway. Since the program cost $2.5 million per year, that worked out to about $46,000 per discharge. Which wouldn't be expensive if the patients that TCM discharged stayed discharged. But it was impossible to find out what happened to them, and I always wondered how it worked out, efficiency-wise.

Because TCM did not discharge our patients to sweet little houses in the suburbs. Our patients went back to the single rooms in skid-row hotels from whence they'd come. And I wondered: What happened to them after they hobbled or wheeled themselves back into the life that got them to us in the first place?

I did find out what happened to four of the eight patients named in *Davis*, and perhaps they are exemplary. Two were so sick that they died before *Davis* was settled. The third patient failed his discharge in less than a month and came right back to us. And the fourth was thrilled with his life outside the hospital and never returned. I knew many patients who, after their TCM discharge, ended up right back in the hospital, and I knew a few who, while they didn't blossom, didn't wilt either. But I could never tell how it worked out in the end, either financially, medically, or morally.

I n any case, Laguna Honda was starting to be an expensive proposition for Dr. Stein.

It used to be that we brought in revenue for the city. But now, what with the DOJ letter and the new building, the *Davis* settlement and TCM, Laguna Honda was requiring an ever larger share of Dr. Stein's budget. And his budget wasn't great to start with. There was the recession; there were all the other demands on his budget—immigrants, AIDS, the uninsured, the elderly—and last but not least, the mentally ill homeless. They were even more of a drain because the newly elected mayor had campaigned on the slogan of "Care, not cash." If elected, he promised, the homeless would no longer get their $360 a month at City Hall but the equivalent in care, in particular, a place to stay. He did win the election, and he had charged Dr. Stein with the job of housing the mentally ill homeless.

Now Dr. Stein should have had an easy time doing this, because he had the city's Mental Health Rehabilitation Facility (MHRF, pronounced MERF) built to fill the niche left by the closing of the state mental hospitals. The MHRF was supposed to provide a place where the city's mentally ill could be rehabilitated: the idea being that they would live at the MHRF, receive psychiatric medications and learn to recognize their symptoms and get help before they became severely ill. The MHRF was successful, but it took a big part of Dr. Stein's budget because the state only paid for the first two weeks of a patient's stay at an institution for mental disease. The MHRF's patients, however, stayed for months, and this created a big hole in Dr. Stein's budget.

He thought a lot about what to do and finally he had a brilliant idea. He would use Laguna Honda to house the homeless mentally ill. He would take over two or three wards as mental-health wards; then he would move the mentally ill patients at the MHRF and in the County Hospital's psychiatric ward over to Laguna Honda. This would kill three birds with one stone. He could turn the MHRF into a cheaper residential facility; he could clear out the County's psychiatry ward; and, since Laguna Honda was not an institution for mental disease but a hospital, he would get reimbursed for those patients.

He called up the head of our admitting team, who was Dr. Romero, and explained his new plan to her.

Dr. Romero had been at the hospital for a long time and had come to love it with a passionate, protective love. When she was medical director, she had also studied the city's health-care system and learned about its politics. Plus she'd become friends with Dr. Kay, who was a righteous man, a man of principle, a man who didn't mind saying no. Although she herself liked saying yes, with Dr. Kay by her side, Dr. Romero said no to Dr. Stein. She was sorry, but she just couldn't do it.

Do what? Dr. Stein said.

Admit the mentally ill to Laguna Honda. Use the beds of the only public long-term-care institution in the city for the homeless. Privilege patients who had a place to stay over those who didn't. Laguna Honda was the almshouse for the city, and she would always first admit the patients who needed it the most. Besides, it would be illegal for her to admit mentally ill patients to Laguna Honda. We were not an institution for mental disease, and it wasn't safe. Not to mention that the DOJ was keeping a close eye on just such kinds of admissions.

Dr. Stein was not happy with her answer. Many of the mentally ill patients did have medical problems, he pointed out; surely those patients could be admitted. Dr. Romero should come over to the County and the MHRF, and evaluate the patients for herself.

So she did. Every morning she went over to the County and the MHRF. But she was able to take only a few of Dr. Stein's psychiatric patients because most of them were dangerous, and the few she did take created a lot of problems. They attacked other patients; they brought in serious drugs; and the number of patients emergently transferred back to the County's psychiatric department tripled.

Things finally came to a head with Larry Charles, a schizophrenic who had previously been in a locked psychiatric facility. One day he began refusing to take his medication, as was his right, and eventually he went into a psychotic rage and tried to strangle his roommate. The facility discharged him to the MHRF; the County got a court order that forced him to take his medication; he reverted back to his unpsychotic, pleasant self; and Dr. Stein asked Dr. Romero to admit him to us.

She refused. Larry Charles had no medical diagnosis, and Laguna Honda was not a locked psychiatric facility. She couldn't guarantee his safety or the safety of the patients around him.

Dr. Stein was furious. He demanded an immediate meeting with the medical director, nursing director, and executive administrator. They must overrule Dr. Romero, he insisted. Larry Charles was fine. He was taking his medications, he was calm and pleasant, and he wouldn't be a problem.

But the medical director, nursing director, and executive

administrator refused to overrule Dr. Romero, who had concluded that Larry Charles was a risk. After all, according to the hospital's admissions policy, Dr. Romero, not Dr. Stein, was in charge of Laguna Honda's admissions.

Dr. Stein saw them out of his office, and the next day we awoke to find that overnight our admissions policy had been hacked. The director of public health, our policy now read, could admit to Laguna Honda whomever he wanted.

Of course, this was quite illegal, and the board of supervisors called an emergency meeting. It was crowded and televised. The supervisors began by asking Dr. Stein to explain his side of the admissions dispute, which he did. Then they asked for the public's response. Dr. Romero, Dr. Kay, Sister Miriam, Miss Lester, several nurses, and our executive administrator stood up and explained their position, which was that the MHRF was the right place for Mr. Charles. Then the board went into a closed session. When they came out, they ruled that Dr. Romero was correct: Mr. Charles was too dangerous to be admitted to Laguna Honda. Dr. Stein was to change the admissions policy back to its former wording.

Fine, Dr. Stein said. That was fine with him. He would send Mr. Charles to that expensive private psychiatric facility he'd been trying to avoid. But since the money to do so had to come from somewhere, he would take it from Laguna Honda's medical budget. As he would do in the future with any other patient that Dr. Romero refused to accept.

Two months later, in a budget-cutting move, Dr. Stein eliminated the positions of medical director and nursing director at Laguna Honda, and dismissed the executive administrator. He sent Mr. Charles to that expensive psychiatric facility out of the county, and he did take the money from the medical department.

Mr. Charles is out there still, I believe, with the cost of his psychiatric care still coming from our medical budget. Or perhaps not. But probably. Because Dr. Stein, as it would turn out, had a very long memory.

A ll these investigations and politics were stressful, not to mention having the director of public health unhappy with our medical department. But at the time I didn't pay too much attention. I had finished my PhD and was planning to walk the medieval pilgrimage to Santiago de Compostela in Spain. I had decided to do this years before, as a present to myself when I finished my PhD.

But what is a pilgrimage? And why did I want to go on one?

A pilgrimage is a journey for spiritual reasons, but with a material goal—a shrine, a church, a mountain. It comes from the Latin word for pilgrim, *peregrinus*, from *per ager*, meaning "through the territory." A pilgrim, therefore, is someone who leaves home to travel "through a territory" that is, by definition, "not home," and so has the wider meaning of alien, foreigner, stranger.

But *peregrinus* (stranger) is different from *hostis* (stranger), which is the root for the *hospes* of hospitality. *Hostis* is the stranger from the host's point of view—the stranger who knocks at your door. *Peregrinus* is the stranger from the pilgrim's point of view—the one who does the knocking. The pilgrim leaves home in order to experience being a stranger—speak a different language, eat different foods, encounter different expectations—to experience otherness *as* the other.

In the Middle Ages, being a pilgrim was a big deal. It was what we all are, the medievals thought—pilgrims on the pilgrimage of life, leaving our true home at birth and traveling through time until we reach the spiritual goal of death; along the way, feeling "other" to what we see around us. To make a physical pilgrimage was to make that metaphor real.

There were three major medieval pilgrimages: to Rome, to Jerusalem, and to Santiago de Compostela, and the pilgrimage to Compostela was the most exotic. Rome was in the Bible and so was Jerusalem, and the medievals felt they knew something about both. But Compostela was mysterious. It had become a pilgrimage site only in the ninth century, when the body of Saint James, the apostle who had Christianized Spain, was discovered at the northern tip of Spain. It was said that the body had arrived in a stone boat that set sail from Jerusalem after the saint was martyred. A church was built for it, and monasteries were constructed across France and northern Spain as stopping places for pilgrims.

The pilgrimage to Compostela became popular; by the twelfth century, hundreds of thousands of pilgrims were walking to Compostela every year. After the Middle Ages, it fell into disuse, but was revived in the 1980s with the rediscovery of its ancient paths and motivations.

I was intrigued by the idea of experiencing pilgrimage in the medieval fashion. I, too, could make a vow of pilgrimage, and though I would fly to my starting point and apportion the 1,200-mile pilgrimage into four yearly walks—which didn't seem quite fair—still, I could do it.

I began to look around for a traveling companion.

This wasn't as easy as I'd imagined. None of my friends was intrigued by the idea of walking across France and Spain. Until I asked my friend Rosalind. We'd gone to medical school together, and I thought she would make a good companion. She was tough but flexible, adventurous but not wild, methodical but not rigid. She never complained and had a dry wit, especially about herself. She didn't know anything about pilgrimage, she told me. She was, if anything, antireligious, but she was ready for a long walk, and she was very good at maps.

So Rosalind and I put together our itinerary; we bought the smallest packs and took the fewest things. Then we flew to Paris, took the fast train to Lyon, and the slow train to Le Puy, the traditional starting point for the pilgrimage to Compostela. It was like going back in time, transportation-wise: from jet to high-speed train to the wooden-train technology of the nineteenth century and then stepping out on our own two feet. Le Puy was a big town, but modernity had skipped it, and it was, concentrically, eighteenth century in its outer ring, then seventeenth, sixteenth, and fifteenth century. Right in the center was its eleventh-century cathedral.

We bought our walking sticks in a little store, and the next morning we went to the special mass for pilgrims. After mass, the bishop presented each of us with a cockleshell, the thousand-year-old sign of the pilgrim, for us to put on our packs, and a "pilgrim's passport" for us to sign. The passport averred that having decided to leave our home to take ourselves to Saint James in Compostela, we would respect the spirit of pilgrimage, the other pilgrims, our hosts, and the nature we would walk through. In return, the bishop confided us to the care of all we met and asked them for the love of God, to receive us with charity, pray for us, and help us in our needs.

We were to have our passports stamped every night, the bishop explained. When we reached Santiago, we would give them to the Bishop of Compostela, who would present us with our Compostela, the Latin document that confirmed we'd completed our vow of pilgrimage and forgave us our sins.

The Way was always an adventure, he added, always a proving. Many were the reasons that put a pilgrim on the path: They were inscribed in the depths of each one's heart. But no matter what the interior quest, the Way was a way of life, and what he wished for us was that, with the sound of our footsteps, whatever we were seeking would fill us to overflowing.

Rosalind and I looked at each other. This was way deeper than we'd expected. We signed our passports anyway, attached the cockle-shells to our packs, picked up our sticks, and walked out the west door of the cathedral. And I think I can say for both of us that the bishop's good wishes for us came true, and to the very sound of our footsteps.

The thing about a pilgrimage is that there is no way to experience it except to do it. In that way it is very much like life. No armchair reading, no movies, no virtual photo albums can substitute.

Pilgriming isn't like backpacking. We didn't carry backpacks; instead, we reserved rooms in no-star hotels, in hostels, and once in a monastery, where nuns still practiced the virtue of pilgrim hospitality. So at the end of each day's fifteen miles, we did not put up a tent and cook Ramen. We had hot showers, good wine, and French meals. But pilgriming isn't like day hiking either, because we were walking not just through nature but through history. So nothing went by us too quickly; we were not tourists but actors in a landscape made to the measure of our footsteps. The scenery changed at the pace of walking, and just when we were ready for a village, there a village was, or a river, or a tree with plums.

There were many stunning moments on that first section of the pilgrimage, but the one I carried back to the hospital was the day it was pouring rain. We were a long way from that evening's shelter, and we would be walking in the rain for a long time. It was cold; I was soaking wet; and Rosalind and I were singing to keep warm. There were mud, fields, and rain; and I was chilled to the bone. Yet I didn't want to be anywhere else than in that muddy field, or doing anything else than walking in the rain, or be anything else except chilled. I didn't want to have arrived at our warm and comfortable destination. I didn't want the rain to stop or the fields to stop being muddy. I didn't want to be dry or warm, or to be one step farther along or one step farther back. I wanted to be just where I was because only by being where I was could I experience what I was experiencing. Which was pilgriming.

As I walked through the field, I thought about how much of my life I had spent trying to make sure I would never be in that place—out in the cold, homeless, and without shelter. I thought about my patients who lived on stoops, slept in doorways, and drank vodka while I was working. Once I'd asked a patient who was eager to get discharged and back to her stoop what the attraction of her life was. From what she told me, I'd thought it was freedom—from work, duties, responsibilities. But in the rain that day I wondered if, homeless, cold, and sheltered only by her stoop, she meant the feeling I had that day. I was happy and knew I was happy, the happiest I'd ever been. Not blissful, joyous, angels-coming-out-of-the-clouds happy, but happy as in "a feeling of great pleasure or contentment of mind, arising from satisfaction with one's circumstances." Happy from *hap*, as in what happens—things as they turn out to be.

When I got back home that year, I put away my things—my stick, my pilgrim's passport and shell, my pilgrim clothes. I wouldn't take them out again for a year. And yet I didn't stop feeling like a pilgrim. Now and then, as I was walking down the wide corridor between wards, the click of my footsteps would remind me, and I would be pilgriming across that muddy field, happy with things just as they were.

Perhaps for that reason, my relationships with my patients began to deepen. When you think about it, doctoring has everything to do with not accepting things as they are, and while I didn't stop doctoring my patients, there was some new way in which I was appreciating them just for who they were.

Which was a good thing for the patients on my other ward, E4.

E4 was two floors below E6 and looked just like it, with a narrow entrance, linen room, nursing station, and big, open ward.

But E4 was not a "dementia ward." It was a "medically complex" ward, which meant that it had patients with serious illnesses who, for other reasons, were unable to take care of themselves. The patients on E4 were paralyzed from strokes or car accidents, had multiple sclerosis, Parkinson's disease, head trauma, spinal cord injury, and cerebral palsy. In addition to their main problem, each patient—and this is what made them "medically complex"—had other problems: diabetes, seizures, chronic pain, lung disease, heart disease, kidney disease. Almost every patient also had a psychiatric diagnosis— schizophrenia, manic depression—and often a personality disorder, too—borderline, schizoid, histrionic, or obsessive-compulsive disorder. Quite a few had been affected by the closure of the state mental institutions; with no place to go, they had done the best they could on the streets. Many had treated their psychiatric illnesses with cocaine and heroin, and then treated the side effects of cocaine and heroin with alcohol, and so had the complications of their drug and alcohol abuse as well.

Not only were they medically complex, but the patients on E4 were complicated nursing problems. Almost every patient had tubes the nurses had to manage—shunts in their brains, PIC lines in their

veins, PEG tubes in their stomachs, nephrostomy tubes in their kidneys, catheters in their bladders. Several patients had open wounds
from a chronic infection or bedsore, and the nurses cared for those,
too, changing dressings three times a day.

Although the men of E4 were complicated and sick, they were
not withdrawn or depressed but open-faced, flirtatious, and handsome. There was a reason for their good looks: No ugly person would
have survived what they had survived. Even in orphanages, on the
streets, and in prison, handsome people get special treatment. And
the men of E4 knew that they were handsome, which is why they were
flirtatious. They rarely complained either, at least not about the hand
God dealt them. They complained about the food and the paucity of
cigarettes, sometimes about the nurses, and occasionally about pain;
but mostly they were stoic and funny.

Like its patients, E4 was a shabby and unregenerate ward. What
with the new Laguna Honda a-building, administration was loath to
put money into the old hospital, although every now and then some
lucky ward would get new paint, new curtains, and, when the pressure
from the investigating magistrates became too heavy, new dressers.
But E4's ticket had not yet come up; its paint was peeling; its curtains
faded; its dressers cracked.

Nor did it have much decoration. Most of the patients had only
the tops of their dressers on which to put the photos that had survived the shipwrecks of their lives. Bill Luckly had a picture from his
navy days, wearing the handlebar mustache he still wore, with husky
shoulders and a white grin. Steve Milton had a pink-and-orange psy-
chedelic poster of his rock band, and Sammy, our Down's patient, had
his photo from St. Patrick's Day; with a green shamrock pinned to his
green vest and a shiny green top hat, he looked like an aging

elf. Occasionally a student from the Art Institute would sketch our handsome men, and a beautiful charcoal drawing would appear above a bed. But, on the whole, there wasn't much decoration on E4.

There was even less after the fire on D3.

A patient set the fire. He'd waited until the day before his discharge, which happened to be the first of the month. He left the hospital and went first to City Hall, where he picked up his $360 of welfare cash that the mayor hadn't yet stopped. Then he went to a gas station and bought two cans of gasoline and a quart of vodka, and came back. D3 was closed for its renovation, but he snuck inside, and as he looked around for towels, he started to drink. Then he dowsed the towels in gasoline, shoved them under the doors, lit them, and fell asleep.

The old building still had a lot of asbestos left and did not burn but smoldered. The fire was extinguished, and Mr. Jax was awakened and discharged to jail, the outcome of the fire being that the day after, fire marshals appeared on every ward. Not to search for potential arsonists, but to remove every piece of paper on the walls—every picture, photo, and drawing. They were fire hazards, the marshals explained.

So after the fire, the walls of E4 were bare. But then another examining magistrate complained that the walls were empty and insisted that patients be allowed to express their personalities on the walls above their beds, which were, after all, their homes. A decree went forth, and a few weeks later, each ward's activity therapist brought in thirty-four corkboards and set to work. They cut out and pasted pictures from old magazines onto the corkboards—*Good Housekeeping, Sports Illustrated, Time*. They were random but efficient, and by the time the next investigation came round, every patient did have a personality expressed above his bed.

The patients of E4 didn't pay much attention either way. There weren't many walls in the shelters, boxcars, and army barracks they were used to, and none on the streets, and most of them had consolidated their memorabilia all the way to nothing, except for their tattoos, those dermal memories so easy to take from place to place.

If the demented men of E6 were bodies without minds, then the patients of E4 were minds without bodies, and sometimes when I went from E4 to E6, I thought it was a pity we couldn't take what still worked in each—the bodies of the patients on E6, the minds of the patients on E4—and combine them, transplanting, for instance, Bill Luckly's still usable mind into Mr. Dell's still usable body.

Although, on second thought, perhaps not. Bill would most likely go back to his drinking, fall off his bar stool once again, hit his head, and end up paralyzed and back at the hospital, only in Mr. Dell's body.

In addition to its handsome patients, what gave life and cohesion to E4 were its staff, especially its charge nurse, Christina; its male nurse, Allen; and Lacy, its activity therapist.

Like many of Laguna Honda's nurses, Christina was from the Philippines; and she was short and stocky, with dark hair, skin, and eyes. But Christina had something special about her. Although most of the Filipina nurses were agreeable, deferential, and warm, they maintained a certain reserve; their polite deference seeming as much a second language as their English. But Christina was warm in both languages. You wouldn't call her beautiful, and yet she had something in her eyes and her smile—a softness, an intelligent kindness. The thing about Christina was—she loved her patients. She knew every one; she remembered everything about them; and she was proud of them. I discovered this on my second day on E4 when she insisted I walk over to see "her" patient, Mr. Jerry Gillon.

Now, Mr. Gillon was one of the few patients on E4 who didn't fall into the category I described. Mr. Gillon didn't have a stroke, multiple sclerosis, or a traumatic brain injury; he didn't have diabetes or schizophrenia or a drug habit; and he wasn't handsome or flirtatious either. Mr. Gillon had a birth condition, no one knew what, and had been in an institution since he was an infant, being now fifty-nine years old. He was blind; he had seizures; and he was mentally retarded, with the IQ of a two-year-old, so Christina said. Although I doubted that. Not the two-year-olds I knew, who were sparkly little devils. "Two-year-old" was Christina's motherly overestimation of her charge's abilities. Because Mr. Gillon could do nothing at all. He was a wonder to me, a mystery, and a question, the question being, why were we taking care of him in the remarkable way we were?

Not that there was any alternative. Besides, I enjoyed taking care of Mr. Gillon—it was so very impractical. He was never going to get better and be discharged; he was never going to marry, get a job, and become a productive member of society. In spite of or because of this, I took pride in taking the best possible care of him.

But over the years, I did get something from him. Something special. Sitting in his chair with his hands in his lap, his face peaceful and alert, his eyes open though blind, Mr. Gillon came to remind me of those Egyptian statues of the Sitting Scribe—silent but listening, blind but aware, noninterfering but observing. Whenever I walked past him in that busy, hectic ward, repository of so much damage, so much sadness, Mr. Gillon recalled me to myself. He reminded me that there were more ways to be of use than to be of use; that there was something to be said for pure existence; that none of us knows what is valuable to God. Isn't the Buddha's description of nirvana "no eyes, no ears, no nose, no tongue, no body, no mind"? And hadn't Mr. Gillon unwittingly achieved it?

Mr. Gillon went to school every day. A bus took him in the morning and brought him back at three o'clock, just in time for his snack of graham crackers and orange juice. In the morning the nurses dressed and buttoned him, fed him, and combed the remaining hair over his bald spot, and did it all in reverse when he returned. I was responsible for his medical care. I managed his complex seizure disorder and his occasional pneumonia; I made sure he had his flu shots, his monthly checkups, and his annual physical examinations, and I can assure you, Mr. Gillon was in tip-top health.

Christina was proud of Mr. Gillon, as she demonstrated for me on my second day.

"Come over, Dr. S., and see what Jerry can do."

I closed the chart I'd been reading and followed her out of the nursing station. Mr. Gillon did have a nice little blind smile, I thought. His clothes were neat and clean, and as we approached him, his head turned a little as if he heard us.

We stood in front of him.

"Jerry! Clap your hands, Jerry!" Christina shouted in his ear. "Clap your hands for Dr. S.!"

She waited.

Nothing happened.

"Jerry! Clap your hands! Show Dr. S. what you can do!"

Mr. Gillon made no sign that he had heard. Christina's words seemed to hang in the air and then one by one float across the three feet that separated us from him. All of a sudden, his face brightened, and he raised both stubby, uncallused hands and moved them together in a sort of clap, three times.

"There!" Christina smiled. "He can clap his hands."

Christina knew things like that about all the patients, which weren't unvaluable to know. For instance, asking Jerry to clap his hands was the best way to tell whether he was sick. It was a mini mental-status examination and a lab panel rolled into one, and over the years I found myself more than once shouting in his ear, "Jerry! Clap your hands!" If they lifted up and moved together three times, then I was safe; he was well. If they didn't, then X-rays, blood tests, and antibiotics were indicated.

Christina knew about the families of the patients—the divorces, the remarriages, the stepchildren. She knew the foods the patients liked and disliked. She knew the medications that had been tried over the years and why they failed; she remembered the tests whose results our overzealous medical records department removed from the chart. If I had a question or an answer, an idea to try, or a concern about a patient, I asked Christina.

On the other hand, Allen, our male nurse, was the peacock of the staff. He was slim, with even features and a proud, self-conscious carriage. He didn't talk much. His pride and joy was the BMW he bought with his hard-earned wages. Which he never drove to work, he confided to me once; he took the bus. On the weekends, he would polish that BMW and take it out on the desert roads at 120 miles an hour. Allen was a peacock in the way that all the male Filipino nurses played peacock to the reserved peahens of the female Filipina nurses, who, though they appeared deferential, were in charge. Perhaps it was the matriarchal culture of the Philippines, but it always gave me a sense of camaraderie with those male Filipino nurses. They, too, were subservient and a little afraid of the more powerful opposite sex.

Allen followed Christina's lead, and they tag-teamed their

vacations, their weekends, and their sick days. It was hard work on E4, and I never knew how much it meant to him until later, after E4 was disbanded, its patients and nurses scattered. Allen was scattered to Dr. Kay's hospice unit, where, I heard, he wasn't doing well. He was slumping, gaining weight, losing his vital force in the same way that the hospice patients did, though they were supposed to. We ran into each other—Allen on his way, I am sorry to say, to the morgue with a body.

"Dr. S.!" His face lit up. He gave me a hug.

"How are you doing, Allen?" I asked.

He raised an eyebrow, rolled his eyes, and looked at the gurney he was pushing. "They're too efficient down there," he said. "I don't like it. I like trying to get patients better, keep them alive. Not the opposite."

"We don't like death much, do we, Allen?"

"No, Dr. S., we don't. I really do miss you and Christina and Lacy and the patients on E4."

Lacy was E4's activity therapist. She was big, with wide hips and big breasts, and quite black, with round, merry eyes, and the resonant contralto that went with her body.

Lacy knew quite a few of the patients, "our boys," as she called them, from some past life she'd led before she came to Laguna Honda. She played poker and blackjack with them. She read them the news and showed them a lot of terrible movies. But mainly she teased them.

"Now, Mistah Bill, why don't you want to par-tic-i-pate in our little game today? 'Fraid ya gonna lose, hunh? 'Fraid Mistah Gillon's gonna win, hunh? Come on, just try one hand. . . . Hey, you got the jack right off!"

It was Lacy who made it possible for Mr. Simon Scurly to get back home.

I can't say I took to Mr. Simon Scurly. The name, for starters, referencing *scurrilous,* and Simon, as in the master of some old Southern plantation, which is most likely how Mr. Scurly got his name. Nor was Mr. Scurly handsome and flirtatious. He was irritable, suspicious, and angry. He didn't want to be in the hospital, he told us, and he didn't have to be. There was nothing wrong with him. His landlord just wanted his rent-controlled apartment, and he was fair game, being eighty-two years old and a black man.

But there was quite a lot wrong with Mr. Simon Scurly, or so the visiting nurses told me. He'd ignored his diabetes for so long that now he was almost blind. He'd lost a leg from the poor circulation that diabetes can sometimes cause. He was anemic with a low red blood cell count. He didn't eat right, and he wasn't able to give himself his twice-daily insulin injections. Worst of all, his diabetes had apparently affected the nerves to his bladder and his gastrointestinal tract, and he was no longer able to control his excretions. Which was, as it so often is, the last straw.

Mr. Scurly, stocky, a freckled brown, and bald, did not agree with any of this. He was fine, he told me, Christina, Allen, and Lacy. He didn't need the insulin, and if we let him go home, he'd manage. It was just those workers the city sent over to his house—he glared at us—interfering women!

I had more time to fuss with my patients on E4 than I'd had on the admitting ward, and for Mr. Simon Scurly this was a good thing. Because, as I realized after a while, he was right about the insulin. The visiting nurses had been giving him just the tiniest amount of insulin, an amount so small that if you need that amount, you don't need insulin at all, and when I stopped it—sure enough—Mr. Scurly

was fine without it. It was the same with his blood-pressure medication. He was taking it three times a day, but in tiny doses, and I
discontinued it, too, without a problem. Mr. Scurly did turn out to
have a bladder infection, but after that was treated, and his gastrointestinal tract tuned up, he regained control of his functions, as my
patients so delicately refer to the condition.

So one day we looked at one another—Christina, Allen, Lacy, and
I. Maybe we could send Mr. Scurly home. We could arrange for visiting nurses, Meals on Wheels, a case manager, a social worker. . . .
What did Mr. Scurly think of that? We asked him at our monthly
meeting.

He didn't need any strange ladies from welfare knocking on his
door is what he thought of that, and, he told us, he wouldn't let them in.

"Just send me home," he insisted. "I'll be all right."

We wanted to send him home, but we were worried. Someone
needed to keep an eye on him, and he had no family. But he did have
Lacy.

"I'll go by and see him, Dr. S.," she volunteered. "He doesn't live
too far from me, and he likes me. He'll let me in. I'll make him a pot
roast on Saturday. You'd like that, wouldn't you, Simon? I'll go by
after work a couple of times a week and check up on him."

We did send Mr. Simon Scurly home, and he stayed home until he
died, two years later. Lacy continued to watch over him, and now and
then she made him dinner in his own kitchen. It pleased me to imagine the scene: that warm, genial woman, young and pretty, big and
black, joshing him in his own kitchen, with him sitting, smiling and
thrilled, at his Formica table.

I did wonder what the Department of Justice and the *Davis* lawyers
would have thought of Mr. Scurly's discharge. Would they have ap-

proved because Mr. Scurly was not in an institution but in the community? Or would they have disapproved because his discharge depended on the unmonitored charity of a staff member? At any rate, Mr. Scurly's discharge meant that E4 now had an open bed, which is how I met Paul Bennett, and how, in a manner of speaking, I fell in love.

Nine

HOW I FELL IN LOVE

O N PAPER, and doubtless on the computerized minimum data set form, Paul Bennett was just another of the difficult patients that Dr. Stein was trying to send over—an abuser of cocaine and alcohol, homeless, angry, and self-destructive, with an incurable physical illness. Which shows you just how wrong a form can be, even one with 1,100 little boxes.

The first time I met Paul, he'd been transferred to E4 from the admitting ward, and he was in bed. As soon as he saw me walking down the ward, he went on the offensive. The nurses weren't changing his dressings correctly, he complained, and his foot was getting worse. He needed to smoke, and he had no wheelchair; plus he had an appointment at the County Hospital. And had it been arranged? Then he glared at me.

He was dark brown and very thin. His cheeks, with their wisp of black beard, were hollow, and his black hair was short, frizzy, and thin on top. He was a tall man and too long for his bed, so that his remaining leg, the one that hadn't been amputated, was pushed against the end with the foot pressed into the railing. He was unshaven and unwashed, angry and irritable.

And yet there was something about him. Perhaps it was the way he held his head straight on his neck or the way his jaw jutted out. Or perhaps it was that he was not flirtatious; his clear brown eyes had grown-up in them; they didn't beseech or seduce; they looked into mine frankly, if irritably, as one deserving Self to another.

I'd already spoken with Dr. Romero, and I knew that Paul's main problem was "peripheral vascular disease." This is a vague but bad diagnosis that means the circulation to the legs is poor because the arteries have been blocked by blood clots or cholesterol plaques. It usually develops in the elderly, and it was rare to have it, as Paul did, at the age of forty-seven.

It all started, he told me, when he was working at the Monte Antique Show, arranging the furniture for a display. A credenza fell on top of him, and his left hip snapped, which was weird because he was strong and healthy and only forty-two. He was taken to the University Hospital, and they replaced his hip, but after that, he had nothing but problems with that left leg. It hurt him all the time, and his doctors discovered that the main artery to the leg was blocked by a blood clot. So he had another surgery, and they tried to bypass the blockage using one of his veins. But that vein clotted, too. The surgeons tried three times, in three different bypass surgeries, and every time the blood vessels they used clotted.

Then the same thing happened to his right leg. Although he didn't break the hip, it deteriorated on its own and had to be replaced, and after that, the circulation in his right leg went, too. He had to have that artery bypassed several times. Yet his hips and legs kept hurting him even after he'd had both hips replaced twice and the blockages in his arteries bypassed four times. Then several months ago, his newest right hip had dislocated out of its socket, and the doctors put him on bed rest. But while he was on bed rest, his left foot got infected, and even with antibiotics, it didn't get better. So he was admitted to the County Hospital, and the surgeons amputated the infected toes. But because of his bad circulation, that amputation did not heal, and they operated again, and this time they amputated his entire lower leg. The leg still didn't heal, and they amputated it high above the knee, leaving him with a stub. The stub healed, but he'd had to spend most of his time lying on his right side, and now he had sores on his right foot and a bedsore on his right hip. Plus, he'd lost his job and his place, and everything he owned was now in storage.

Did he have any family or friends? I asked him.

Divorced. He didn't know where his ex-wife was, and he had a son somewhere.

What about drugs? Alcohol?

A long time ago. Not anymore. Heroin, cocaine, alcohol, but he'd worked hard on that.

How did he get the bullet in his back? The one Dr. Romero had seen on X-ray?

Oh, that. He got that driving a cab, and he didn't want to go into details.

I examined him. The stub had healed, but the right leg was a mess. I couldn't feel a pulse in the right foot, and there were several soupy sores on the sole and along the side; the skin over the right hip was gone, and there was a deep, infected hole instead.

It was tragic, and yet it was predictable: In trying to keep him off his left leg so that it could heal, his doctors had had him lie on his right hip, which had developed a bedsore. And here he was on E4, for us to try to heal it and get him home.

Paul did not do well those first few months.

All he liked to do was sit outside in his wheelchair, rain or shine, and read and smoke, although he knew nicotine and sitting were bad for his circulation and the healing of his sores. He read even more than he smoked. He read all the time and everything, but especially science fiction, and he went through the books in the hospital's library one by one. He was angry and irritable and way too smart for the staff; he wouldn't let the nurses clean his bed or the space around it; and he had stuff everywhere: CDs and DVDs, brown paper bags, books. It drove the nurses, nice as they were, crazy; there was stuff everywhere, and they needed to straighten up, but when Christina tried to speak to him about the mess, Paul's eyes would narrow; and he would refuse. He wouldn't let them bathe him; his hair was dirty and his body unclean. He slept most of the day and stayed up all night, and he ate very little.

The first thing Christina asked me to do when I was back from the first section of my pilgrimage was "Dr. S., go talk to Paul about his sores. He won't go to plastic surgery or orthopedics, and they are looking very bad."

She was right. Paul's wounds looked awful. Despite the antibiotics he'd been taking, the sores on his right foot and the big sore over his right hip were slimy and smelly and infected, probably down to the bone. It took quite a bit of persuading, but he agreed to see our orthopedic surgeons. They were not happy with what they saw. They told him that his prosthetic hip was infected and would have to be removed, that the sores on his right foot would have to be surgically debrided, and that some kind of skin covering would have to be fashioned for the huge sore over his hip. He would have to go back to the County Hospital.

Things did not go as planned. He did go over to the County and was there for three months. The surgeons removed the prosthetic right hip, but Paul's bedsore still did not heal. They debrided the sores on his right foot, and the foot did not heal either, most likely because of his peripheral vascular disease. So Paul's lower right leg had to be amputated. Meanwhile, the sore over his right hip widened and deepened, and the surgeons finally gave up and took the whole leg off, including the right hip. They tacked the skin that was left back over the open area of his buttock and sent him back to us.

Paul was not better, I saw, when I examined him. He was very thin, edgy, and depressed; and the new amputation was astonishingly deforming—he had no legs. But the most disturbing part was the skin flap itself, which was tacked over the five-by-eight-inch open area of his missing right buttock and was starting to turn black at the edges. Now all of this was scary—to be a no-legged, ex-handsome, ex-independent black man—but it would be nothing compared to having that skin flap turn gangrenous, as it seemed to be doing. Because if Paul lost that skin flap, if it finished turning black and sloughed off, then there would be nothing to protect his body from progressive gangrene. The gangrene would spread, and he would die a slow death.

Even he was subdued. Not that he stopped smoking and reading, or staying up all night in his wheelchair watching television. But subdued in that now he let the nurses change his dressings and thanked them; he tried to eat; and when he was in bed, he tried to stay off what remained of his right hip.

But the wound worsened. The skin that had been tacked down turned black, and the wound it covered was draining and malodorous, despite antibiotics. So I went with Paul to see our plastic surgeon and learn what else we could do. The surgeon examined the wound. There was no way to cover it or graft the area because Paul had no extremities left from which to take a large enough skin graft. He didn't say anything, though, until Paul left the surgical suite. Then I asked, "What do you think?"

He shook his head. "It's a catastrophe. There's nothing for me to do. If that wound doesn't heal on its own, well . . . He needs to stay off that hip, and he needs to stop smoking."

It was impossible to imagine what would happen next, and I couldn't think of anything else to do. But if nothing else was done, Paul would die, in the twenty-first century, of an old-fashioned, a medieval diagnosis—an open wound. And though I suppose you could blame it all on Paul—he did, after all, keep smoking and reading and sitting up in his wheelchair all night—I didn't believe that if he stopped smoking and took to his bed, his wound would heal. It was just too far along.

So I left the hospital and went for a walk at the beach. I wanted to think. Surely there was something left for me to do. "Remove obstructions," I remembered from Terry Becker, but the obstruction in Paul's way was not a simple obstruction. It was a malevolent and active closing of his blood vessels, a lack of flow, a blockage. As I walked, I went through my list. He was already on antibiotics. There wasn't anything left of him to debride and remove. He already had a special bed and good nurses. He could stop smoking, but he wouldn't, and even if he obeyed the plastic surgeon and went to bed, there wasn't much left to lie on anyway. I couldn't think of anything else to do.

As I walked I thought about the pilgrimage, and I thought about Hildegard. What would Hildegard do, I asked myself, if she had nothing left to do? She would pray. What would she pray for? For

Paul's healing—body, mind, and soul. So I did. Pray. Not to anyone in particular, though. I didn't have to. I was, after all, walking on the beach, in the sand, with the salty wind coming off the water and the waves coming and going.

Then I went back to the hospital. As soon as I got back, that instant, Dr. Bart paged me. And while I wouldn't say that her call was miraculous, it did mark the beginning of Paul's healing—physically, mentally, and spiritually.

"I've been just thinking about Paul," she said. "How's he doing? I saw him outside. We talked; he was reading and smoking as usual."

I told her.

Then Dr. Bart had an idea I hadn't thought of. "Why not try hyperbaric oxygen?"

Hyperbaric oxygen is 100 percent oxygen administered under pressure to the patient while he lies inside a clear plastic chamber, the idea being that the high concentration of oxygen somehow helps the healing of wounds. It isn't a common or a proven treatment, and I had never used it before.

"You think?"

"I've had it work for a few other patients. It's a hassle to arrange, but it just might work. Let me tell you how to make it happen."

She did, and I arranged an appointment for Paul at the only hyperbaric chamber in our city. We went over together to meet the hyperbaric specialist in charge. He talked to Paul, examined his wound, and thought it might work. So Paul began going over to the hyperbaric chamber every day.

It did work. It was amazing. In a few weeks the black skin over the wound began to turn pink, and the gangrene began to flake off. After eight weeks, Paul's wound was healed.

During those few months, other things healed, too. Paul had been estranged from his family—sister, ex-wife, son—but one day while he was sitting outside smoking, he recognized his niece, who happened to work at the hospital. She began to visit him in the evenings, and she let the rest of his family know where he was. They began bringing in his favorite foods, and he began to gain weight.

Pretty soon Paul was just another of the patients on E4. Only with a twist because, as it turned out, he had a gift. He knew how to build computers out of parts and pieces, and while he was healing on the ward, he built himself one. The patients around him were fascinated, and from his bed, he taught them about computers. Soon the nurses were coming to him with their computer problems. Often, especially in the evenings, I would see them, small and pudgy and giggling, surrounding Paul, who, in bed with his sheet pulled up, looked like the full man he really was.

Paul became a popular person. Not least because his cousin, James, brought him bootlegged versions of the newest films, which Paul copied onto DVDs and sold around the hospital for three dollars each. He made enough money to buy himself an LCD television and keep himself in cigarettes. He and Donald, one of the starstruck patients across from him, started to make plans to open a DVD store after they were discharged.

He did have a few setbacks. There was an episode of pneumonia. There was a computer breakdown that required a new motherboard and a soldering iron to connect it. But he recovered from the pneumonia, and from somewhere acquired a soldering iron, which he used one night near someone's oxygen. He didn't start a fire, but the nurses were pretty upset, and they took the soldering iron away, though not before Paul's computer was once again operative. He had phantom-limb pain from the amputated right leg. But the bedsore over his hip had healed; he was bright and alert; and he was looking forward to reconnecting with his son.

We began to think about discharge.

It would not be easy. Although Paul was resourceful and independent, managing his own finances, doing his own care, establishing businesses, and building computers, the last time he'd been out in the community, he had been a six-foot-tall handsome black man. Now he had no legs and could barely balance himself in his wheelchair. Nevertheless, the social worker began scheduling interviews for Paul at various hotels—the kind of hotels our patients went to, that is.

I t was around Christmas. I'd known Paul for more than a year, and I liked him a lot. Was there something he wanted, I asked him, from Santa?

He looked up at me from the depths of his wheelchair. Sometimes, sitting in that chair with only half his body left, he looked so small.

"I want a fishing vest," he told me. "One of those fishing vests with all the pockets. And I can't get hold of one here."

"A fishing vest? Why?"

"I can't keep the stuff I carry with me organized. 'Cause I don't have legs I don't wear trousers, and the only pocket I have is here on my shirt. Not enough. I figure with a fishing vest I'll have places for everything."

So one lunchtime I went over to the Big Box Store. Fishing vests were over in the manly section, I was told, by the fishing rods, and I found lots of them in grays, beiges, taupes—manly colors. They were not expensive, and they did have pockets—big and small, zippered and open, square and rectangular—all over. I picked taupe because it would look good with Paul's skin tone, and medium, which would fit. I had the vest wrapped, and I wrote him a note, signed SANTA. When I got back to the hospital, I gave the present to Christina and asked her to put it on Paul's pillow Christmas morning.

When I woke up that Christmas, the first thing I thought about was Paul getting his vest. I hoped he liked it, and I hoped it fit. And I couldn't help but notice the pleasure I was getting out of him and that vest. It didn't seem quite right, somehow, but there it was. This got me to thinking about charity—its motivations, its emotions, and how, after hospitality and community, charity was the third principle of Laguna Honda.

The charity I meant was nothing organized. It was not in the hospital's mission statement, on its new website, or in the PowerPoint presentations of middle management. And yet charity, in the medieval sense of a "personal action evoked by dearness and contributing to the well-being of its giver as well as its receiver," was as much built into the place as its arches, bell tower, and church.

Charity came into the West when Saint Jerome translated the Greek word *agape* by the Latin *caritas*, which became the English *charity*. Today *agape* is usually translated as "love," but *agape* was more nuanced; in ancient Greek it meant "to treat with affectionate regard." *Caritas*, charity, is closer because the root of *caritas* is *cara*—"dear"—as in expensive and cherished. So *caritas* has the sense of "dearness"—of a love that is precious and sweet.

In English, *charity* evolved over the centuries. At first it meant "the love of God"; later it meant the actions that expressed that love— in specific, caring for the sick poor. In the Middle Ages, charity was accepted as doing as much for the giver as it did for the receiver, the "goodness of charity being a bond of love that draws us to God."

And even when the monasteries in England were disbanded, this insight—that caring for the sick poor was a spiritual good for the giver—continued to inspire charitable institutions. It was one reason why the state built hospitals to care for the sick poor, and why we still believe and act as if taking care of the sick poor is something that a society should do. Charity built Laguna Honda in the first place, and charity was why the bond for the new Laguna Honda had passed by a margin of three to one. At Laguna Honda, charity was in the air.

There was our volunteer organization of nearly one thousand members. It ran the little store where patients could buy candy and shaving cream, and staffed the clothing department, where patients could "shop" for clothes (donated, cleaned, and mended), such as the Armani suit Mr. Teal wore at his wedding. It put on dances that supported the Patient Gift Fund, and it sponsored the monthly outings that got every patient out of the hospital to a ball game, a restaurant, or the horse races.

But in addition to this organized charity, and at least as important, was personal charity, and the longer I was at Laguna Honda, the more of it I saw. There was the nurse who roasted an entire pig on his Sunday off for a homesick Tahitian patient with breast cancer. There was the doctor who took a music-loving patient to the opera. There were the birthday dinners for patients that staff paid for themselves; clothes brought in, cats adopted. All simple acts, not expensive, not cumbersome.

But why? I asked myself that Christmas morning. What was the motivation? And was the pleasure charity gave me good or bad?

The Greeks called that emotion *eleos,* I later discovered, and defined it as the "feeling of pain caused by the sight of some evil that befalls one who doesn't deserve it." The pleasure I felt was, in part, the relief of pain by giving. *Eleos* gave the Latin *eleemosyna,* the French *aumone,* and eventually even our English *alms.* The emotion of *eleos* was why Laguna Honda had been built as an almshouse in the first place and why it was still an almshouse despite its name, because *eleos*—alms, charity—was still one of its main motivating forces.

Charity assuages *eleos* and it is selfish, at least in part. And there is more selfishness in it than simply the relief of one's own pain; there is a complicated pleasure in it, which is what gave charity its bad name and what made it, as the third principle of Laguna Honda, a secret. Its motivation is always suspect—acts done not necessarily for the good of the receiver but of the giver. That was why at Laguna Honda charity was hidden; and although I saw a lot of it, I never heard it mentioned. It was passed along only in actions. But it was passed along. If I hadn't seen charity all around me, I don't think I, as Paul's doctor, would have gone out and bought him a vest. Yet at Laguna Honda, buying that vest seemed natural; everybody did that sort of thing.

Paul wore that vest for a good long while. And propped up in his electric wheelchair, cigarettes in the left pocket, matches in the right, he looked manly and imperturbable.

In the meantime, while Paul was healing and I was taking care of my patients on E6 and E4, the new hospital was in the planning stages. And then we saw the architects taking measurements around the grounds. Like the administrators, they wore real shoes and real clothes, but it was easy to tell them apart. The architects were small, neat men, and their shoes were brown loafers with no socks; their uniform, a charcoal gray jacket, black T-shirt, and pleated slacks; their look, a short haircut and silver rimless glasses. In fact, they were as different from all the denizens of Laguna Honda—doctors, nurses, patients, and administrators—as their virtual health care and rehabilitation facility would be from the hospital we knew so well.

It took about a year, but finally they were ready to present their designs to us, the doctors, in the medical library on the eighth floor. The library wasn't much, but it was ours—shelved journals around the walls, sofas, and a conference table, and the big open windows that were almost a signature of the place. The architects had been working for quite a while on their plans. What they would show us today was preliminary, and they'd like to hear our thoughts.

The head architect began. The patients, now called "residents," would be housed in three identical six-story buildings, he explained. Two would be built in the valley between the present buildings; the third would be on the site of the 1910 Clarendon Hall, which would be demolished. The patient buildings would be connected to one another by a three-story glass "link" building; it would contain the lobby, a new aviary, two swimming pools, the library, and the auditorium, as well as the X-ray department and the dialysis units. The four buildings would surround an open space that would have the new greenhouse and animal farm. Gardens, perhaps a maze, would be placed outside the buildings, and everything would be built to the highest ecological standards.

Then the lights went down, the PowerPoint came on, and we went on a virtual tour of the new Laguna Honda-to-be.

With the valley and the old Clarendon building gone, I can't say I recognized anything. The general effect was very green, with computer-simulated vegetation and new trees. The three patient buildings were square and windowed, and along with the glass "link" building, seemed to grow out of this green, like office buildings out of a new suburban development.

Then we went inside, starting with the lobby.

Inside it was light and airy. The lobby was high and wide; the aviary was glass, with bamboo around it and a ledge for sitting. There were simulated patients enjoying themselves—slim, smiling, and sitting in immaculate wheelchairs with their legs crossed, or leaning on their canes, peering out at green vistas. We saw the new dining area, which was nothing like the old dining room. It had curved booths, halogen lights, and a long shiny grill; and outside was a deck with wrought-iron tables and Cinzano umbrellas.

Then we went into one of the virtual patient buildings. There were lots of windows and glass doors that opened to a balcony where other elegant, simulated patients gazed out at the sky and down into the gardens six stories below. The space was beautiful and calm, with cream-and-coffee-colored walls, and I found it hard to imagine our Fourth of July goat or our Thanksgiving turkey making a visit, no matter what hat and sunglasses they wore, not to speak of Mrs. McCoy, yellow and swollen, really quite messy and actually diseased, at least when she first arrived.

The lights came on. Did we have any questions? Comments?

I spoke up. The drawings were beautiful, yes, thank you, but . . . Had they ever toured the existing hospital? Met with any of our patients? Discussed with them what they liked and didn't like about their current living conditions?

They had not, no, not yet.

Would they like a tour? Sometime? At their convenience?

Yes, of course. They would give me a call when they had a chance.

The architects did give me a call, and I did take them on the tour. I introduced them to patients and nurses, and showed them the open wards, the open hall for playing poker, the church, the breezeways, and the stairwells.

They were intrigued, if a little stunned. As we walked around, they seemed to retract into their charcoal jackets, and though they didn't touch anything, they made sure to wash up after we finished.

I didn't expect much from them. I knew they had a thousand regulations to follow, a hundred people to satisfy, but I did hope they would take to heart the idea of making the new hospital as pluripotential as the old, where patient rooms could become offices when needed or where, in a pinch, we could store wheelchairs in a solarium when sunning had gone out of fashion. Who knew what medicine would be like, I told them, what fads might come and go in the hundred years their buildings would stand. The principle of privacy giving way to company? Style to comfort? Aesthetics to sturdiness? Could they try to build a place that, like the old hospital, would go with the punches, change with the tides of thought?

They smiled and nodded, but did not seem convinced.

When they made their next presentation, at the first of our newly instituted Town Hall Meetings, I made sure to go.

The presentation was almost the same as the one they'd shown the medical staff months before. Once again I saw the gardens and grounds, the lobby and the grill, although this time their rendering of the patients' buildings was more detailed. On every floor there would be two "neighborhoods"—the new term for ward—of thirty patients each; in the center of each neighborhood would be an open nursing station, around which the fifteen double-bedded patient rooms would fan. Each patient room would have two flat-screen televisions and, perhaps, cameras, to allow distant family to see their dear ones without having to visit. Each neighborhood would have its own kitchen, where patients could cook, and its own common room, where patients could mingle. All the floors would be carpeted to help with the noise, and there would be a computer-adjusted air-flow system so that each kitchen, common room, and patient room would have its own closed environment.

A stir of unease went through the Town. We were used to something simpler, more open, and more neighborly than the architects' neighborhoods, if neighborly meant running next door for a cup of coffee, a missing form, or just to chat. Still it wasn't the computerized air flow, the carpets (a bad idea), or even the overall design of the buildings—stacked up, one identical floor on top of the next, with elevators the only access to fresh air—that made everyone worry. It was the wheelchairs.

Now everyone knew that the architects had spent a lot of time designing and that it was not easy for them to keep within their budget. Laguna Honda was, after all, a public hospital, at best nonprofit and usually antiprofit; our budget was fixed; and there were many regulations. A hospital had to have computerized air flow, we knew; the patients had to be in semiprivate rooms; there had to be so many bathrooms, elevators, sprinklers per patient; and the architects had to follow every rule. It was just that they forgot the wheelchairs.

"Are there any questions?" the head architect asked after he finished his presentation.

The audience was quiet. Then one of the nurses raised her hand. It was Christina.

"Where is the room for the wheelchairs?" she asked.

The architect looked blank. "Wheelchairs?"

"Yes. The wheelchairs for the patients. They have to be stored someplace. When they're not being used, or at night; and the electric wheelchairs have to be charged."

"Oh, well," he mumbled. "How many are there? One or two?"

"Well, how many beds are there?" Christina asked.

"Sixty on each floor."

"Well, then, sixty wheelchairs."

That's a lot of wheelchairs. They take up a lot of room. In the old hospital they were stored in various places, depending on the ward and its kind of patients. Sometimes in the unused kitchen; sometimes in the big room with the ice machine; most often in the solarium. Because when the old Laguna Honda was designed, wheelchairs were rare, but a belief in the value of sun and fresh air was common. A large solarium for taking the sun was put at the end of every ward and bed-bound patients were wheeled into it daily so they, too, could get sun and fresh air. Later, after the sun fell out of fashion, the solarium was used for whatever was needed—as a bingo room, an isolation room, a room for making private phone calls, but especially for storing wheelchairs.

I wish I could say that the architects thanked Christina for her observation and incorporated it into their plans. But they did not. I'm sure there was a reason; still, to this day there is no special room for the wheelchairs in the new health-care and rehabilitation facility, and little enough space in the new patient rooms, and we don't know what to do with them.

Meanwhile, the conflict between Dr. Stein and us was escalating. Although at the board of supervisors meeting he had agreed to revert to our former admissions policy, whereby the doctors would decide which patients we could safely take care of, Dr. Stein did not reinstate that policy. How could he? His budget was no better than it had been before the board meeting, and there were more demands on it every month. He still had no place to send the unreimbursed psychiatric patients who lived at the mental health rehabilitation facility or the homeless psychiatric patients at the County, and there were more and more days when the County Hospital was full and closed to new admissions. On those days, the private hospitals had to admit the County patients, and this was bad for their budgets. It was usually bad for the patients, too, because the private hospitals were far away from their homes and stoops, had no records of their care, and discharged them as soon as possible. It was good for Dr. Stein's budget because he didn't have to reimburse the private hospitals, but still, it wasn't a long-term solution.

And when he looked across town, what did he see? He saw Laguna Honda, with its 1,100 beds, its doctors and nurses, and its patients, most of whom, according to Targeted Case Management, could be discharged. Dr. Stein couldn't help but think that this was the best place to send those patients at the MHRF and the County. So instead of going back to the old admissions policy, he started his "Flow Project."

He called it the Flow Project because it was going to increase the flow of patients from the County to Laguna Honda by acting as a substitute for our admissions committee. He handpicked its members, and the idea was that it would pass along its preaccepted patients for Dr. Romero to rubber-stamp. To ensure its success, Dr. Stein replaced our executive administrator with a friend of his, Mr. James Conley. It was a big promotion for Mr. Conley, whose training had been in marine engineering.

Dr. Stein came over to the hospital to introduce Mr. Conley. Mr. Conley would preside over Laguna Honda's evolution from the out-moded "model of medical care" to a new, modern "model of social rehabilitation," he told us.

"What does that mean?" someone from the audience asked. "What is 'social rehabilitation'?"

It meant, Dr. Stein replied, that at the new facility, three hundred beds would be reserved for homeless psychiatric patients.

Now, most of the staff didn't care which patients we admitted as long as we had the resources to take care of them safely. But for some, the idea of the hospital becoming, even in part, a locked psychiatric facility was unacceptable. There were few enough places in the city for the elderly and disabled; and if three hundred beds were given to the homeless, what would happen to the citizens who'd supported Laguna Honda over the years when they needed its services?

It especially bothered Sister Miriam, our resident nun. She contacted the newspapers with her concerns, and she made an appointment to see Mr. Conley as soon as he'd settled in.

The meeting did not go well. Sister Miriam began her speech with nunlike modesty, but pretty soon her Irish got the best of her. She raised her voice, and then she lost her temper. We have a moral obligation to care for our elders, she told Mr. Conley. If he put younger able-bodied patients in with elderly disabled patients, neither would receive the care they deserved! It was wrong! It was unjust!

But Mr. Conley was Irish, too. He listened, and then he interrupted. To the contrary, he said, the hospital had to help the County out during difficult budget times—everyone had to do their best. Sister Miriam was a member of the staff; she had no right to involve the media in Laguna Honda's affairs. It would be better for her and for the hospital if she just piped down.

That was the wrong thing to say to Sister Miriam. She left his office and immediately contacted the community of well-connected professionals around the hospital. They were startled to learn about the new plans to turn the genial old almshouse into a psychiatric facility for the homeless. Then she met with the newspapers; with

Dr. Romero, Dr. Kay, and Miss Lester. Last she met with the mayor, who agreed with her that moving the psychiatrically disabled homeless to Laguna Honda was a bad idea. He ordered Dr. Stein to revert to the old admissions policy and to stop the Flow Project.

S o Dr. Stein changed his strategy.
     Its first prong was Mirene Larose.

The position of director of nursing having been involuntarily vacated by Ellen Mary Flanders, Dr. Stein appointed Mirene Larose, RN, MS, CNS, as our new director of nursing. She'd been a nurse at the Mental Health Rehabilitation Facility and was in favor of turning a large part of Laguna Honda into a similar social rehabilitation facility. In fact, she had a grant proposal all ready to hand that proposed using the BioPsychoSocialSpiritual model for the rehabilitation of the psychiatrically disabled, drug-abusing homeless. Dr. Stein was delighted to let her try out her model on two wards at Laguna Honda, with a view to expanding it to all thirty-eight of our wards.

The second prong was hiring a health-care consulting firm, Health Management Associates, to advise him on the appropriate use of Laguna Honda. It spent months at the hospital, the County, and the community clinics, and its report was brilliant.

The city provided remarkable health care to its citizens, it acknowledged; the main problem being that there was no continuum of care. The County Hospital was separate from Laguna Honda Hospital, and the community clinics separate from both. All three had distinct administrations, clinics, and staff, and Dr. Stein was preoccupied with their operations. So its first recommendation was that he should hire a Chief Operating Officer.

Second, Laguna Honda was too big. It was old-fashioned to have such a large institution. Instead of going ahead with the rebuild, Dr. Stein should downsize the new facility by one-third and use the savings to provide long-term care in the community. If the city did need more long-term-care beds, he should contract them out to private hospitals.

Last was the problem of the unreimbursed patients at the mental health rehabilitation facility, for which Health Management Associates had a solution. The reason that the city did not receive payment for those patients was that the mental health rehabilitation facility was licensed as an institution for mental disease, and Medicaid only paid for the first two weeks of hospitalization for patients in an institution for mental disease. Laguna Honda, on the other hand, was licensed as a long-term-care facility and did get paid for psychiatric patients with medical problems. Dr. Stein had been prevented from transferring patients to Laguna Honda from the MHRF, true. But if he simply merged the mental health rehabilitation facility under Laguna Honda's license, then its patients would, ipso facto, become Laguna Honda's patients. So Laguna Honda could bill for them, and Medicaid would pay for them. Then, once the new Laguna Honda was completed, Dr. Stein could put it under the County Hospital's license and the resulting "continuum of care" would not only allow for payment for its patients, but also put him in charge of admissions and the Laguna Honda medical staff.

It was brilliant, and Dr. Stein immediately began planning how to put it into effect.

A few weeks later, a new political committee appeared: Citizens for Laguna Honda. Its founders were Sister Miriam and Miss Lester, and its goal was to reserve the hospital for the elderly and disabled, not for psychiatric patients. The committee set to work to put an initiative on the ballot and slowly gained steam and money.

Then Dr. Stein had a setback. For the first time in its history, Laguna Honda failed its recertification as a hospital. It didn't just fail; it was humiliated, if an institution can be humiliated, by the 274-page report of the State Licensing Bureau.

Every year the state came to the hospital to recertify it. But until Miss Lester retired, it hadn't found much to dislike about the place except for our open wards. After she retired, it did begin to find many problems, however, all related to the budget cuts that Dr. Stein was making: the halving of the head nurses, the decrease in staff, the deferred maintenance of the buildings. But that year its report was scathing, although patience was required because, like all the investigative reports I've ever read, it lumped together the irrelevant with the shocking, the inevitable with the unacceptable, the nuisances with the catastrophes, and it started with the trivial.

Laguna Honda did not deliver mail on Saturdays, it began, in violation of Federal Regulation F170. The daily menus were not translated into Chinese, and this violated Federal Regulation F242. An open bottle of disinfectant had been found in a kitchen refrigerator (F252), and three pairs of slippers on the floor of ward D3 (F253). Next, there were problems with maintenance. Paint was peeling from the walls of ward E4 (F253); microwave ovens were not clean (F371); there were dusty vents in the bathrooms and mildew in the shower stalls. So for the first one hundred pages the report read like the report of a picky, shortsighted mother-in-law in white gloves, come to your big, rambling farmhouse to inspect. She would never want to leave.

You had to wait until page 100 for the real disasters to appear. The investigators had found alcohol and drug abuse at the hospital; unsafe sex between patients; even the selling of drugs. Patients had started fires; fought with each other; gang members had shown up and threatened and attacked patients. Many patients had decompensated, going back and forth between Laguna Honda and the County Hospital's psychiatric department. Patients had fallen, and their call lights had gone unanswered; bedsores had developed. Although the investigators acknowledged that the staff was doing its best, they were also clear that the hospital had accepted patients it could not manage, was not being well maintained, and had insufficient staff. Until administration resolved all these problems, it concluded, the hospital would be fined one thousand dollars per day, and would not be reimbursed for new patients.

It was a pretty devastating report. And it begs the question: Why? Why couldn't the hospital prevent falls and bedsores and keep the microwaves, gurneys, and windows clean?

There were reasons the hospital could not, but the usual culprit, the budget, was not really one of them, because the budget had never been cut. It had gone up each year, even as the number of patients decreased, and the staff-to-patient ratio was now higher than ever. The problem was that this additional staff was all administrative, hired to produce the assessments, policies, and procedures the Department of Justice and HCFA demanded. And, unlike Miss Lester, who toured each ward daily with set mouth and eagle eye, none of the administrative staff ever toured the wards. But without that scrutiny, all the plans, policies, and procedures didn't clean any gurneys, turn any patients, or pick up any slippers off the floor.

What about alcohol and drug abuse, unprotected sex, fights and fires; why were they so difficult to prevent?

There were reasons, but again, not the budget.

First was our almshouse architecture—our hidden hallways, stairwells, and linen closets. There were just too many places where patients could go to do whatever they wanted to do. Although the architecture wasn't the only reason. When the nuns ran the almshouses, there were incidents involving sex, drugs, and alcohol, but if you were caught, something happened. You were thrown out of the almshouse, or if you were too sick, you were punished in some way—confined to your ward, your cigarettes taken away. As for thefts, fights, and fires, the nuns of the Hôtel-Dieu simply called the gendarmes, who took the ex-almshouse patient to prison.

Our city's gendarmes used to do that, in the old days, but no longer. Our patients were too sick and would not have enough medical care in jail, the police almost always concluded. Patients, even those who committed a crime, were almost never arrested. Even Mr. Jax, who set the arson fire on D3, had been ordered back to Laguna Honda, and he would have been sent back, too, except that he disappeared.

Of course, the hospital did have a policy against drugs, sex, setting fires, and attacking other patients, which patients signed when they were admitted. But if they contravened the policy, there were few repercussions. They were too sick to be discharged. Instead, the nurse manager would formulate a "contract" for the patient to sign, such as: "I will not smoke with my oxygen on"; and a behavior plan, such as: "If I do smoke with my oxygen on, my cigarettes will be taken away for twenty-four hours." And even that kind of contract, according to the state's report, contravened regulations, and the hospital received a citation for that, too. Anyway, demented patients who smoked, drank, and set fires did not understand contracts or repercussions.

As for other ways of preventing patients from such activities—restraints, tranquilizers, and locked wards—they were no longer allowed either. The only thing that was allowed was a "sitter"—a staff member to sit with a patient all day. But sitters were expensive. They threw the budget off, and Mr. Conley had decreed that there would be no more sitters.

So the only way to prevent sex, drugs, and violence was not to admit the patient in the first place. Or if he was in your hospital, to discharge him as soon as you could. Which was why Dr. Stein and the County Hospital had their Flow Project, and why Sister Miriam and Miss Lester founded their citizens' group. Because in one way, at least, Laguna Honda was just like the almshouse of yore—it was the last resort. Once a patient was admitted, there was no place else to send him.

With all this going on—a new director of nursing, a new executive administrator, the BioPsychoSocialSpiritual program, a ballot measure brewing, and the new kind of patients from the County wreaking occasional havoc—the hospital was ever more chaotic. I was happy that I had my pilgrimage to go back to.

Rosalind and I began to organize the second section. We would walk for two hundred miles through the south of France, and we would begin in our footsteps of the year before. We flew to Paris, took the fast and slow trains to our starting point, and spent the night in the hotel we'd left the year before. Then we put on last year's clothes, fastened our shells to our packs, lifted up our walking sticks, and took the next step.

As soon as I heard the click of my stick on the cobblestones, I was right back in that space of pilgrimage, right back where I'd been a year before, as if only a night had passed. The swing of my legs, the slide of my stick through my hand, the click as it landed, had a cadence as rhythmic as a heartbeat.

The second section of the pilgrimage starts in the area of France known for its white limestone, the *causse*. The *causse* makes beautiful churches and castles, but hard stone paths that heat the pilgrim's feet and reflect white hot light into the pilgrim's face. It is also a depopulated part of France. Its villages are nearly empty, each one with a World War I monument that explains the emptiness: entire families of sons wiped out at the Battle of the Marne, the Battle of the Somme. Rosalind and I could walk for hours without seeing anyone, although the countryside was still cultivated somehow, with green farms and truffled oak forests.

The experience that most stayed with me that year was our longest and hardest day. It was twelve miles to our lunch stop and eight miles to our evening shelter, which was a monastery that still offered pilgrim hospitality. It was the middle of a heat wave and hard going, and we didn't get to our lunch stop until two PM. We lunched on the bread and cheese we'd carried, drank some water, and then hurried along. Because the rules of the monastery were strict: Supper was at seven PM. If you weren't there by seven PM, our guidebook warned, well, there was always breakfast.

We struggled through the heat, but around six o'clock we realized that we would never make it in time. We would have no supper. And as we stumbled along, although I can't say I felt sorry for myself, I did keep imagining a Styrofoam ice chest with cold beer that the nuns kept, perhaps, for late-arriving pilgrims. That wouldn't be so bad, I thought. With an ice-cold beer, the bread and orange I had left would be fine. Then, click, click . . . my imagination would present a different scenario—a sink of lukewarm water, a dormitory with rows of iron cots. I would be hungry. There would be no privacy. It would be a tough night.

Those eight miles took a long time. It was way past seven PM when we arrived. As we walked through the monastery's gates, flushed and thirsty, out of the main door came a tiny, very old nun in a dark blue habit and white wimple. She, too, was flushed and sweating. But she was smiling. Her eyes behind her glasses twinkled. She said in French, "You made it! We were so worried! Come in."

We followed her inside. With its stone floor, stone walls, and stone ceiling, the monastery was cool.

"Put your things here," she said, showing us the stone washroom. "Wash up . . . and hurry. We've delayed dinner for you."

We washed up while Sister Monique waited, and then she led us to the dining room. There were other pilgrims seated at a long table, which was set with carafes of red wine and cold water. We sat down, and then we were served one of our best meals ever. Soup, potato-and-caper salad, French lentils, cheese, and for dessert, fresh-cooked plums from the nuns' own trees. It turned into a party, and the pilgrims we met that night interwove themselves with us for the rest of the walk to Compostela.

After dinner Sister Monique showed us to our rooms. There was no dormitory. I had my own room, whitewashed and plastered, with a sleigh bed of walnut and a rope mattress. In the night, there was a thunderstorm; in the morning, there were the monastery bells; and out of my window I could see the nuns' medicinal herb garden down below. The longest and hardest day turned out to be the opposite of what I'd expected. And over and over again, for the rest of that second section, that's how things would turn out. That was the main lesson I took from the pilgrimage that year.

During that second section of walking I began to see that a

pilgrimage had a rhythm, a dailiness, just like at home. Every day I awoke, ate breakfast, started walking, and things happened. People showed up; I had adventures. Some I liked, some I didn't. Some I expected to like and did not like; others I expected not to like and did like. I began to see that the unexpected—the *inattendu,* the unwaited-for, as the French have it—was the only thing I could expect. One was presented with an experience, a person, whose value one did not know in advance. What seemed to be good might be bad; what seemed to be bad, good. One didn't know; one had to wait.

That waiting to see how it would turn out was what made pil-griming different from ordinary life, I began to see. And that year I learned I didn't have to leave it with my last footstep. If I wanted, I could take that kind of waiting home and have my daily life become a kind of pilgrimage.

With that open expecting, I discovered that a day at the hospital was even more interesting. One never knew. All one knew was that there would be a beginning and a middle and an end to the day, just like on a pilgrimage. And just like on a pilgrimage, characters would appear—patients, nurses, deliverymen, doctors—with spiritual and moral messages, if I chose to decipher them. Sometimes in words, sometimes in actions, sometimes in silence.

That year there was Paul, especially.

After Christmas, Paul reached a kind of equilibrium. His wounds had healed; his social worker was looking for a place; he was selling DVDs, smoking and reading outside, and making friends with many people.

Then he fell.

Now, to be independent there are surprisingly few things you need to be able to do, but transferring yourself from bed to chair and back again is one of them. It doesn't seem like much. It's not reading or thinking or fixing computers, but if you can't transfer, discharge is almost impossible. With his strong arms and the trapeze bar set over his bed, Paul could transfer himself: he would hoist his half body above the bed and swing himself into his chair. But it wasn't easy, because all he had to land on was the stub of his left thigh. And that day he missed the chair, and he fell.

He didn't hurt himself. He kept his wits, cushioned his fall and slid to the floor, but once on the floor, he couldn't get back into his bed or chair. He had to call the nurses. They got him up and put him in his chair, but they asked me to tell him not to transfer himself any-more without asking for help.

I didn't tell him. He was an independent man; he would figure something out for himself. And he did.

What he did was avoid going on any of the interviews that the social worker arranged for him at the skid-row hotels. After he fell, there was always something that prevented him. He was sick; he was busy; he was late and missed his ride. He never admitted that he couldn't manage outside anymore, and the social worker kept setting up interviews, and he kept missing them. She asked me to remind Paul to go, but I didn't do that either. Because I began to see what Paul saw, that he couldn't make it on the outside anymore, in those skid-row hotels, with only half a body. He'd lived in them, and they were tough, especially the first of the month, when the vulnerable and disabled got their cash. He would be an easy mark.

Still he and Donald continued to plan their DVD store: where it would be, what they would stock. He didn't tell the social worker to stop looking for places, and he continued to read, smoke, work on his computer, and transfer himself from bed to chair and chair to bed.

Then he got a cough. I ordered a chest X-ray and went upstairs to look at it. I didn't expect to see anything. But when I put that X-ray up, there was something. In his upper right lung, a crab-shaped spot, with legs spiraling out of a central body. It was, perhaps, an infection. But I didn't think so. Most likely it was cancer, and, given his smoking, it was probably lung cancer, one of the worst.

I looked at that X-ray for a long while.

I thought about telling Paul. I thought about all the procedures he would have and I would go through with him: the surgeries, radiation, chemotherapy, and the 3 percent survival rate of lung cancer.

I just didn't want to do it.

And this being Laguna Honda, I didn't have to.

Because on my way down from X-ray, I met Dr. Benicia, the doctor in charge of our schedules. She was looking for me. She wanted to ask me: Would I consider returning to the admitting ward? As I knew, Dr. Dan had already left it for greener or maybe just more peaceful pastures, and Dr. Romero had been making do, somehow, more or less alone. But now she was tired, exhausted from fighting about admissions with Dr. Stein, and she wanted to leave.

I raised my eyebrows. Dr. Stein, did he have anything to do with this?

Dr. Benicia shrugged. Maybe. It was better for him if Dr. Romero wasn't in the way of admissions, and he knew how much she liked the admitting ward. Anyway, she, Dr. Benicia, was hiring two fresh new young doctors from the university for it, but she also wanted to have a senior physician there who knew what the place was like. Would I come back?

I would.

So Dr. Romero and I exchanged places. I returned to the admitting ward, and she took over E6 and E4 and Paul, whom she knew well.

Ten days later Paul died.

t was a Paul kind of death.

Quiet, efficient, and when you come to think of it, very intelligent. He didn't get sick, cry out, or cause any problems at all. It was an ordinary day, and he did his usual things: ate lunch; went out for a smoke; fell asleep in his wheelchair, head back, dozing. When the nurse tried to wake him for his afternoon medications, he was dead.

I heard the Code Blue to E4, and as I ran over, I went down my list of patients, wondering who it was. The last patient I expected to see, surrounded by anxious staff, was the legless mound of Paul, straddled by one doctor pushing on his chest, and surrounded by nurses trying to find a vein. They couldn't find a vein, but it didn't matter. He was dead, and we stopped the Code Blue very soon. Everyone else left, and I picked up his chart. Had there been mistakes? Had I missed something? No, there was nothing. Paul had simply died, probably from a heart attack due to his untreatable clotting disorder.

A week later Christina called to tell me that Paul's memorial service would be that morning in the chapel. It was just for E4, because his family was making its own funeral arrangements. I kept track of the time, and at eleven o'clock I walked over to the chapel, sat down in a pew, and watched as the patients, staff, and nurses of E4 arrived. The patients rolled in and sat next to the pews in their wheelchairs. Christina, Allen, Lacy, and the other nurses and therapists from E4 hurried in and stood. No one said anything while we waited for the minister to appear. He didn't appear, though, and after a while Christina looked at me. Would I say something?

I did say something, but I don't remember what it was. It was short, and it was not eloquent.

After I finished, the minister was still not there, and we all looked at one another—patients, nurses, therapists, and I.

Then Lacy broke the silence. "Mr. Zed wrote a poem for Paul, didn't you, David? Why don't you read it to us?"

"Okay," David said, fumbling a bit and unfolding a crumpled piece of paper.

Remember how I told you that Laguna Honda had one of just about every kind of patient? Well, Mr. Zed was our manic Jewish New York intellectual. I should really title him Dr. Zed, because before his mania got the best of him, he'd completed a PhD in linguistics.

David was a big man, tall and wide, with the thick, weepy legs that had been his ticket to the hospital. He had a square face, brown curly hair turning gray, and narrow brown eyes. His voice was husky, with a light Brooklyn accent. He cleared his throat and read his poem:

> *Farewell, Captain Bennett, now Paul, Human Star-Man.*
> *The stars are yours; you may enter any Stargate.*
> *You shall explore 7,000 galaxies, which is only your beginning.*
> *All the magic of Jupiter, Andromeda, and the Clingon Empire are*
> *   yours to explore.*
> *And, Captain Paul, you shall return happily as both a Monolith*
> *   and a Child-of-the-Stars!*

After he finished, it was still. No one stirred. His vision of Captain Paul—Human Star-Man, with legs back and even with wings, exploring galaxies and planets and the Klingon Empire—was irresistible.

The minister never did show up, and after a while, we all left the chapel—patients, nurses, doctors—on our crutches, in our wheelchairs, or, if we were lucky, on both our sound, strong legs.

A few days later Christina found me in my office. With tears in her eyes, she handed me a color-Xeroxed piece of paper folded in two. It was Paul's funeral notice.

A photo of Paul was on the front, with the dates of his birth and death underneath. He must have been very young when it was taken; baby-faced and handsome, he stared out of it with clear brown eyes and long black lashes. What I didn't expect was that he was dressed in full-dress Marine uniform—white cap with black brim set on his forehead, dark blue jacket with red piping and gold buttons. He'd never told me or anyone that he'd been a Marine, and how Mr. Zed had pictured him as Captain Paul was a manic mystery.

As I looked into his eyes, so clear, so unwavering under the white cap, I understood finally what I'd felt from him. He'd always approached me with that same clear gaze. At first, irritably and angrily; later, openly and expectantly; toward the end, quietly. I can't say I knew what made him tick, who he was or what he thought about; and yet I knew that clear Self behind his eyes, that proud, uncompromising Paul Self, different from all others. Even as a young man it was there. In the eyes of that proud Marine, I could see my Paul.

What he'd taught me, I understood at that moment, was integrity—from *integer,* wholeness—from *integro*—untouched, unhurt. It wasn't that I'd lacked integrity before I knew him, but I'd accepted the teaching that a good doctor does not get too close to his patient. He or she does not jump into the mix, but keeps some distance, watches for the "countertransference," does not get drawn in.

There is much truth in that wisdom passed down by generations of doctors. The Hippocratic physician does not fall in love with his patients, or in hate either. He keeps their secrets no matter how heinous; he does not have dinner with his patients or buy them presents. He remains "other" to their lives, their families, their neuroses.

It is a good ground rule. For a patient to be able to turn to someone kind but distant, caring but calm, wise but not attached, is important, is necessary. But it requires that the doctor maintain a certain distance, and this means not quite being yourself.

Paul didn't operate that way, and with him, after a while, I didn't either. His integrity evoked mine, and it was not something I wanted to give up any longer. I didn't want to reestablish distance; I didn't want to be a Hippocratic physician; with my patients, I wanted to be myself.

Whether that was possible for a doctor, I didn't yet know.

I would soon find out.

Ten

IT'S A WONDERFUL COUNTRY

T WAS A THRILL to walk through the doors of the admitting ward once again. I hadn't been inside it for years. After Dr. Romero went back to it from her medical directorship, she shut its doors, and what had once been a place everyone went to for a second opinion, or maybe just for a late-afternoon chat, became off-limits.

Dr. Romero herself became kind of off-limits. She had closed the doors, and no one knew what was up with her. All we did know was that no one worked as hard as she did; no one gave of herself as much. I fixed glasses and bought Cokes for patients; Dr. Curtis bought shoes; all of us brought in food from home. But Dr. Romero did more. When necessary, she became medical director and dealt with the seamy side of the hospital, which was not its patients but its politics. When a doctor was needed to spend the night, she volunteered. She fought against the changes she thought were bad for the hospital, and mostly she was right. She was relentless in her ideals.

After she became a devotee of Dr. Kay's project of Edenizing the hospital—of making it more like the garden of Eden, with plants, animals, nature, and quiet—she did as much as she could to Edenize the admitting ward. She obtained headphones for the televisions of the patients so that the ward would be quiet; she lined the corridor with green plants; and she put caged birds in the television room and the doctors' office. But until I was walking down the corridor once again and got to our office, that was all I knew.

The door of the doctors' office was locked. I didn't even know it had a lock. But I found the key and opened it.

It hadn't changed much. The yellowed shade, half drawn over the window, was still there; so was the computer and the counter desk. Mrs. McCoy's plant was still there, grown all across the wall, and was now over by the bookcase, which appeared to be a still life of Dr. Romero's years there. The bookcase was filled to overflowing with books, conference folders, patient charts, expired medications, suture removal kits, and boxes of gloves. The only thing that had changed in the office was a huge old oak desk that had replaced our rickety ones, and the oak cabinet next to it, which was covered with bird droppings.

I didn't think we would need a file cabinet, and I telephoned Facility Management to have it removed. Then I fetched some garbage bags, cleaned out the bookcase, and brought everything down to Dr. Romero's new office. Last, I called in Rose, our long-suffering, gentle Chinese janitor.

Rose looked around the office. Her face lit up. "Ah, Dr. S.! Bird gone! I clean floor now! And window! And walls!" She shook her head. "Bird not belong in hospital!"

Then I left Rose to do her job and went out to see how the admitting ward had fared in my absence.

It, too, hadn't changed much.

The nursing station was just as crowded as ever, with the patient charts in their rack by the door. Larissa was still there, with her Russian accent, her irony, and her competence; her thin gold necklace, good haircut, and Italian slacks. The head nurse and most of the nurses were the same, and while they were sad that Dr. Romero and Dr. Dan had gone, they were happy to have me back.

The patients hadn't changed either, in style if not in substance. I walked down the ward to take a look. I introduced myself, sat on their beds, shook their hands, and said hello. Although I didn't know anyone in particular, I knew them all in general; they were nice; they were funny, interesting, and quirky. Then Larissa handed me a set of stamped-up index cards and a cup of fresh coffee, and I went back to our little doctors' office, which was once again looking the way a little doctors' office should look.

Although the doctors' office was the same, the nurses were the same, and the patients were the same, there was something different about the admitting ward.

What was different were the doctors I worked with, the medical students I taught, and everything outside Laguna Honda. During the years I'd been studying Hildegard, I'd been protected from those changes, but medicine was different—the practice of medicine had become the delivery of health care.

I had changed, too, but in a diametrically opposed way. Back on the admitting ward, meeting my old self, I discovered I did things differently; I saw things differently.

I took back to the admitting ward the lessons I'd learned from Mr. Bramwell and Mr. Bramwell's sister-in-law, from Mr. and Mrs. Teal, from Paul, and from so many others, and, somehow, medicine no longer seemed so complicated. There were not so many different things that could happen to a body after all. There were many ways that things could happen, but there were only a handful of organs and a handful of mechanisms of disease, and the 2,630 pages of *Harrison's Principles of Internal Medicine* no longer seemed so daunting. So many of them were extra, I knew now, not important, and the complicated edifice of medicine seemed to collapse upon itself. I began to enjoy my patients and know that I enjoyed them and that they enjoyed me. Because I didn't have to do very much, I knew now. With just a little bit on my part, my patients would get better.

I used to wonder about the old doctors. They would do—hardly anything at all. They would come in, say hello to the patient, ask him his name, and then lean forward for his reply, all the while watching the patient's face and body. They would give him their hand for a handshake and then hold the patient's hand in theirs. They would ask just a few questions. Then they would tell us what the diagnosis was. It was maddening. And now what I was doing was more like that, and it was no longer burdensome or stressful.

Mr. Steven Harp, for instance.

Steve was not my patient.

He belonged to Dr. Rajif, one of the two new doctors on the admitting ward, who had, along with me, replaced Dr. Dan and Dr. Romero. Dr. Rajif was the doctor who admitted Steve and did his workup, and he had concluded that things were as the County Hospital said they were: Mr. Harp was a Bad Boy with bad luck. At the age of thirty-four years, while using cocaine, he'd had a stroke; and now at thirty-eight years, while using cocaine, he'd had another. He could no longer walk; his speech was muffled; and he had so much trouble swallowing that he couldn't manage his own saliva. Also, he had heart failure. There wasn't much to do for him, but Dr. Rajif ordered physical, occupational, and, especially, speech therapy, because Mr. Harp was so difficult to understand that he had to write down whatever he wanted to say.

Now, in the past, Mr. Harp, not being my patient, would never have come onto my radar screen. In the old days on the admitting ward, with Dr. Jeffers, Dr. Romero, and Dr. Fintner, I stayed out of other doctors' patients unless invited in. Too many doctors spoiled the patient's broth, I knew; every doctor had a style, with medicines and ways that worked for him or her. Some doctors were aggressive, doing everything for everybody all the time, and their patients improved. Other doctors did as little as possible, and their patients improved, too. Some doctors used one medicine for a certain disease, while another found that very same medicine ineffective and swore by a different one. Which made the evidence-based, data-driven people crazy and demonstrated that medicine was not only a science but an art. What did not work, I'd learned, was to step into one doctor's studio or kitchen and add a dab of blue and some cumin for good measure.

That was in the old days.

But in the new days we had new doctors who didn't seem to mind my keeping an eye on things. So when I walked past Steve's bed, I paid attention to him, although he was not my patient. And when he flagged me down, I stopped.

He looked much younger than his thirty-eight years. He had a dark brown, round, smooth face, unlined and unwrinkled, with round, button-black eyes, and short, thick black hair. His shoulders were heavy and muscular, and so were both his arms and legs. But he was drooling and impossible to understand, his voice being so low and his words running together softly, insistently. Somehow he didn't seem quite like the stroke victim that I'd heard about from Dr. Rajif, and I was curious. So when I got back to our office, I opened his chart and began reading about him.

Steve had been admitted to the County Hospital four years before because of a sudden neurologic change. He was weak on his left side; he drooled; he had trouble talking; and he'd taken cocaine. A stroke, it was thought, most likely. But his brain scans had been ambiguous, and so many other studies were done—looking for AIDS, for a brain infection, for an autoimmune disease, a clotting disorder. Nothing panned out. His doctors therefore concluded that he must have had a stroke and they discharged him to a skid-row hotel with all necessary services. Then he'd been stable until five weeks ago, when his social worker noticed he'd taken to his wheelchair and was spending all day in the lobby, watching television and drooling, and when he tried to eat, he choked. So she contacted the County and arranged for him to be admitted for another workup. Once again it wasn't clear what was wrong, but most likely another stroke. Certainly he had deteriorated, presumably from taking cocaine, and in any case, he could no longer manage for himself. So he was sent to us.

At the end of his first week there was a meeting with Steve's team of nurses, therapists, social worker, and family. Since Dr. Rajif was on vacation, I attended in his stead. The meeting intrigued me further.

First, there was Steve's sister, Bonnie. She told us that Steve was the thirteenth of eighteen children by eleven different fathers and that both his mother and his father had been alcoholics. Nevertheless, he finished high school and attended college. He married, had a daughter, divorced, and became a commercial truck driver. Steve loved driving trucks, she said. In fact, he stopped driving trucks only this past year, when he took to his wheelchair and became impossible to understand.

"He was driving trucks up until a year ago?" I asked.

"He sure was."

That seemed impossible.

What did she think was going on, then? If he had a stroke years before and was still driving trucks until a year ago, what had changed?

"He's just lazy," she said.

I looked at Steve, who was listening attentively.

He nodded and got out "Yeah, I'm just lazy."

Then the nurses discussed his nursing needs; the social worker described the unfortunate state of his room in the skid-row hotel; and last the speech therapist reported. Steve's problems with speaking and swallowing were much greater than warranted by his stroke, she told us. Even she couldn't understand him and had to have him write down his answers to her questions.

"Look." She passed around his answers.

Steve wrote a nice hand, I saw, when his answers got to me. His letters were small, carefully formed, and neatly printed; and he wrote in full sentences, with a sophisticated vocabulary. To the therapist's question about why he left a previous rehabilitation facility, he'd written: "I was asked to leave because I was a single parent and they could not accommodate me." And, my favorite: "I used to love writing."

Neatly printed, sophisticated sentences did not go along with what seemed like a dementia from multiple strokes any more than Steve's symmetrical, well-muscled body or his ability to drive trucks—even badly—as recently as a year ago.

So after the meeting I sat down with all his records and began looking for a unifying diagnosis.

It popped out pretty quickly. Someone at some time had ordered a CPK on Steve—a blood test that measures the amount of creatine phosphokinase (CPK) in the blood. It is an enzyme mainly found in the muscles of arms, legs, and heart; and the test for it is usually ordered when a heart attack is suspected, because a heart attack damages the muscles of the heart and causes them to leach CPK into the blood. Steve's CPK had indeed been high—one hundred times normal—which was too high to mean he'd had a heart attack, because a heart attack that big would have killed him. A CPK that high could have come only from injured skeletal muscles.

This is not rare. If a patient receives an intramuscular injection just before the CPK is drawn, then the result can be very high. Or if he is taking statins to lower his cholesterol, it can be high. Steve must have had an intramuscular injection before his CPK was ordered, I thought, or he'd been taking statins. But when I looked through his records, there was no evidence of either an injection or a statin.

Which left the rare diagnosis of muscular dystrophy.

Muscular dystrophy is a genetic disease: a faulty enzyme causes the muscles to deteriorate. It runs in families. The girls are carriers; the boys are affected as children and usually die in their teens. Since Steve was in his thirties and since his sister hadn't mentioned any family history, muscular dystrophy would be a very surprising diagnosis. On the other hand, muscular dystrophy does cause exactly what Steve had. It would explain his big shoulders and thighs, which were, however, weak; his drooling, choking, and low voice. It would explain his clinical course—his gradual deterioration and his heart failure. And there was a rare form that did affect adults—only three people out of 100,000—but then, this was Laguna Honda.

I ordered another CPK. It, too, was one hundred times normal, and since Steve wasn't taking statins and hadn't received an intramuscular injection, this meant he did have the diagnosis of muscular dystrophy.

It was satisfying to have made the correct diagnosis, but it wasn't a good diagnosis to have made. It was not a better diagnosis for Steve than stroke. With a stroke, even with two strokes, if he stopped using cocaine and dedicated himself to his rehabilitation, he would stabilize and improve. But muscular dystrophy was progressive. Steve might improve a bit with the care he would get at the hospital, but over the long run he would only get worse. The diagnosis did prove that he wasn't lazy, and it did mean that our focus could change from stroke rehabilitation to dealing with an ongoing muscular process. Also, since muscular dystrophy was a sex-linked disease, passed along from mother to sons, it was also something the family should know about.

I thought for quite a while how I would explain this unusual genetic diagnosis to Steve and his family. With his permission, I started by telephoning Bonnie.

"I think we've discovered what's wrong with Steve," I began.

"I thought we knew. I thought he had a stroke."

"Well, he might have had a stroke, too. But a stroke doesn't explain what's been going on this past year. Steve has a rare muscular problem." I took a breath. "It runs in families and . . ."

"You mean—like muscular dystrophy?"

"Uh . . . huh . . . yeah . . . How do you know about muscular dystrophy?"

"Well, one of our brothers has muscular dystrophy, and he died of it. And one of our cousins has it, and an aunt, or maybe it's an uncle."

I had been rather proud of my diagnosis, and when I heard Bonnie's "You mean—like muscular dystrophy?" I was nonplussed. The diagnosis had been there, right out in the open, all along.

"Well, then, yes. Exactly like muscular dystrophy. So it hasn't been a stroke that caused Steve to deteriorate this past year but muscular dystrophy. Along with his lifestyle, of course—the cocaine, the not eating well, the not taking care of himself. As you know."

"Maybe you can talk to him about that, doctor. I've tried, but no way he's gonna listen to me."

"The main thing is: The family should understand—this does run in families, mainly in the boys."

"Uh-huh. You gonna tell him?"

"Of course."

I did tell him, but Steve didn't seem to care. He didn't mention his brother, cousin, or uncle; all he talked about was that he wanted to keep trucking and would I fill out the form he needed to get his driver's license back?

I temporized on the license and called Dr. Hanes, our rehabilitation doctor, to persuade him to take Steve for a course of rehabilitation. He could learn some strategies for dealing with his weakness, I said; he could learn about his disease and how to take care of it, and perhaps some of the deterioration due to his lifestyle could be reversed.

Dr. Hanes was a good-looking doctor, with wide-open, though small, blue eyes, blond hair with a cowlick, and a square face. He wore buttoned-down, pressed white shirts, colorful ties, and a starched white coat he made sure not to put through our laundry. He'd graduated from the University of Virginia School of Medicine and had the noncommittal smile of a Southern gentleman. Dr. Hanes did not approve of our city's attitude toward Bad Boys. And when he went to see Steve, and Steve asked him to sign his trucker's license, Dr. Hanes's mouth went up at one corner and down at the other; he raised his eyebrows and rolled his eyes. He didn't even say no.

Dr. Hanes was skeptical of the diagnosis of muscular dystrophy, and he was skeptical of Steve's improving. Still, he did accept him on the rehabilitation ward.

Dr. Hanes turned out to be half wrong and half right. A muscle biopsy confirmed the diagnosis of muscular dystrophy, but, as Dr. Hanes predicted, Steve didn't improve much. After a few weeks of therapy, he was able to walk again, but that was about it. Then he stopped going to his therapies, and became annoying, disruptive, and manipulative, as Dr. Hanes documented in his notes. Steve perseverated on his trucker's license. He swore at the staff. He ran his electric wheelchair full speed into crowds. He smoked marijuana; and no matter how many contracts he signed, he broke every one.

I don't know what the final straw was: when Steve began antagonizing the bedbound patients on rehabilitation by turning off their televisions; when he urinated in Dr. Hanes's plants; or when he pushed into Dr. Hanes's face the four-page truck driver's form he'd somehow acquired. At any rate, after five weeks Dr. Hanes had had enough. Steve could walk; he could take care of himself; he no longer needed our care. So Dr. Hanes called a van. Then, as the state's regulations required, he informed Steve, Steve's family, and his outside physician of his imminent discharge, and Steve was reintegrated back into his community. To wit: A van dropped him off at the lobby of his skid-row hotel.

I could see Dr. Hanes's point. Steve was a Bad Boy with bad luck, and he wasn't even charming. And yet I kind of liked him. True, he didn't do what was good for him, and he did do what was bad for him; he wasn't stupid, but he ignored his diagnosis, and he did go on about that driver's license. Still, I couldn't help but respect him, just a little.

He was determined not only to live until he died, but to live as himself until he died.

Besides, he'd taught me something unique. The sound of his sister's voice, "You mean—like muscular dystrophy?" echoed in my ears for years, and even to this day, as a reminder of how much we don't know about our patients or, for that matter, about one another. There's so much experience in a single life, in a single day. Even with all the questions in the history, there was so much I would never know about my patients.

I learned something else from Steve: I was becoming like one of the old doctors. I hadn't done his workup or examined him; I had done nothing but listen to him and look into his eyes. The fact was that he didn't fit the pattern of all the stroke patients I'd ever had, which was why I'd gone through his records. In medical school they'd taught us: "If it looks like a duck and walks like a duck and quacks like a duck, it's a duck." What I learned from Steve was that the inverse was better and truer: "If it doesn't look like a duck and doesn't walk like a duck and doesn't quack like a duck, it's not a duck." If it doesn't look like a stroke, it's not a stroke.

In thinking about Steve, I realized that there was something special about how those old doctors looked at the patient. They were quiet. And now for me also; since medicine was no longer complicated, burdensome, or stressful, when I saw a patient, I, too, was quiet. I had lots of time. There was no emergency.

It was in this way that the admitting ward had changed for me. It was just as hectic, chaotic, and noisy as ever; its patients were as sick or sicker, but somehow—perhaps it was the pilgrimage—I'd learned to key into the calm, order, and quiet that lay underneath its hecticness, chaos, and noise. That quiet was the opposite of interruption. It was the quiet of walking, the quiet that underlies all activity. It's where

everything is connected. Once you key into it, there are no emergencies, and you have all the time you need.

O
utside the admitting ward, it was not quiet. There were a lot of
politics.

First, there was Proposition D.

The Committee to Save Laguna Honda had come up with a strategy to prevent Dr. Stein from turning the hospital into a psychiatric
facility—Proposition D, a ballot measure sponsored by a second,
related group, San Franciscans for Laguna Honda. Proposition D
would rezone the hospital as a "special use zone," its special use being
that it would care only for the chronically ill and never for the psychiatrically disabled, drug-abusing homeless. It was a clever strategy, but
it had two problems. In order to fund the campaign, the committee
took money from the Builders' Association and had agreed that the
proposition would also allow the building of for-profit residential
care facilities on city lands. Second, if the proposition passed, the
zoning administrator, not the doctors or the hospital, would henceforth have the last say on admissions.

The mayor and Dr. Stein took advantage of these flaws. In their
arguments they said that Proposition D was "probably the most
poorly drafted proposition" in the city's history. It would put the
zoning administrator in charge of admissions, allow residential care
facilities everywhere in the city, and require Laguna Honda to discharge hundreds of its Alzheimer's patients.

The committee tried to defend the measure, but they ended up
simply attacking the mayor and Dr. Stein. The mayor was "deceptive"
and "despicable," they wrote. Dr. Stein was driven not by the needs of
patients but only by his budget. Sister Miriam lost her temper once

again and declared that voting against Proposition D would be actually "immoral." Even I was not convinced by these ad hominem attacks, and Proposition D went down to defeat three to one.

To their credit, Dr. Stein and the mayor did not immediately retaliate against Sister Miriam, Dr. Kay, Dr. Romero, or other supporters of Proposition D for the attacks against themselves. Nor was it a full rout on the patient-admission front. Perhaps Dr. Stein was chastened. But whatever the reason, we were no longer getting the psychotic, drug-abusing criminals that Dr. Romero had tried so hard to stop from being admitted. Most likely, Dr. Stein had a longer-term retributory plan in mind. I think, as a matter of fact, he did. Certainly the next years would prove difficult for Sister Miriam, Dr. Kay, and Dr. Romero.

The next thing that happened was the *Chambers* class-action lawsuit against the city. It alleged that by keeping patients at Laguna Honda, the city violated the civil rights of the disabled.

If this sounds familiar, it was. *Chambers v. City and County of San Francisco* was a continuation of *Davis*. *Davis* had won its demand that the city review every Laguna Honda patient for discharge and inform them of community alternatives. *Chambers* went three steps further. It demanded that the city provide those community alternatives to any patient who wanted to be discharged; that the city cut the new Laguna Honda by one-third; and that the hospital change its mission from long-term care to short-term rehabilitative care.

To find the six patient-plaintiffs for *Chambers*, the lawyers strolled around the hospital for months, putting up flyers and encouraging patients to join their suit. Most of the patients didn't want to leave the hospital, the lawyers discovered, but eventually they found six who did. Two were not, perhaps, the best choices for a case alleging the hospital's failure to discharge patients because they had already been discharged from Laguna Honda twice. The family of the third patient opposed his discharge and fought his inclusion as a plaintiff. But the other three plaintiffs were good examples of patients who could have been discharged if we had money enough for housing and the panoply of services each one needed.

Because *Chambers* was right: Disabled patients are best cared for at home. And if money were no object, every patient at Laguna Honda could have been discharged. But money was an object. The lawyers for *Chambers* argued that caring for our patients at home would be less expensive than in the hospital, but their calculations worked out only because they estimated the cost of the patients' medical care at zero. Yet it was precisely their medical problems that brought patients to Laguna Honda in the first place, and it was their medical problems that made them so complicated, so expensive, and so difficult to discharge. And although Laguna Honda was expensive, it was still cost-effective, because with our daily doctor visits, careful nursing, and open wards, it was rare for a patient to get so sick that he needed to be admitted to the County.

The lawyers for *Chambers* also argued that Laguna Honda was big, old, and old-fashioned. Which was true. But with its faults, it had its virtues. In fact, its faults were its virtues. Its very bigness, oldness, and old-fashionedness provided play in the city's health-care system. At Laguna Honda we knew we could always find a place for someone with no other place to go.

So we all worried about *Chambers,* although the mayor and Dr. Stein seemed sanguine about its demands and settled the suit without a fight. The board of supervisors agreed to provide whatever money was needed so that any patient who wanted to leave the hospital could leave. It also provided funds for still another new program, the "Diversion and Community Integration Program," to monitor admissions and discharges. And last, it cut the new Laguna Honda by one-third.

No one knew how much this *Chambers* settlement would end up costing. Rumor had it that discharging the lead plaintiff alone came to $78,000 per year, not including his medical care or housing. But Dr. Stein seemed happy about it. And in his next budget, he cut the position of Dr. Kay's hospice chaplain, which Sister Miriam had instituted so long ago and was still so very proud of.

During all of this—my return to the admitting ward, Proposition D, *Chambers*—Rosalind and I continued our pilgrimage to Santiago de Compostela.

The third section of the pilgrimage goes over the Pyrenees and halfway across Spain. That walk was even more varied than the first two, and there were many more pilgrims. What I took back to the hospital that third year was the day we got ahead of "our group."

Not that we had a formal group. Rosalind and I traveled as the two of us; nevertheless, groups formed, just as they had for Chaucer at the inn of *The Canterbury Tales*. Because, starting out from the same place every day, most people walk about the same distance—a kilometer every fifteen minutes, or about two miles an hour. Some walk quickly, arrive at their destination early, and take a siesta or drink a beer. Others take their time, though they still arrive at the same destination by the end of the day. So groups naturally form: the two Americans, the French singers, the flirtatious divorcée, the talkative Spaniards, the friendly Dane, the two serious Germans.

But that particular day we somehow got ahead of "our" group—a whole day ahead, though we didn't know it. That evening we went out for dinner, sat down at a table, and ordered. As we waited for our meal, I noticed that right next to us, at the next table, were two other American women—pilgrims just about our age. They even looked kind of like us. Then I sat back in my chair and looked around. Sure enough. Over there were the two somber German pilgrims, engaged in their serious discussion, except they were not our serious German pilgrims. There was the French singing group—true, they were Belgian and they didn't sing but played recorders, but still. Way in the back was a dour Norwegian, taking the place of our friendly Dane. And the little group of Spaniards, talking loudly, just not our Spaniards.

It was uncanny. It was a whole group of pilgrims traveling together, just like our group of pilgrims, but not our group of pilgrims. All the time I'd thought we were unique, walking on the pilgrim path; I thought it was our pilgrim path, walked by us for the first time, opening its adventures, stumbles, and stones for the first time—to us. But no. Ahead of us, all the time, was a near-identical group, and, doubtless, behind us, too. For lo and behold, there "they"—that is, "we"—were, in the restaurant that night, a version of ourselves and our group. Unaware that just one day's walk behind them were their adequate replacements. And, two days ahead of them, and two days behind them, too.

That is what I brought back to the hospital that year.

I'd already begun to realize something like that. On the admitting ward, I'd noticed there was a way in which my patients were almost, if not quite, interchangeable. I always had a kind of "group," it seemed: two Bad Boys, one Bad Girl, one querulous old woman, one stroked-out Chinese, one aging hobo, one new and miscellaneous. But after that third year of the pilgrimage, I began to see that it was also true about the nurses and the doctors and everyone else at the hospital. My group, individual as each of its members was—Dr. Jeffers, Dr. Fintner, Dr. Romero, Dr. Kay, Larissa, Christina, Mr. Conley, even Dr. S.—was not unique. After us, as before us, would assemble some other group, with our approximate equivalents. It might be in a different building, in a new Laguna Honda, even in a different century, but such a group would arise; the nature of the hospital required it.

My patients and I and the doctors and nurses and administrators were just as accidental a group as a group of pilgrims on their way.

I found that to be a very relaxing thought. It meant I was off the hook. If I weren't the perfect Dr. S. this time—well, eventually someone would come along who would be.

It also meant that the parts we were playing were, in some sense, parts; as if this time, I'll be doctor and you'll be patient; next time, we'll switch. And so, after that third section of the pilgrimage, I began to look much more closely into the faces and eyes of my patients and the janitors and the nurses and the bus drivers. Which parts were they playing? I wondered. And I found they were looking back at me in the same searching, intimate way.

I n the meantime, Mr. Conley, our new executive administrator, was trying to figure out how he could implement *Chambers*, especially its requirement that the new Laguna Honda be one-third smaller.

How was he going to do that? The obvious thing would be to stop admissions and just let the census dwindle down to 780, which would take more than a year. But there was a long waiting list of patients, and he would be pressured to admit them. It would play hell with his budget, too, which was based on revenues for 1,030 patients, not for

780. Plus, he would have to lay off staff and that would be tricky, because it wasn't like whole wards would be emptied; each ward would just dwindle.

So Mr. Conley decided to do nothing. He would wait until the new facility opened. Then he would transfer the sickest 780 patients over, and leave the other 250 patients at the old facility, from which they would gradually be discharged. Of course, that would mean keeping two hospitals, two kitchens, and two policy-and-procedure manuals going at the same time, and he couldn't imagine how it would all work out, but he couldn't come up with any other possibility.

Now, Mr. Conley was a bluff, hearty fellow, with an energetic, gravelly voice, red hair, and a red beard. He reminded me of the youngish Henry VIII around the time he fell in love with Anne Boleyn, and he was, as they said in the Middle Ages, Dr. Stein's Man. His orders were to change Laguna Honda from an old-fashioned almshouse to a modern health-care and rehabilitation facility, and he had been warned by Dr. Stein about the obstructions he would face—the balky doctors, the obstreperous nun, the ex-director of nursing. Mr. Conley was prepared. But Mr. Conley, with the best will in the world, eventually made a fatal mistake—he stepped out of the administration wing and met the patients of Laguna Honda.

I don't know how it happened, but I suppose it had to do with the crashing of our computers—every computer in the hospital, and everything about them—e-mail, printing, all the laboratory data, all the MDS forms. The computers went down and stayed down for months. It was fortunate that the hospital was as big and sloppy as it was, because not everything was on those computers. Most of us still had our books; the telephones were still plugged into the walls; we still had our wooden mailboxes, overhead paging, and clocks.

There was no e-mail, however, and so instead of sitting in his

re-redecorated administration wing and shooting out electronic mis-
sives, Mr. Conley had to scribble his messages on pieces of paper
and, when they were important and confidential, deliver them himself. Huffing and puffing the whole long length of the hospital, himself praying that the elevator would start and not stop midway, himself
passing the tattooed smokers in Harmony Park—like the rest of us,
Mr. Conley fell under Laguna Honda's spell. He began to say hello to
the patients he passed. He began to know some of them. He began to
visit them in their rooms and on the open wards. And he softened. He
got a bit confused. Perhaps there were patients at Laguna Honda and
not simply "residents." Perhaps Laguna Honda was a hospital and not
a health-care and rehabilitation facility.

And so, even after the computers were fixed, which took four
months—and I was surprised at how much less work I had while they
were down, even including telephoning the lab for my lab results—
Mr. Conley continued to step out of the administration wing and visit
the patients. Not with Miss Lester's compressed mouth and eagle eye,
but still, he sat on beds; he talked; he listened; and he learned about
the hospital from the patients' point of view.

Which would prove to be fatal.

No, Mr. Conley was not a lucky man. At least not as far as Laguna
Honda was concerned and especially not as far as this particular
time went.

Almost immediately after *Chambers* was filed, and while the
computers were still down, Mrs. Han fell to her death from a second-
or possibly third-story window, and no one knew how. She was
demented, to be sure, and one afternoon she was more agitated than
usual, wandering around her ward and trying to get out of the hospital

to visit her family. The nurses put her to bed and gave her a sedative. Mrs. Han fell asleep, and they went about their other tasks. But a few hours later when they returned to check on her, her bed was empty. They found her bracelet on the ledge of an open window and her body two, or possibly three, stories below. She was dead.

Naturally, the state began an investigation.

Next, *The Wall Street Journal* contacted Mr. Conley. It was doing a piece on the anachronism of old-fashioned institutions like Laguna Honda and was sending out a reporter to interview him. The very same week, the Department of Justice arrived and handed him five pages of questions to answer about the status of their minimal remedial measures. And then came a TV journalist with coifed hair and jutting jaw, to interview him on camera about Mrs. Han's death and the several investigations taking place.

Now, Mr. Conley was a nice man and a marine engineer, but in that interview he was out of his depth. When the reporter asked him how it happened that such a confused, restless woman as Mrs. Han, who was trying to get out of the hospital, had been left alone long enough to get out the window, Mr. Conley kind of put his foot in it.

"She was clearly supervised," he answered.

"Oh, come on, Mr. Conley," the reporter said. "She was supervised to the point she went out a third-floor window?"

"It wasn't a third-floor window," Mr. Conley corrected.

What was he going to do to prevent further incidents?

"I think you improve staffing," he replied. "You look at your procedures, you look at your quality measures, and you stay focused on them; you try not to get distracted by external factors."

The reporter followed up by interviewing a former Laguna Honda doctor, who told him that Mrs. Han's death had everything to do with the mayor's budget cuts to the hospital. Mrs. Han needed someone to sit and watch her, which she hadn't had. Had a sitter been with her, she would not have gone out that window. But sitters were expensive, the doctor pointed out, and Mr. Conley had all but cut them from his budget.

Then the reporter tried to get the mayor's response to this accusation. He sent in a request for an interview; he telephoned; and finally he waylaid the mayor coming out of a meeting. Did the mayor agree that his budget cuts had caused the death of a patient?

The mayor, who was just as well-coifed as the reporter, had no comment.

But right after that, Mr. Conley's luck changed. One hundred thousand dollars turned up in his budget, earmarked for hiring a public relations firm to "support the hospital's journey from institution to community." Also, he had a new position to fill, a director of government and community relations, to "handle negative publicity and improve Laguna Honda's community and media relations." Mr. Conley did not have to look far for either one. For our first public relations firm, he selected the firm that the mayor used. For our first director of government and community relations, he hired the mayor's spokesman, Adrian Serf. Also, at Dr. Stein's request, he hired back Dr. Dan as assistant medical director, to help him out with all the new paperwork, questions, and decisions.

t was more and more difficult for us to take care of patients. With the computers down for so long, I had to depend even more than before on my physical examination and on Hildegard's *methodus medendi*, and with the investigators, the media, the articles, and the press all so confident that our big old almshouse was not the wave of the future, it was easy to get demoralized.

Eventually, however, things seemed to settle down. Perhaps we were getting used to the changes. The hospital passed its next licensing and certification review; the computers came back online; and the new Laguna Honda finally began to emerge from the filled-in valley.

It had been so quiet over there for so many years. I'd gotten used to the parade of trucks up and down the hill, arriving with dirt, leaving with dirt; the wire fences; the tree removals; the swaths of earth replacing meadows. And so I was surprised one day to see real buildings, with steel girders and glass walls, rising out of the dirt. Suddenly—there was the Link Building, green-glassed and handsome, just as the architects had shown us years before. There was the South Building next to it, square and tall and wrapped in white. There was no East Building because *Chambers* had eliminated it; and construction of the West Building was delayed until Clarendon Hall could be demolished. Nevertheless, it was interesting. Sudden. Disconcerting.

But the barred window of our little doctors' office did not face the new structure. It looked backward onto the parking lot, with the ambulances coming and going, and even farther back toward the forest, where patients still went to smoke, drink, and have unprotected sex. And I continued to admit the remarkable patients we still welcomed. There were many such patients that year. But Radka is the one I want to tell you about.

Radka Semonovna was a beautiful woman.

I saw it at a glance the first time I met her, despite the dark circles under her eyes, her pale skin, and her bald head. And when I met her daughter, well, I knew for sure. Right off the plane from Bulgaria, she walked past the open door of our office, and I stopped talking. She was tallish and slimish, with dark hair cut short, thick eyelashes that cast a shadow on her cheek, a straight nose, and a finely drawn, full mouth. It was a beautiful face, an open face, and a puzzled face, I realized, as we talked an hour later at her mother's bedside, and she tried to understand what was wrong.

She knew that her mother had had cancer for the last two years and was now dying. But as I talked, and she concentrated on understanding my English, I could see that it wasn't easy for her; her thick-lashed brown eyes followed my lips, and a crease appeared in her brow. Radka also listened to me closely. Then she translated for her daughter what I'd said. She spoke Bulgarian, which I'd never heard before—sensual syllables that moved the inside of her mouth in all directions, front to back and side to side, and had a cadence like Russian.

"I know, doctor," Radka told me between breaths. "The cancer has spread to my lungs, and it is in my bones and my spinal cord. That is what I told my daughter."

Then Radka looked up at me from the bed, having stated the facts, and I sat down on it. I had her daughter sit down in one of our few remaining Naugahyde chairs. She took off her leather jacket and put it on the back of the chair.

"I'm going to give you antibiotics, as well as more chemotherapy," I explained, "because there may be some infection behind or inside the cancers in the lungs; and although the antibiotics won't kill the cancer, they will kill the infections, and you will breathe better."

"Okay, doctor, thank you," Radka said.

Radka's daughter still looked puzzled, but didn't ask any questions. She said, simply, "Thank you, doctor, thank you," in a tone of voice that doctors don't hear that often anymore, ever since we became health-care providers. Then I left them together, quietly speaking Bulgarian.

Originally Radka had not been my patient; she'd been Dr. Chang's.

Dr. Chang was the other of the two new health-care providers on the admitting ward, along with Dr. Rajif, and she did them credit. She was pleasant, reliable, and well trained. She came in on time, stayed all day, and worked hard. She seemed to like her health-care consumers well enough; and her workups were almost as elegant as Dr. Rachman's long ago. Although she did prefer a computer, she also wrote her workups longhand; and they were neatly scripted and intelligent. Reading them, I had no idea that, as Dr. Chang confessed to me one slow day, she did not know how to fully examine a patient.

"They don't teach us any longer. There's too much else for us to learn."

Radka started out as Dr. Chang's patient: The County Hospital sent her over to die and, in the meantime, to have chemotherapy. She'd been in excellent health until two years before, when cervical cancer was diagnosed. She had surgery and chemotherapy and felt well, but then, on a trip to meet her son and daughter in Yugoslavia (she was not allowed back in Bulgaria), she'd become short of breath. The doctors in Yugoslavia took X-rays and told her the cancer was now in her lungs, so she came back to the city and went to the County Hospital for a workup.

The news had not been good. The cancer was now in her lungs, bones, and spinal cord. The doctors at the County recommended additional chemotherapy and, since she lived with roommates, worked as a house cleaner, and her family was in Bulgaria, they sent her to us. Dr. Chang admitted her and scheduled the first round of her new chemotherapy, but the next day was Dr. Chang's day off. I was taking care of her patients, and that was when I met Radka and her daughter. The new chemotherapy made Radka's heart race, however, and so that very day she was readmitted to the County Hospital for monitoring. And when she returned, she became my patient.

Radka and her daughter were my first and so far only encounter with Bulgarians.

Bulgaria, Radka explained to me one day, was a very old country on the Black Sea. It was settled by slim, dark people but invaded regularly by Greeks, Turks, and Russians. The invaders were met quietly; they came, they saw, they conquered, and eventually they went home. Except for the Germans. The Bulgarians did not like the Germans, Radka said, and the Germans did not make out well in World War II Bulgaria. They did invade and conquer it; the king did shake hands with them; and the parliament did agree to enact certain new laws. But non-Jews as well as Jews showed up on the streets wearing yellow stars; broken windows in Jewish shops were somehow mended; and anti-Semitic graffiti was painted over by someone. Neither the Jews nor the Gypsies were transported from Bulgaria to concentration camps, and eventually the Germans, too, went home.

But the Russians must have been different, judging by the freezing of Radka's beautiful face when I asked her why she didn't go back for a visit. I knew that she'd been in America for several years; that, in spite of her PhD in economics, she cleaned houses for a living. She didn't answer.

"Political problems?"

She moved her head—just a little jerk—yes. Nothing more.

I tried to fill in what she was not saying. The nineteen seventies—printing clandestine newspapers on mimeograph machines late at night, passing them hand to hand on the streets? Or the eighties—an essay written on the efficient economy of private business, followed by reprimand, transfer, job loss? Or the nineties—Radka's husband, now in South America, an unpopular politician? Or a tax evader, a businessman who didn't pay the right bribes?

She never told me.

The nurses ended up liking Radka as much as I did, and when she returned from the County Hospital after one of her relapses, they gave her a quieter bed in the corner of the ward. The corner bed was a prime bed if you were a person who needed silence and privacy, who loved Mozart and *The Wall Street Journal*, which you read with serious, black-framed glasses. In the corner, you only had one roommate, not counting the patient across the aisle. True, the telephone on the ward was also in the corner, which meant that people stopped on the other side of your curtain to answer it and to talk. Still, it was a prized place, and Radka knew it and was grateful for the move.

Soon there were flowers on the windowsill by her bed, and herbal remedies and vitamins in her bureau, and though her sleep was broken by the sounds of other patients, when we finally had a truly prized bed for her, a single bed in a private room, Radka was wary. That was when I began to see, behind her face, some long-ago shock, some long-ago decision.

"It sounds very nice, thank you," she told me when I spoke of this new room she could move to. "But what happens if you need the room for someone else? Will I come back to my corner bed?"

She was right; she was exactly right; it was a politically astute and systemically wise question. But it was a question that no native-born American would have thought to ask or ever did ask. In America we know, for the most part, and especially in a public hospital, that the race is not to the swift nor the battle to the strong nor riches to men of understanding, but time and chance happen to them all. In order of arrival. And that once time and chance have awarded you your room, it's yours and cannot be taken back.

But Radka was more careful, strategic, and stoic than a native-born American. She declined the private room and suffered in silence her nights of broken sleep. A few weeks and several occupants later, however, the private room was free again, and this time I pushed her in the direction of health and sleep, if not eternal security.

"I think, Radka, you should move into the private room. You need the sleep. I can't promise, but we'll do our best to make sure you keep the room."

Silence.

There was some worry she wasn't telling.

Then I understood.

"You know," I explained, "this is a public hospital; it's run by the city for the poor. In my mind I call it God's Hotel because that's what we used to call hospitals for the poor, and what they're still called in France."

Radka nodded.

"It's old-fashioned; it's funky; it's not fancy—but it's free."

"You mean, doctor, that the private room doesn't cost more than this bed?"

"No," I told her. "It's all the same. Laguna Honda is a hospital for those who have nothing. We have some private rooms, some double rooms, lots of ward rooms, but all the beds cost the same—nothing."

Radka got even quieter than usual.

"America," she said. "America is a wonderful country."

And by that she meant a generous country, a rich country of generosity, in the true sense of the word *generosus*—noble.

America, especially these days, in its role as everyone's younger

sibling, focuses on its faults. Like the Puritans, its stone-faced founders, America is sternly self-unforgiving. We see only what we do not
do, have not accomplished, have done badly or even wrongly. And
seen from the perfect eyes of the perfect God, this vision of ourselves
may be just and accurate, but seen from Radka's eyes, America is
almost unbelievable. Hunted by her own country for some right or
wrong that she did; stoically, with tight lips and quiet mind, cleaning
houses, with little hope of ever going home. . . . Why should America
take account of her? And yet it does. Freely and with goodwill. America keeps Radka warm in the winter and cool in the summer, gives her
food, treats her cancer, and surrounds her with kindness, if not luxury. And asks for nothing back, not even gratitude.

America is a wonderful country. We should be proud.

Not long after that, we found Radka an even better room, in
doomed Clarendon Hall, across the filled-in valley. There she
would have only three roommates, and even better, she would have
Dr. Lydia, who spoke Russian, as her doctor. Radka was sad to leave
the admitting ward, and I was sad to see her go, but it was for the best.
I would visit her now and then, and her daughter could call on me, if
she needed. So she went.

Radka's turned out to be a long Calvary, as so many deaths by
cancer are. She wasn't ready to die. She wanted to see her son pass his
boards, finish his internship; she wanted to make sure her daughter
stayed safe; and she took the chemotherapy, which, at first diagnosis,
she thought about not taking at all. She took the carboplatin, which
made her beautiful hair fall out and her fingers go numb; then she
took the Taxol, which made her heart race nigh unto death. And
when those failed, Dr. Lydia found her something else to take, and

she took that, too. She didn't complain, but she wasn't ready to die, to leave, to shove off for that next unknown continent. Eventually, though, there wasn't anything else for her to take, and she sent her daughter over to find me.

Her daughter was as beautiful as ever, except for the new line between her brows, her sadness, her helplessness, and her resignation. Would I come over to Clarendon to see her mother, who was not doing well?

Now, Dr. Lydia was an old doctor, old and old-fashioned, and stood up, I knew, for the old protocols of politeness. So I telephoned to ask if it was all right for me to visit.

It would be helpful, Dr. Lydia told me. Radka was withdrawn, and the psychiatrist thought she was depressed, but she wouldn't take anything for her depression. Perhaps I could convince her. It was sad, so sad, Dr. Lydia said, such a sad case.

I walked over with Radka's daughter to Clarendon. Down around the worksite of the new building, then through the doors of the old Edwardian. We went up the stairs, down the hall, and into Radka's four-bed room. She had the corner bed nearest the door, and when I came in, she was lying down, so flat and thin that she disappeared into the covers. But there were herbs by the bed, a radio, books, and her black-framed glasses. Her hair had grown back and was thick, curly, and gray.

But she was very sick. It was a struggle for her to move, talk, or even breathe; and she wasn't coughing because it took too much energy. She seemed dim, her flame of life low and flickering, dying down; her lamp running out of fuel, just as the medieval metaphor had it. She was suffering mentally and physically, with her usual silent but oh-so-expressive stoicism.

Then I left the room to go to the nursing station and look

at Radka's chart. Dr. Lydia was old, but she was good—thorough, careful, and kind—and there was the report of the lung scan showing even bigger cancers; there was the report of the oncologist, who did have one more medication to try, although she wasn't optimistic. There was the report of the psychiatrist, who recommended an anti-depressant; and there were her lab reports, documenting the ebbing of her life force as so many fewer milliliters of blood and bone.

Then I went back to Radka's room, which, except for her, was empty of other patients. It faced north, and natural light must never have quite hit her corner.

Her daughter stood up. "I have to go to work now. . . . Thank you, doctor." She looked at me. Her beautiful light had dimmed, too. Her face was tired and tense and sad. But she was cleaning Radka's houses, and so she left.

There was just us.

I sat down in the chair by the bed. Radka sat up, leaning against the pillows at the wall. She queried me with a look.

"It's not great," I said. "But there is something else to try. It will help."

She nodded.

"Also, the psychiatrist wants you to take some pills to help you feel better, more lively."

"Yes, he told me. Should I?"

"I think so. They don't have many side effects, and after a few weeks, you'll feel better, stronger, more able to deal with—all this. How's your son? Is he coming to see you?"

She brightened. "He can't come. He's studying for his boards. But we talk on the phone every week. Maybe in the summer if he can get . . . you know . . . permission . . . a visa."

She stopped talking to breathe, and we sat together for a while.

She leaned forward. "Would you like to see some pictures . . . of Bulgaria?" She looked at me, and I nodded. "There, in the top drawer . . . Would you get them, please?"

I opened the top drawer. There wasn't much in it, but there was an envelope, and it had the pictures. I moved my chair so I was sitting right next to Radka, and she took out the yellowed black-and-white photos, with their creased, shiny surfaces. She looked at the first one, then handed it to me.

"This is my house in Bulgaria."

I took it. We were out in the country; there was a big, one-story wooden house, and the photo was taken from across a garden looking toward the house. The garden was not like my garden—small with some roses, dahlias, and vegetables. This garden was cultivated; it was serious; and it had a purpose. It was probably an acre of leeks and staked beans, cabbages, squash, tomatoes, and potatoes, orderly, in many rows.

Radka watched me look at the photo.

"We had many things but no money," she said.

She handed me the next photo. Vivid and smiling, with a shock of dark brown curls, standing next to the house was . . . Radka. Next to her was a large, laughing man. Sleeves rolled up; black hair; black, thick mustache.

"Me. My husband. I was strong."

"When was this taken?"

"Five years ago."

I could imagine the two of them, living a not-so-easy but well-populated life. Other intellectuals visiting; dinner outside in the summer darkness, with candles, fireflies, crickets.

"Our house wasn't far from the city, just an hour or so. We went out for the weekends and the summers."

Card games; working in the garden; frustration with the System; anger, a decision, repercussions, flight to another continent.

I looked at the other photos, different views of the house and the garden, then I handed them back.

"Thank you." I stood up. Despite, or perhaps because of, her vulnerability, Radka was not a person to hug. "I'll speak to Dr. Lydia," I told her.

"And my daughter?"

"Yes."

didn't see Radka again. A few months later, her daughter came over to the admitting ward to tell me that Radka had decided to go to Dr. Kay's hospice unit; her son had graduated and passed his boards. After that she died very quickly. Her daughter came to find me once again, thanked me, and once more invited me to Bulgaria, which was a beautiful country.

I do plan to go sometime. I'd like to find the pilgrimage route across it, through the mountains, and then down to the Black Sea; and I'd like to meet the rest of the Bulgarians.

But in the meantime, a big change was coming to Laguna Honda. It was packing up its bags in Hawaii; it was flying back to our city; it was finding a place to live, and then I heard it walking, in its elegant, soft brown leather shoes, which were nicer than the administrators' shoes, the architects' shoes, even the lawyers' shoes.

It was Dr. Dan, come back.

Eleven

RECALLED TO LIFE

D R. DAN AND I had never been properly introduced.

What had happened was this: He'd arrived at Laguna Honda for the first time during the year I was in Switzerland, which was a tough year for Dr. Romero as medical director. The Department of Justice visited thirteen times, each time grilling her about the workings of the hospital, and the admitting ward had been chaotic. She didn't like being medical director anyway, with its demand for negotiation and compromise. It was easy for Dr. Romero to lead with one of her two sides—the sweet, compliant side or the sardonic, righteous side—but compromise, having to start from some place in the middle, was almost impossible. She didn't believe in it.

Finally she'd had enough. She decided to resign as medical director and return to the admitting ward, but not to Dr. Jeffers, Dr. Fintner, and Dr. S. She would start over. She would find a new, fresh, untouched physician, one who was willing to work with her full-time on the admitting ward. She sent out feelers, and Dr. Dan came over for his tour and his interview. She liked him right away.

He was tanned and brown, with a 1950s flattop and sideburns, and he was beautifully dressed, from his Armani jacket to his Gucci shoes. Also, he was meticulously groomed, with his nails manicured and his thick brown eyebrows trimmed. Although not a handsome man, being too tall and too thin with a head just a little small for his body, he had done a lot with what nature had given him. Dr. Romero thought he would make a good medical director and that she would groom him for the position. So she offered him the job, and by the time I came back from Switzerland, he was on the admitting ward with the Welcome! sign up and the doors closed.

Consequently, I was never properly introduced to Dr. Dan. I knew him by sight on the evenings when I passed him in my car, as he loped down the hill to the streetcar. I knew him by rumor, which had it that the doctors' part-time schedules drove him crazy and that he monitored our comings and goings with janitorial spies. But I knew him best by his workups, which were neatly printed backhand, clear, readable, and short.

Dr. Dan liked his patients, and they liked him, but he did not delve into their problems, I saw by his workups. He did not call their former physicians, review all their records, or do a detailed physical examination. He prized efficiency above all and had not found that an extensive workup added much to his patients' care. Instead, he transferred into his own workup the diagnoses and medications his patients arrived with, which was why he could see a patient faster than any physician I've ever known and couldn't fathom what took the rest of us so much time. What Dr. Dan did think worth his while were procedures. He could put in a needle just about anywhere—

spinal canal, lung, abdomen, veins, arteries—quickly and efficiently. For procedures, Dr. Dan was the man to call.

For several years he stayed behind the closed doors of the admitting ward. He did become co–medical director. He never was able to replace the part-time doctors with full-timers as he had planned, nor persuade a quorum of doctors to attend his early-morning meetings, but he did install cameras in the doctors' parking lot and was about to put in a time clock when . . . he disappeared. We came in one day, and he was gone. He'd taken a more lucrative position in Hawaii, and sold his house, packed up his clothes, and taken ship for the Big Island, all in two weeks' time.

We didn't hear from him again until two years later, when Mr. Conley telephoned to persuade him to return. He could have his old job back as co–medical director, Mr. Conley offered, and his office on the admitting ward. He would assist Mr. Conley with implementing *Chambers*; he would respond to the medical concerns of the Department of Justice; he would help organize the move to the new Laguna Honda after the facility was finished; and he would keep the doctors in tow. Particularly Dr. Kay and Dr. Romero, who were infuriating Dr. Stein by their persistent questioning about the hospital, the County, and the budget. Mr. Conley could guarantee Dr. Dan carte blanche because the medical director was now Dr. Sonnen, who mostly stayed in his office upstairs.

Dr. Dan was interested. He did make more money in Hawaii, and it was a more prestigious position, but he missed Laguna Honda. The thing was, he told Mr. Conley, he wouldn't work with Dr. Romero. They'd had a falling-out. He wouldn't go into the details.

What about working with Dr. S.? Mr. Conley asked. She was back on the admitting ward.

Maybe. He would see.

And so when I heard Dr. Dan striding down the hallway on the day he came back, it was with some trepidation.

His stride did not break until it came to the open door of our doctors' office. Then it stopped. I was reading a chart at my desk and turned my head. Soft brown shoes, gray silk socks, creased linen pants, dark green, open-collared shirt, cream-colored Armani jacket—Dr. Dan was, I saw, just as well-dressed as ever. And even more perfectly tanned. He stood in the doorway and looked around. Then he walked in, pulled the chair out from the counter desk, sat down, spread his long arms along the desk, and put his head down.

"It's still here!" he murmured.

"So you love this place, too," I said.

Then he sat up and turned his chair partly around. He had a remarkable profile. It was the profile of a French knight in the Bayeux Tapestry—high forehead sloping back, strong nose that started at his eyebrows—perfectly shaped to wear a medieval Norman helmet.

"Oh, I missed it so much when I was in Hawaii!"

"How was it? What did you do there? What didn't you like?"

"Well, it was a great job, on paper. I was head of subacute care for the Kaiser system on the whole island. Paid well, almost twice as much as here. The beaches were great, and James was pretty happy. But it was a mess. There were hardly any beds for the subacute patients—the ones ready to leave the acute hospital but not ready to go home; you know—they needed IV antibiotics, wound care, or just time to recover from the intensive care unit. But the utilization review managers were always on our case to discharge them as soon as possible, even when there was no place to send them, and at the same time the hospitals were sending us their sickest patients, with tubes, trachs, vents—you name it."

Dr. Dan stood up and walked out. I followed him. He meandered down the corridor and looked at each of the metal brackets, now empty of the plants he'd abandoned two years before. Then he went into the nursing station, took the ring of keys from above the file cabinet, and walked through the ward almost to the solarium. There was a door I'd never noticed, and he unlocked it. I saw a narrow room, five or six feet wide, with a steel counter along the wall and a dirty window at its end.

Dr. Dan smiled.

"What's this for?" I asked.

"I don't know what it was for originally. But I use it for my plants and my flowers. It's perfect. When the plants aren't looking well, I bring them in here and mist them. And I use it to arrange bouquets for the ward. Looks like I'm going to have to run out later today and bring in a whole new set of plants and a lot of flowers."

Which he did. In the mid-afternoon, he asked me to watch his new patients, and he walked down the hill and took the J trolley to his favorite florist.

Before I left that day, I saw Dr. Dan's Armani jacket hanging in the office, and I walked over to the little room he'd shown me that morning. Its door was open, and so was its window, now clean. The counter was crowded with green plants in pots, and in the sink were dozens of irises, roses, and gerbera, and various greenery. Dr. Dan, wearing an apron and with scissors in hand, was clipping and cutting and arranging them all into vases he'd found, only he knew where.

When I came in the next morning, the metal brackets were once again filled with green plants, and there were bouquets in the solarium and on the ward. But the doctors' office was empty and so was the nursing station; the chart rack was gone and the door of the lounge was closed. It was Wednesday, and the team meeting for the patients had started.

I needed a patient's chart, though, so I knocked on the door and then walked in. There was Dr. Dan, lounging in a peeling deck chair, legs straddled out in front of him, open chart on his lap. He was flipping through it, scanning the notes, and talking about when the patient might be discharged and what medications he would need. After a bit, I realized he was talking about one of my patients.

"What are you doing?" I interrupted.

Dr. Dan did not look up. "I'm discussing Mr. Eks."

"Mr. Eks is my patient."

"I know. You weren't here."

"Why didn't you start with your own patients then? You don't know anything about Mr. Eks."

"You weren't here."

The room got very quiet. Dr. Dan did look up from the chart then, and we looked right at each other. His eyes, I saw for the first time, were narrow and a flat gray-green. They were cold. Then he turned back to the chart and continued to present Mr. Eks.

I left.

About an hour later he came into our office, but he didn't sit down.

"Do not present my patients when you know I'm in the hospital," I told him.

"If you aren't around, I will present your patients, and if you raise your voice to me, we won't be able to work together," he retorted.

I looked up at him—his flat face and flat eyes, and felt his flat, determined will. I took in a deep breath and let it out slowly. Working with Dr. Dan was going to be quite different from working with Dr. Chang, Dr. Fintner, or Dr. Jeffers.

Dr. Dan was one of the few doctors at Laguna Honda—perhaps the only doctor—who was ambitious about a career in health care. As an old almshouse, the hospital was not mainstream, and the ambitious who came to it were ambitious in other areas— in physics, surfing, history—but not in health care. Except for Dr. Dan. And his ambition was limited; he just wanted to be medical director.

He was a farm boy from upstate New York, and though you could take the farm boy out of the farm, you couldn't take the farm out of the farm boy. Although he dressed with exquisite taste, his time was farm time; his view, a farm view.

He woke at dawn and took the streetcar to the foot of the hospital, then walked up the hill. He left late in the evening, walking down the hill and taking the streetcar home. He didn't drink or smoke or play around with women or men. On winter evenings at home, he went over hospital reports and went to bed early, and on his days off he came in anyway, strolling in his long-legged way through the wards, reading other doctors' charts, talking to the nurses. Or he took long walks through the city, over the bridge and out into the country, many miles. And yet, with all his Franklinsonian living, Dr. Dan wasn't even boring. He told a good story. He had an eye for detail, especially vestimentary, an ear for the ridiculous, and a taste for mockery, which extended to the patients, doctors, and administrators, though not, by and large, to the nurses.

Dr. Dan came from a long line of nurses and probably should have been a nurse himself but, tall and the only son, he went to medical school. Still the stories he told me were of visiting his mother, Head Nurse Stanislaus, in her hospital on Sundays when he was just a little boy, and feeling the romance of her white uniform and cap, her rigorous schedule, and the nursing camaraderie. And though I never met his mother, I couldn't help but imagine her as cousin to Miss Lester and descendant of those fierce nuns of the Hôtel-Dieu in Paris. He himself was the closest thing we'd had to Miss Lester since Miss Lester.

Dr. Dan loved the nurses and the Way of Nursing, although he didn't nurse much, not in the way that Dr. Bart did, who, before she was a doctor, had been a nurse—plumping pillows, helping a patient drink through a straw. Dr. Dan didn't sit on beds, shake hands, or touch patients all that much, but, then, neither did Miss Lester.

And he had the nurse's attitude toward the doctor: the nurse's impatience with the doctor's attention to such small details as a certain pulse and blood pressure, a slightly elevated copper level, or the particular shape of a red blood cell. Dr. Dan, too, suspicioned that medicine was overblown; its careful histories and physicals pretentious and unnecessary.

After a while I began to realize that Dr. Dan was an amazing guy—a whirlwind—and what is that about sowing the wind and reaping the whirlwind?

He was everywhere at once, quick and confident, but also hasty and hotheaded. If he saw his patients, it was in the early morning. He wrote his notes while listening to nursing rounds, and by eight AM had moved on to his duties as co–medical director, conducted at his counter desk.

Hence, for the first time in my years at the hospital, I was privy to its politics—its meetings and secret plans, its backbiting and incompetence. All day long, while I was seeing patients, people showed up at the door of our office with complaints and concerns. Dr. Dan would listen for a minute or two and then prescribe. He didn't mull over or investigate, but he did cut Gordian knots, order babies partitioned in two, deny, approve, and legislate.

He did not give up his duties as physician on the admitting ward either. He piled up televisions and headphones under his counter desk, and now and then he could be found fitting a patient with a headset. Every Wednesday afternoon he left the hospital to buy flowers, and in the early evening he arranged new bouquets. He ordered furniture for the TV room and solarium, and had the lounge repainted. He spent quite a while with the furniture swatches and paint samples, sitting first in the lounge, then in the TV room, then in the solarium. He wanted to get the colors just right.

He loved the hospital even more than I did and knew it better. It was Dr. Dan who showed me the priest's flat in the turret, with its heavy wooden door and barred window. It was Dr. Dan who, at Christmas, gave each staff member on the admitting ward, including Rose, our gentle janitor, a hundred-dollar gift certificate and a thank-you note from him. He was never sick; he was devoted and engaged.

It took us a while, but gradually he and I got to know and use each other's strengths and weaknesses. He covered for me on my days off; I covered for him while he was in his administrative role. Slowly he began to appreciate that my way could be useful and even efficient, and, with the case of Janice Gilroy, he changed his mind about the value of the Way of Medicine.

Somewhat.

D r. Dan was not the first doctor at Laguna Honda to take care of Janice Gilroy.

At fifty, Ms. Gilroy had come and gone and come back to us many times. She was of the rare breed of Bad Girl and had been saved by modern medicine from the worst consequence of her badness— namely death—but preserved for quite a bit of suffering, as she resided just this side of death. Laguna Honda had always had a few patients like her, but now it had many more, as medicine became more and more amazing, bringing patients back—but just a little back—from the brink.

Ms. Gilroy was a drug abuser, and she would use anything, especially cocaine, marijuana, heroin, and alcohol. Cocaine is especially hard on the body, and Ms. Gilroy had the high blood pressure, kidney disease, and poor circulation to show for it. She had the poor memory of the chronic marijuana user, the bad liver of the heroin user, and the weak heart of the alcoholic. This was in general.

But in particular, she'd had a stroke in the right side of her brain. Now, a stroke on the right side of the brain is both easier and harder than a stroke on the left side of the brain. It is easier because a stroke on the right side of the brain does not injure the left side of the brain, with its capacity for speech. Also, because the brain is cross-wired, a stroke on the right side of the brain does not paralyze the right side of the body, with its usually more dexterous abilities, but the left side, and so is usually less disabling.

But a stroke on the right side of the brain is harder than one on the left because the right side of the brain has something special about it, indefinable and unnamed—a kind of centered cheerfulness— and with a stroke on the right side of the brain, a patient often becomes depressed. So that in addition to being paralyzed on her left side, and in addition to her other disabilities, Ms. Gilroy was also despondent. As an antidote to her depression, she used drugs whenever she could get them, which would upset the delicate balance among her many medications and diseases, and put her right back in the hospital.

When she wasn't in the hospital, she lived with her daughter, who did not quite understand her mother's disabilities nor the imperative of keeping her away from drugs. So Ms. Gilroy would stabilize at Laguna Honda, and then her daughter would take her home on a pass or even against medical advice, where she would eat, drink, and be merry, and end up back in the intensive care unit and then back with us. I'd admitted her myself in the past.

But this time it was Dr. Dan who admitted her, and he'd done a good job. He had told her daughter off—there's no other way to say it—and she'd made herself scarce. Hence, Ms. Gilroy had no access to drugs; she wasn't eating food that threw her system off; nor was she being taken home clandestinely, though with the best intentions in the world. And she'd improved. Everything about her was just a little bit better—heart, liver, kidneys.

Until this afternoon, Dr. Dan told me, when she'd deteriorated. Actually, it had started three days earlier. At morning nursing rounds he'd heard that Ms. Gilroy was different somehow—moaning, confused, and complaining of pain. So he'd ordered pain medications. But the next day she was worse—agitated and still complaining of pain. So he'd ordered more pain medications and added something for restlessness.

Did he examine her? I asked him.

Not exactly. But he had checked her blood and urine and didn't find any infection or illicit drugs. Then he asked the psychiatrist to

see her, because perhaps the change in her mental status was psychiatric. The psychiatrist did see her and he increased her antipsychotic
medications, but still she was no better. She was worse—more restless,
agitated, and confused. Dr. Dan had a meeting to attend; would I take
a look and try to figure out what was wrong with her?

Wow.

Trying to find the cause for the change in mental status that Dr.
Dan described was daunting. Especially in someone as ill as Ms. Gilroy. There were endless possibilities. She would need a brain scan and
a bone scan, a spinal tap, perhaps biopsies, and even after those, the
complexity of her medical problems would doubtless require another
prolonged hospitalization at the County. But Ms. Gilroy came after
Steve Harp. So instead of first going through her records, talking to
her family and the nurses, and then examining her, I went over to see
her for myself. I'd learned from Steve that seeing the real patient was
worth a thousand words.

The nurses had moved Ms. Gilroy from the open ward into one of
the private rooms, I learned, which meant she must have been very
agitated. When I came into her room I saw that they had also turned
off the lights, pulled down the shades, and set up a large fan, blowing
full blast. Although it was quiet, dark, and cool in the room, Ms. Gilroy, nevertheless, was lying on top of the sheets, stark naked. She was
restless, tossing and turning and picking at the sheets, and sweat was
beading off her body. When I tried to talk to her, she kept her eyes
tightly shut and didn't answer my questions, and when I tried to
examine her, she screamed. I couldn't examine her, not with my usual
questions and answers, stethoscope and reflex hammer. It made me
wonder how the nurses could have been getting her blood pressure,
pulse, and temperature.

After Mrs. Han, Mr. Conley was a little looser about sitters, and

Ms. Gilroy did have a sitter, who was reading a magazine in a chair at the foot of the bed. But I wanted to sit myself. So I asked her to go out on break, and after she left, I pulled the chair right next to Ms. Gilroy and sat down.

I sat for quite a while.

The hospital was often hot but with the shades down, the lights off, and a fan on, it was cool in the room. At first. Yet as I sat there and the minutes passed, and I watched Ms. Gilroy toss and turn, shake her head from side to side, and throw off anything that touched her naked body, I, too, began to feel hot and restless. I began to feel as if I wanted to crawl out of my skin; as if there were something in my body—some toxin, some poison—that just had to get out. And at that moment, I realized that Ms. Gilroy was acting as if she'd been poisoned, as if there were a toxin in her body that had to get out.

I wondered. Could she have been poisoned?

An actual poisoning didn't seem likely. Despite its checkered history, Laguna Honda had never yet had a poisoner. If Ms. Gilroy was being poisoned, it was by something internal: an obscure infection, a hallucinogen she'd gotten hold of, or, most likely, by some medication she was taking.

So I left the room to get her chart; it was time to take a look. I brought it back, sat down again, and began to review what she'd been prescribed.

Dr. Dan had not added any new medications to her regime; all he'd done was increase the ones she'd already been getting—the pain medications, sedatives, antipsychotics, and antidepressants. Nevertheless, Ms. Gilroy was being poisoned, I was more and more certain, and by something that made her hot, restless, agitated, and confused.

Suddenly it occurred to me.

Serotonin syndrome.

I'd never seen it, but I'd read about it. Serotonin is a natural chemical made by the brain, and each one of Ms. Gilroy's medications increased it. Taken all together and in escalating doses, they could have raised her brain serotonin to a toxic level, which would provoke the symptoms she had—agitation, confusion, hyperthermia. I sat and thought about it, while Ms. Gilroy moaned and picked at nonexistent bedclothes.

My problem was that there was no test for serotonin syndrome— no blood test or X-ray. The only way I could diagnose it would be to take her off her medications, and this could be dangerous, because if she did have something else instead of serotonin syndrome—an unusual kind of stroke, for instance, or an infection, or something I hadn't thought of—taking her off her medications would make her more, not less, agitated, and make her worse. But if she did have serotonin syndrome, then I had to stop her medications immediately because serotonin syndrome is fatal.

I was sure enough, and after I explained my thinking to Dr. Dan, he agreed. I decreased Ms. Gilroy's sedatives, antipsychotics, antidepressants, and pain medications just a little; within a few hours, she'd improved. I took her off all of them, and she calmed and cleared. Eventually she even went home again to her daughter, for a while.

Like so many of my experiences at Laguna Honda, that sitting with Ms. Gilroy in her dark and cool room as she tossed and turned changed me and stayed with me. I thought about it a lot. I'd done so little for her, even less than I'd done for Steve. I hadn't looked into her eyes, held her hand, or reviewed all her records. I'd done nothing at all. Except sit. But how effective that had been! The diagnosis had appeared without me sending her to the emergency room, without additional tests, scans, or biopsies. Somehow, just by sitting with her, I'd understood what was wrong.

I began to try it with my other patients. Just sitting.

Just sitting was not the same thing as sitting, however. It's a little hard to explain. It was sitting, but it was not sitting and doing something—reading or talking—and it wasn't the "just sitting" of Zen either, which is a strenuous, focused vacancy. It was, I decided, like the mental state of knitting, but it was most like waiting for a train in Switzerland. I remembered that well. Sitting on a bench, with ticket purchased and in your pocket, knowing that the train will arrive on time; there is nothing more to worry about and nothing more to do. The activity of the train station flows around you, and you observe, but not intently; you are aware, but not focused. People come and go; there is a hustle and bustle; but it is not your hustle and bustle.

That was "just sitting," and after Ms. Gilroy, I took the time to "just sit" in this way with all my patients. Especially if they took a turn for the worse, or if a nurse or a family member was worried that something wasn't quite right. I would leave my cell phone in the nursing station, turn off my beeper, move a chair next to the patient, and sit down. Not for long—five or ten minutes. Sometimes the patient would want to chat, and we would chat, and sometimes I would study the patient's face, bedclothes, and bureau. But mostly I would just sit. And something, somehow, would happen. It would become clear what, if anything, was wrong with the patient and what, if anything, I could do about it.

I can't say for sure that Dr. Dan was impressed after Ms. Gilroy, but he did look at me differently. He never again presented one of my patients when he knew I was in the hospital, and during the many hours of meetings he sat through every day, he had me take care of his patients.

I t didn't take Dr. Dan long to catch up with the politics at the hospital.

He met with Mr. Conley; he went over the last year's budget and the dicey budget for the next year. He studied the *Chambers* settlement, the latest state survey, and the investigations of the Department of Justice. He met with the new marketing department and began going to the Health Commission meetings, the administrators' meetings, and the builder's meetings.

There were many decisions to be made, Dr. Dan decided, and one that had to be unmade. Because of *Chambers*, the hospital had to downsize from 1,030 patients to 780, and Mr. Conley's idea of doing that over several years did not make sense. The downsizing had to happen before the new buildings were completed, and the only way to do that was to stop admitting patients. It took him a while, but finally he convinced Mr. Conley that at the beginning of the next year, admissions to Laguna Honda would cease. The only new patients would be to rehabilitation, hospice, or the AIDS wards.

Next he turned his attention to planning. Every patient should know in advance where he or she was going to go, he decided, and so the organization of the new hospital had to be thought out in advance. Which floors would house men, which women, which the hospice patients, the AIDS patients, the demented patients? To do that, however, he had to know every patient's disabilities and medical conditions, age, gender, and sex preference (it was San Francisco, after all). Dr. Dan did not organize a subcommittee to do all this; he did not consult with administration or nursing. Instead, he put together a form, typed it up, printed out 1,030 copies, and went to every ward himself and filled out a form on every patient.

I was amazed when he told me this, one slow afternoon in our office. He went and examined every patient in the hospital?

No, of course not. He couldn't do that. He got the information he needed from the charts.

In only a few weeks he'd sketched out each floor of the new facility and assigned every patient to his or her future bed there.

Then he took on the problem of Clarendon Hall, which was to be demolished the next year to make way for the new buildings. Its 180 patients had to be moved to the old hospital as soon as possible. Had Dr. Dan tried to maintain the nursing model of clustering patients together by diagnosis, this would have been impossible, but he did not. Instead, whenever a bed opened up, he filled it with some patient from Clarendon, regardless of diagnosis, disability, or gender. Soon, men and women, the ambulatory elderly and the demented, the drug-abusing psychotics, and the developmentally disabled were right next to one another on the same ward. It wasn't optimal, or maybe it was; at any rate, it was very efficient, and Dr. Dan was able to start closing down Clarendon right away.

His last problem was the budget.

Of course, the budget was an issue every year. But with so many fewer patients, in the next year's budget real cuts would be necessary— in theory, one-third fewer patients should mean that one-third of the staff would be cut. In practice, though, one-third fewer patients did not make for one-third less work for the quality assurance team, the marketing team, or administration. Given the upcoming move, the Department of Justice's demands, and the *Chambers* settlement, the demands on nonclinical staff would only increase, and Dr. Stein had already given Mr. Conley an additional ten million dollars for more administrative staff. However, the clinical staff who took care of patients could be decreased, and Mr. Conley gave Dr. Dan the job of cutting the medical staff by one-third.

Dr. Dan didn't want to. He went over the budget many times—the medical staff's budget of 2.5 million dollars and the hospital's budget of 170 million dollars—looking for cuts that wouldn't cut. He found only a few. Finally he had an idea. If the daytime doctors covered the hospital at night and on weekends, using some of their daytime hours to do so, he could lay off the night and weekend doctors and that would make his one-third. True, many of the night doctors had been at the hospital for decades, and it would be difficult for the daytime doctors to take care of the same number of patients during the day and also come in at night. But it would be better than cutting the regular staff, and he would take quite a few of the night shifts himself.

We would manage somehow, he told us at our next medical staff meeting. Besides, our new schedules wouldn't start until the middle of the next year, when the new budget cycle would begin.

He did have one piece of good news. The Department of Justice had accepted the *Chambers* settlement and was closing its ten-year investigation. It still had two additional demands, however. First, the city would agree never to use the new Laguna Honda for its homeless, even if the homeless needed its care. Instead, the city would provide whatever it took for the homeless to stay in the community—housing, medical clinics, community centers, outreach teams, mobile behavioral teams, whatever. Second, the city would agree to implement the Health Management Associates recommendations, and that, Dr. Dan said, concerned all of us.

Everyone at the meeting looked blank.

Well, maybe no one but he had ever read them, Dr. Dan

admitted. Health Management Associates was the group that Dr. Stein had hired years before, and their original report had had many recommendations. Although it wasn't clear which recommendations the Department of Justice meant, Dr. Dan thought most likely the recommendation to create a "continuum of care" by merging Laguna Honda with the MHRF, and then, after the move to the new facility, merging the County Hospital with Laguna Honda.

So?

Well, that would mean that we would lose our independence as a separate hospital, Dr. Dan explained. After those two mergers, Dr. Stein would be in charge of Laguna Honda as well as the County Hospital, and we would have to apply to him to be on the medical staff.

A frisson went around the room. There were quite a few doctors there whom Dr. Stein did not like, all that much.

These were a lot of changes, both actual and potential. Fortunately, another year had passed, and it was time for Rosalind and me to pack our bags and finish our pilgrimage to Compostela.

The last section starts with a ten-day walk across the meseta, a high plateau in northern Spain known to be physically and spiritually challenging. In the pilgrimage literature, walking the meseta was compared to those times in life when life is just a drag—tiring, dispiriting, depressing. Rosalind and I had read about it; we knew about it and were prepared for it.

The thing was, the meseta was tedious. Dry, dusty, and hot. Long. The villages along the way were not nice; the churches were locked; and our fellow pilgrims! We were very disappointed. They were not the spiritual, solemn, and singing pilgrims of our last three years. They were partygoers, and they hurried across the meseta to the day's stopping place to drink. Some of them even gave up on the meseta and went from place to place by taxi.

After a few days, I began to have doubts. Why was I walking across France and Spain in this medieval way? It was not comfortable; it was not pleasant; it was not spiritual. Why not take a taxi? We'd still get to Compostela, and we'd still get our Compostelas. Rosalind felt the same way, and so we talked. We didn't want to skip anything, we decided. You never know. Perhaps walking across the meseta was necessary. Perhaps we would miss something important by taxi.

It turned out I did get something special from the meseta. I got more accustomed to the heat and more muscled. I also got more determined. My goal was fixed: I would walk to Compostela—no matter what. And with my goal fixed, without self-doubt and the minute-by-minute attention to frustrations and disappointments, I discovered something. Underneath the surface actions, events, and partying of the path was silence. Even when it was noisy, that silence was underneath activity. That quiet was solid and always accessible. I could depend on it; I could return to it at any time, in any emergency. It was the quiet of pilgrimage, and it was worth the meseta.

Finally, after nine days of walking through dust, we saw the cooling mountains ahead. We attained them, walked over them, and entered a different country, a country you can only get to by walking.

On the day we arrived at Compostela it was raining. The outskirts of the city were modern, but we crossed a bridge and then it became the Middle Ages. We passed a bearded, smiling pilgrim and his smiling dog, who'd come the whole way, too. We walked under a stone arch and began to hear the bagpipe music of Galicia. Then the path opened up into a cobblestoned square and, looming over us, was Saint James's twelfth-century cathedral.

We did the usual pilgrim things.

We touched the marble foot of Saint James. Behind the altar we put our arms through two holes and hugged the thirteenth-century statue of Santiago, which was dressed in gold and jewels. We went to the Pilgrim's Mass and saw the Botafumeiro fall. We walked over to the bishop's office, where our Créancial was scrutinized and where we received our Compostela, the Latin scroll that forgave us our sins. And we went to the evening vigil.

I'd read in our guidebook that on Saturday night there was a special pilgrim's vigil at the cathedral at ten PM. That's late for a pilgrim, and it was raining; our hotel was comfortable; still we went out. We didn't find anyone in front of the cathedral, but when we walked around it, there was a group of pilgrims in the rain, standing in front of the south door. A few minutes later, the door opened, and a little monk appeared and beckoned us inside.

Us?

We all looked around.

He nodded.

He walked inside, and the small group followed him. Except for us, the cathedral was empty. He took us through another side door into the dark cloister. A charcoal brazier was on the stones, and he gestured for us to sit down around it. Then he handed out black cards and told us they would symbolize the sins we wanted to get rid of. He would light the brazier; we would go around the circle and, in whatever language we spoke, tell the sin we were casting into the fire.

Is worry a sin? I asked myself. I sure would like to get rid of it. I decided that it was. Worry about the future seemed uncharitable somehow, toward God, after everything I'd experienced on the pilgrimage—so many days I'd worried would be bad had turned out so well! And so many days when my good anticipations had turned out so bad! I didn't know whether worry was a sin, but I threw it in the brazier.

Although our pilgrimage to Santiago was over, our pilgriming was not, because there was one last bit we wanted to do—to walk to Finisterre, Land's End, the end of the medieval earth. From the medieval perspective, this was the farthest west you could go in Europe; after Finisterre, nothing got in the way until Cathay and India. I wanted to see it. So we set off.

It was a three-day walk, and though it wasn't lonely exactly, it was quite isolated. There were no other pilgrims on the path, no towns or villages, and the forests we walked through had been burned that summer. There were lots of patches of blackened, acrid-smelling ground and blackened tree trunks.

We smelled the ocean before we saw it, moist and salty. Fog was rolling through, but when we climbed up a ridge, it lifted, and there it was. The ocean. Silver blue, stretched out forever, nothing modern to remind us, just a little fishing village on the edge, one fishing boat hugging the coastline. We climbed down to the beach and gathered cockleshells, and then we walked the very last bit to Finisterre. A pole marked the spot, where other pilgrims had left their walking sticks. We left ours.

Then I went off to sit for a while at the edge.

It was very satisfying. We had made it. To the very end of the medieval earth. There was no place else to go. The ocean stretched out as far as I could see, all the way to the shores of a continent that the medievals had no inkling of. When they'd sat where I was sitting, looking out at the ocean, they'd imagined Cathay and its silk, India and its spices. It was land's end because for them there was only one land, with Europe at one end and Asia at the other. They knew the earth was spherical, and they knew that if any sailor had been brave enough to leave the sight of the shore, he would, eventually, have come to the other side, to Asia.

They had had no idea. Not an inkling. A whole continent. Huge, as vast as the world they knew. A new world was out there, but not for them.

I wondered what it had been like, to hear about this new, undiscovered world that no one had even imagined. It was the biggest difference between me and them, I thought. Everything else that had been interposed between me and the medieval experience on our pilgrimage—airplanes, electric lights, cell phones—would not have surprised them so very much. They'd imagined all of it: flying carpets, magic light, invisible voices—their magicians could do such things. But that new world was completely unimaginable and unimagined. I knew it was there, and knowing it was there in their future made it impossible for me to imagine it not being there, to imagine their world as they saw it.

It made me wonder especially, what new world was in our future, unimagined, unimaginable, and completely unexpected?

When I returned to the hospital, having completed my vow of pilgrimage, I felt somehow carefree. Perhaps it was all those days of walking and watching bad turn into good and good turn into bad, or perhaps it was burning that black card of worry. At any rate, I felt carefree. Whatever was going to happen would happen, according to its time and the seasons. Which was a good way to feel, because the real and irrevocable changes at the hospital were beginning.

Dr. Dan stopped the admission of new patients. With no new patients, the admitting ward was not needed, and Dr. Dan closed it. He moved himself into Dr. Major's office; he moved me into the doctors' offices downstairs, and he sent Larissa and the other nurses to other wards. While I was away, he packed up my things—papers, books, and index cards, including Mrs. McCoy's plant, which he tried to prepare for its move. He took it into his special room, pruned it, and watered it, but when I got back from the pilgrimage, it was dead.

That seemed symbolic because Dr. Dan was not closing the admitting ward temporarily but permanently. He was not going to reopen it in the new hospital. It was too inefficient. In the new facility patients would be admitted to the wards where they would stay, and the doctor of that ward would admit them, so from the beginning the doctor would know his or her new patient well. In theory. But in practice, admitting patients on other wards would be stressful, another duty to add to what everyone already had to do. The other wards were not prepared for the patient who was much sicker than billed; who had to be sent back to the acute hospital right away; who had the wrong diagnosis or was on the wrong medications. The admitting ward was an investment that paid off in correct diagnoses and discontinued medications and in the diminishing of stress throughout the hospital.

The admitting ward was also a symbol of medicine's place in the hospital. Dr. Curtis used to call it the brain of the hospital, because if you had a question about a patient, all you had to do was ask the admitting doctors. The admitting ward was where you would go for a second opinion on a patient, an X-ray, or a lab test, about a difficult family or a confusing diagnosis. Without it, I wasn't sure that medicine would have a central place in the hospital any longer.

Perhaps Dr. Dan felt the same way.

Now I began doing something I'd never done before: I was what physicians call the "covering doctor" and what nurses call a "floater." I held the hospital beeper, I ran the Code Blues, and I floated on the tide of every day to whichever wards lacked their sick or vacationing doctor.

I liked my new position a lot. I saw patients I'd admitted long before and how they were doing. I visited all the wards in the hospital and learned how unique each one was, despite their superficial similarity.

I had many adventures. I diagnosed a case of pseudopseudohypoparathyroidism, that bizarrely named rare disease I had vowed to diagnose at least once when we learned about it in medical school. I explored the obscure wing of the hospital where the podiatry students still lived, receiving board and room in exchange for their services as had been done for a hundred years. I discovered Room Eleven. But above all, I met Mr. Meng Tam and experienced what resuscitation really means.

Even now, years after his Great Event of Death, Meng Tam remains a mystery to me. Like the Cheshire Cat, his smile is all I know of him for sure.

It's a sweet smile, though slightly askew now from his recent stroke. It's a wide smile, for Mr. Tam still has all his teeth, and a wise smile, with eyes crinkling down at the corners. It's a shy smile, a child's smile or a bodhisattva's smile, and behind it is a whole life and chosen way of being, though to this day I don't know what that way of being is.

Here's what I do know about Mr. Meng Tam.

He was picked up by the paramedics and brought to the County

Hospital for the first time after he totaled his new white Toyota Camry. He wasn't admitted, but that is how he got his social worker. It was she who noticed how neglected Mr. Tam's basement apartment was and decided he must be moved into a board-and-care home. In the meantime, she found him a new apartment. He moved into it on the first of April, and on the second of April the paramedics found him wandering in the rain.

So they took him to the County Hospital for the second time. In the emergency room, he told the doctor he was just trying to get back into his old apartment because he couldn't get into his new one, and a neighbor had called the police. The doctor thought Mr. Tam seemed fine enough but, while arranging to send him home, asked him a few more questions, and discovered that Meng Tam did not know his address or his phone number, his doctor or where his family lived, except that they all lived in China. Further questioning revealed that Mr. Tam did not know the day, date, or year, or where he was. So he was admitted to the hospital to find out why he was demented and whether he could still live alone.

He was given a complete dementia workup, with all necessary blood tests and X-rays, and he was evaluated by a psychiatrist. The blood tests were fine; the brain scans showed a lot of little strokes; and the psychiatrist decided that he was demented and possibly psychotic, because Mr. Tam told him that he was a professor of literature and had come to this country for his PhD and to inform people about counterrevolutionary activities. Psychiatric testing confirmed that Mr. Tam could no longer manage for himself, and so he came to us.

This was before the admitting ward was closed, and when I met him for the first time, he was sitting in the chair next to his bed. He had a full head of graying hair and a calm, proud demeanor, and he looked like the professor he'd said he was. An easy smile lit up his otherwise stolid and forbidding face, which, with just a wisp of added beard, would have been the classic face of a Chinese sage.

But he was certainly demented. When I asked him who was governor, he said "Reagan," and when I asked him who was president, he said, "Reagan, too." He took a long time to answer the simplest question, if he answered it at all. Worst was when I asked him to draw a clock, which is a usual question in the mental-status exam. I watched as he laboriously drew a circle with a center, put in lines that went out from the center, and then connected them to one another like a web. It was a bizarre clock and the sign of a severe dementia.

What was the cause, or causes, of his dementia? I found the signs of untreated high blood pressure when I looked in his eyes, which would account for the little strokes on his brain scan, and pointed to multi-infarct dementia. His walk was shuffling and wide-based, which meant some additional neurologic condition, perhaps B_{12} deficiency, which can also cause dementia. His stolid face and slow movements suggested Parkinson's dementia, Lewy body dementia, or depression. So most likely Mr. Tam's dementia was multifactorial: three parts stroke, one part depression, one part Parkinson's, one part Alzheimer's, and one part . . . something else. There must be something else, I thought, because the course of Mr. Tam's dementia had been so rapid. After all, two months before he'd been well enough to buy a car and drive it, albeit into a wall. So Mr. Tam was a mystery.

This being Laguna Honda, however, I had the time to wait and see—for family and friends to show up and fill me in on the details; for Mr. Tam to get better or worse or stay the same; for a trial of medications to treat his possible depression, Alzheimer's, Parkinson's. In short, for Slow Medicine to do its job.

I would begin by tapering him off all the medications he didn't need. Then I would give him an antidepressant, an Alzheimer drug, and a Parkinson drug, one after the other, and we would see.

But we didn't see, because a few days after he was admitted, a bed became available out in Clarendon Hall, and Mr. Tam was transferred. Nevertheless, over the next year and a half he did get a trial of antidepressants, an Alzheimer drug, and a Parkinson drug. But nothing worked, and he was worse. He stopped talking and walking; he stayed in bed and refused medications and blood tests. Sometimes he spit at the nurses. And no friends or family ever showed up.

He was so demented that he was assigned a public guardian to make decisions for him, and she was able to find out more about him. Much of what Mr. Tam had told the psychiatrist turned out to be true. He had come to this country for his PhD, although she couldn't confirm his counterrevolutionary activities. He did become a professor at the university and, until two years before, had been investing in real estate and the stock market. His dementia, therefore, was quite rapid, and it was all the more remarkable that during the year and a half at Clarendon, it hadn't progressed very much. He should have been way worse than he was and probably dead. So Mr. Tam was still a mystery.

But Dr. Dan was emptying Clarendon, and Mr. Tam was transferred back to the main building and into the care of Dr. Mack.

I liked Dr. Mack a lot. He always reminded me of a television doctor, but in a good way. He had thick, short, silver hair parted on the right, a tanned face, and a smile that creased the corners of his blue eyes all the way down to his cheeks. He usually carried a stethoscope and wore a white coat, white shirt, and silk tie. He was polite but ironic, widely experienced, and a good doctor; and Mr. Tam's rapid deterioration worried him. So after he met Mr. Tam, he went over all of the records, examined him, and then began fussing with the colorful bunch of medications that Mr. Tam had collected over the eighteen months of his hospitalization.

Which is how I met Meng Tam for the second time.

t was late in the afternoon, and I was covering the hospital. It was quiet, and I was in my office reading medical journals when my beeper went off. It was Dr. Mack.

"I have a patient who is dying," he said. "He's a Do Not Resuscitate and, don't worry, you won't have to do anything; I'll stay with him until he dies, which should be in about twenty minutes. But he's going in and out of ventricular tachycardia and has an intermittent pulse and no blood pressure, and I thought you might be interested."

I wasn't sure why Dr. Mack thought I'd be interested. Perhaps he'd read one of my essays on the care of the dying or perhaps he knew I was always ready to see something I'd never seen before. Or perhaps there was some other reason. It didn't matter and I told him I'd be right up.

As I climbed the stairs, I went over what I knew about ventricular tachycardia. It's a tachy cardia—a fast heart rhythm—from the Greek *tachys*, meaning fast, and *kardia*, meaning heart; and it comes from the ventricles, the heart's main pumps. It is usually a predeath heart rhythm. Normally the heart beats in its steady, organized way because of a few hundred cells in the sinus node of the heart. Those cells have a specialized membrane that slowly leaks out calcium and sodium. That leakage decreases the voltage inside the cell; and the moment that voltage gets down to a certain level, those cells twitch;

their membranes open up in the opposite direction; and the calcium and sodium flow back inside. That twitch is what sends an electric current through the heart, and that current is what causes the heart to beat.

Those cells start their leaking, twitch, and electric current when we are fetuses of forty days, and they continue to twitch once a second or so for the rest of our lives, unless something goes wrong—a heart attack, an electrolyte imbalance, a drug toxicity. When they stop twitching, we die, unless a different group of cells somewhere else in the heart takes over. If that group of cells is in the ventricles, it produces a "ventricular rhythm"; and if that rhythm is very fast, it is a "ventricular tachycardia."

But ventricular tachycardia is not a stable rhythm. It is too fast to pump the heart properly, and after twenty minutes or so, it usually deteriorates into "ventricular fibrillation," a disorganized wiggling of the heart muscle that does not pump blood at all. A few minutes after that, the heart stops.

There are, however, treatments for ventricular tachycardia. Often a simple electric shock or certain intravenous medications will convert it into a stable rhythm. Of course, as Dr. Mack told me, his patient was a "Do Not Resuscitate" (DNR): in the event of a cardiac arrest, he was not to be resuscitated. But did that mean that we were not to try to convert his predeath ventricular tachycardia with electric shock or medications? Dr. Mack was a good doctor; more important, he was a wise doctor, I thought as I walked into the ward, so there must be a reason why we were going to simply wait for his patient to die.

It was early evening and the nursing station was cool and empty except for Dr. Mack. I sat down and he handed me the EKG and rhythm strips he'd just obtained. Mr. Tam was a new patient to him, he explained, and over the past month, he'd been decreasing Mr. Tam's medications, many of which were not needed. He had monitored the functioning of Mr. Tam's liver, lungs, and heart as he did so, and they had all been fine. So he couldn't understand why Mr. Tam, that afternoon, went into this predeath rhythm of ventricular tachycardia. Was it one of the changes he'd made in Mr. Tam's medications? Was it some obscure interaction among his many medications? Was there something he'd missed?

"Most likely he just had a heart attack," I reassured him. "He's the right age."

Then I spread out Mr. Tam's EKG on the counter. His EKG was impressive. The shark-tooth line of ventricular tachycardia was there, although it was a healthy and strong ventricular tachycardia, with sharp QRS waves marching across the grid of the EKG paper. It wouldn't be so crisp shortly, I knew. Even now those sharp peaks of Mr. Tam's heart rhythm must be starting to sag, getting rounder and shorter, faster and less regular, as the life force they were sparking dribbled out of them. Soon, like mountains wearing down into foothills and then into flat land, they would begin to merge with the flat line of death. Looking at the EKG, I imagined how Mr. Tam's pulse would feel, bounding up for a few beats, then stopping, then sputtering up again, like a car running out of gas. Sometimes even after a patient is dead, you can feel an occasional beat of pulse or see a blip on the EKG strip.

It was quiet in the nursing station, with that particular quiet and calm you expect as night begins to fall. It was so quiet that it disturbed me, and I lifted up my head from the EKG. Almost everyone had gone home. The day nurses and nurses' aides, the social workers and utilization review managers, who all, somehow, found a place in that small nursing station during the day, were gone, and the

cacophony of voices, buzzers, and beeps gone with them. The charts
of the ward's patients were all back for the night in their rack. Only
Mr. Tam's chart was not back where it belonged, where it would never
be again; it was open on the desk in front of me. My attention fell back
to his EKG, and I wondered if he was dead when Dr. Mack asked,
"Would you like to see him?"

I would, so Dr. Mack and I walked through the ward. We came to
the second-to-the-last bed on the right, and there was the body of
Meng Tam. His head was propped up on several pillows, and his face
was the sallow gray of no circulation. His eyes were half closed and
rolled back so that the whites showed, and his mouth was beginning
to tighten into the *risus sardonicus*—the twisted smile—of death. The
nurse had pulled the sheets up to his neck and tucked them in around
him, and when I pulled them back, they were wet and cold from some
last sweat.

I touched the body. It was doughy, clammy, and cold as ice—
colder than ice really, because ice is, after all, still alive in its own
way—it melts and changes, it warms and flows. But the flesh of the
dead body is thick and doughy, cool where you expect it to be warm,
doughy where you expect it to be resilient. The body was still as well
as cold, and when I felt Mr. Tam's clammy wrist, there was no pulse.

I looked up at Dr. Mack, who was standing on the other side of
the bed. Behind him was the evening nurse, who was watching the
scene while he handed out medications to the other patients, waiting
for the signal to cover the body and call the morgue. But just at that
moment, out of the corner of my eye, I saw a movement from Mr.
Tam's body.

It was his chest, rising and falling. Although he had no pulse and
no blood pressure, Mr. Tam was still breathing. Quite evenly, as a
matter of fact. And when I looked back to his face I saw that, though

his eyes were rolled back and only the whites showed, they seemed somehow aware of me. I stared at his chest and so did Dr. Mack. How long would it keep moving?

I thought about the ventricular tachycardia on the EKG strip in the nursing station. It would be so easy to just shock that ventricular tachycardia back to life. All it would take was a little jolt of electricity. There would be the shock of the shock; the body rising out of the bed, then falling back; then the flat line of the EKG, signifying death, but only for a few seconds. Suddenly would appear those little marching soldiers of a normal sinus rhythm, in calm order, once every second from those amazing sinus cells, and the corresponding steady pulse, blood pressure, and circulation of the living.

But Mr. Tam was a Do Not Resuscitate, a DNR. He had an order that he was not to be resuscitated and Dr. Mack had interpreted this to mean that in the event of a cardiac arrest, which this was, Mr. Tam was not to have any defibrillatory shock. And so I stood by the bed, holding his cold wrist, staring at his stiffening visage, and waiting for his breathing to stop.

As I did so, I realized that Mr. Tam was no stranger to me—he was Meng Tam, who'd wrecked his new Toyota Camry and who thought he was a professor, and I knew him from the admitting ward. I tried to think how his DNR had been obtained. While he was at the County Hospital, on the basis of medical futility? I didn't think so. In the months after he left the admitting ward? I didn't know. Had his mind cleared enough to voice his wishes? Had his public guardian decided on the DNR?

I wondered: Whoever had requested or assented to Mr. Tam's DNR—what did they mean by it? Did they mean this particular case?

Not that it mattered, because there was the DNR, neatly written in the Advance Life Directive section of Mr. Tam's chart, and here he was, dying. He was pretty much dead, actually, which seems an odd thing to say, like saying someone is pretty much pregnant. But it turns out that someone can be pretty much pregnant at first, just as the fertilized egg starts to divide, and in the same way, Meng Tam was pretty much dead.

Or was he?

He had no pulse, true. His circulation had failed, and he was getting colder by the second, but he was still breathing, calmly and smoothly.

Then Dr. Mack said, "You know, if I move his leg a little, he goes into atrial fibrillation and his pulse comes back."

Dr. Mack did move Meng Tam's leg, and I felt a pulse at the wrist, irregular and weak, but still, something. He put the leg down; the pulse disappeared; and Mr. Tam recommenced dying.

Not only that, but with that movement and pulse, Mr. Tam's eyelids fluttered open; his eyes rolled down; and he looked right at me. I looked back at him and for a moment we looked—really looked—at each other. And it was as if I saw him, all of him, present at the back of his eyes—not just his face, but his whole person, there in the back of his eyes—and as if he saw me, in my eyes, in the same way.

We looked at each other, and Hildegard's lines about dying came into my mind: "It is as if the soul, the *anima,* stands with one foot in this world and one in the next, uncertain whether to stay or go." That was just it. Meng Tam was undecided. He was halfway between life and death. And as I looked into his eyes, which were soft, shining, almost a greenish color, I saw them become clear and still, like a shallow mountain pool after a rain, and I knew that he had decided to stay. I can't tell you that I nodded, but I knew, and Meng Tam knew that I knew, that he was coming back.

But he was a DNR, and Dr. Mack's interpretation of DNR was

that, in the event of a cardiac arrest—which this was—no resuscitative measures were to be used. I had a different interpretation of DNR, but Meng Tam's bedside was no place for a philosophical discussion of the point.

So I took an inventory of what we had—consciousness and breath; of what we didn't have—the warmth and animation of the body; and of what we had in part—a pulse, now and again. Then I remembered how, in the days before Code Blues, at this point—at least in those old black-and-white movies—the doctor would slap the patient's face, call his name, and shake him, as if you could slap, call, or shake someone back to life, just like you wake someone up.

So that was what I did.

I called Meng Tam's name, and I shook him, and Dr. Mack started to move his legs. I even slapped his face a few times. And sure enough, Meng Tam's pulse returned; it became quite steady; and then his eyes opened and stayed open, staring at me.

Next I thought about the relationship between neurologic and cardiac function—the head and the heart. The nurse had positioned Meng Tam comfortably for death with his head on several pillows. This was fine for death but not for life because, although his pulse was now steady, his blood pressure wasn't much, not enough to push the blood up against gravity into his brain. So I cranked the head of the bed all the way down until Meng Tam was as upside down as he could be, with gravity in his favor. Blood started to flow from his legs into his dusky face, which began to lighten from gray to almost pink, and his pulse became quite strong.

Dr. Mack and I looked at each other. "Blankets," I remembered from those same old movies and, what else? Ah, yes—hot water bottles; and so the nurse, who had been watching our nonresuscitation efforts, hurried to get warmed blankets and fresh sheets, and an IV pole and fluids. Now that Meng Tam was alive and not dead, we could use IVs.

The nurse tucked the warm blankets around him and started an IV, while Dr. Mack and I jiggled him whenever his pulse faltered or his attention wavered. Slowly he pinked up and warmed up, and then, all of a sudden, he opened his eyes completely, looked at me, and smiled.

The nurse shook his head and muttered, half to himself and half to me, "I've never seen anything like this."

Neither had I.

I'd been at many resuscitations, some of them successful, but never in the quiet and stillness of Meng Tam's; never with the time and space to watch the soul, the *anima,* stop in that dark tunnel with the light at its end and waver. Being with Meng Tam when he heard my voice, watching as he weighed forward or backward, Death or Life, and seeing the flicker of decision in the back of his eyes. Feeling that moment of turning and then observing him revivify—pulse, blood pressure, color, consciousness, smile.

It was more than catching life as a force or substance; it was catching life as a particular energy, as Meng Tam's energy. About to disappear, implode, pass through an impenetrable door; see its hand on the door knob and, half out the door, stop, turn back to say one last thing, and then watch it all in reverse. The pulse pick up, the blood pressure elevate, the color go from dusky to pink, the brightness come back into the eyes. It was an experience of pure life, as distinct from anything life does—move or talk or be—except, of course, for breathe, which was the one thing that Meng Tam did very well.

In my first autopsy I'd been surprised by the difference between the dead body and the live Mr. Baker I'd known. There was something missing—that I missed, and that I'd missed. And now with Mr. Tam I'd caught it; seen it go toward death, stop, change its mind, and come back. I'd seen the *anima*—that which animates the body and the mind.

Hildegard has an illumination that shows the *anima* as a ghostly blur leaving the mouth in that last breath of death; and she has another illumination of that same ghostly *anima* flowing into the fetus in the womb. What she meant was that when the *anima* leaves the body is the moment of death and when it enters the body is the moment of birth. Which, according to medieval medicine, was the moment that the heart starts to beat; the moment, from our point of view, when those few hundred cells leak calcium and sodium for the first time, twitch, and send that electric current around the heart, and the heart makes the first of its two billion usually perfect beats.

Meng Tam survived and even flourished.

Dr. Mack kept me informed of his slow but steady progress. He began to talk a bit and walk a bit, and Dr. Mack had extravagant hopes that one day Meng Tam would talk enough to tell us about his life and walk enough to walk out of the hospital. On the anniversary of his nondeath, I went around to see him. He looked well. He was calm, alert, and attentive, and when I greeted him, he looked at me and smiled.

Not too long after Meng's resuscitation, workmen began taking apart Clarendon Hall. Mr. Conley announced that they would start on the inside, removing any reusable, transplantable items—pipes, sinks, stoves, lights. Once that was completed, they would disconnect the utilities: water, gas, and, last, electricity. Then they would begin on the outside, taking away windows and window frames, doors, brass fixtures, copper—anything useful or salable. When they had finished, the building would be demolished, and we were all invited.

Twelve

THE SPIRIT OF GOD'S HOTEL

THE MONTHS PASSED.

Dr. Dan, now freed from admitting patients, grappled with the surrounding chaos like the flawed knight he was. He arrived at the hospital even earlier and left even later. After he laid off the nighttime doctors and assigned the daytime doctors to their shifts, he himself took the most shifts and the worst. On Christmas Day he came in to the hospital to hand out the presents, one by one.

The daytime doctors did start coming in at night, with covering doctors taking care of our patients on the days we were on nighttime duty, and the clear lines of command about whose decision should prevail began to blur. Some days patients had one doctor, and other days another. Medications were changed frequently; important details—laboratory reports, clinical changes in patients—began to be missed. The nurses were confused about whom to call when a patient got sick; the families were confused; we were confused. Pretty soon,

Dr. Dan started rehiring the night and weekend doctors he'd laid off. Fortunately, this being the city, he was able to use a different part of his budget to rehire them, so on paper it still looked like the medical department had been cut by one-third.

The city accepted the Department of Justice settlement, and the ten-year investigation was closed. The new marketing department began formulating our first branding campaign, and the destruction of Clarendon Hall was about to begin. Soon the old hospital I'd known would be gone. I started to ask myself: What could I take with me? How could I pass its lessons along?

I could think of two ways. First was the ecomedicine project I'd been musing about for so long. It could test my hypothesis that Slow Medicine provides as good a medical outcome as does Modern Efficient Health Care, while being less expensive and more satisfying for patients, families, and staff. I would set it up as a separate ecomedicine unit—the ECU—and apply what I'd learned over the years to a two-year group of patients: a careful workup, minimal medications, tincture of time, and the little things. I would track the savings from correct diagnoses instead of incorrect ones, and the consequent decrease in medications—with their costly side effects and adverse reactions—against the expense of well-staffed medical and nursing care, plus excellent food and drink. It would be a proof of principle.

I told Dr. Dan about my idea. He liked it and was delighted to anoint me "director of the ecomedicine project." Although, he warned me, my project wouldn't be the next thing. The move to the new facility would take up everyone's time and energy for a few years. It might be the next next thing, though, after everyone had settled in, and the health-care pendulum reached its apogee and began to swing back.

I could think of a second way to pass along the lessons of the old hospital. I could tell its stories and its story. So I began putting together a timeline of my years there, which soon wrapped itself around the four walls of my study.

was just starting to write *God's Hotel* when workmen began demolishing the century-old Clarendon Hall.

They started with its west and south wings, harvesting windows and window frames, faucets and sinks; then they moved to the East Wing. They took Clarendon Hall apart the way termites take things apart, leaving the outside intact until the end. Then they disconnected the water, gas, and electricity. It reminded me of what happens when a patient is declared brain-dead: The healthy organs are harvested, then the oxygen is disconnected, the IV taken out, and the EKG turned off. After that, the workmen began on the outside, taking away copper pipes and clay tiles, sculptural elements, landscape. Finally Clarendon Hall was ready.

Since I'd missed the barbecue for the blowing-up of the bridge that once connected Clarendon to the main building, I made sure to be present for its demolition. When the day came, I walked over. From the outside, the building still looked as elegant as ever, an Edwardian one hundred years old.

With a few others, I stood behind the wire fence and watched. The greenery around the building had been taken away, and in the dirt that remained was a machine that looked like a praying mantis made out of metal. It lumbered with neck jutting out and jaws open until it came to a corner of the building. It stopped, took a bite out of the tiled roof, tore a piece off with a little jerk, and threw it on the ground. Then it lumbered to its next position, took another bite, and threw the next piece on the ground. It went all round the building like this, and the insides of Clarendon were gradually exposed. It was a tough old building, though, and pieces of cement and old steel rebar stuck out of its walls for quite a while. But bit by bit it diminished. By the end of the day, Clarendon Hall was rubble; by the next week, the rubble had been cleared, the foundation filled in, and the ground made ready for whatever would come next.

Two weeks later, Sister Miriam resigned. She did not go gentle into her good night, however. Instead, she wrote an article for the local newspaper about how it broke her heart to say good-bye to the beautiful spirit of Clarendon. It was a symbol of the unique and warm atmosphere of Laguna Honda that for so long had served the city's most vulnerable population, she wrote. And she warned: Draconian cuts were being made to the hospital, though oh-so-quietly. The number of patients had already been cut by a third; the hospice chaplain laid off; the day program terminated—all due to the "budget crisis." Yet there was still enough money to hire Wide Angle Communications—the mayor's communication consultant—to support "the hospital's journey from institution to community." Citizens should keep a close eye on what was going on at Laguna Honda, she ended.

In addition to her article, Sister Miriam nominated her successor, Sister Margaret. In appearance, Sister Margaret was as different from Sister Miriam as she could be. Black skin, black hair, dark eyes, lilting Jamaican accent, small blue and white veil perched modestly on her head. But in temperament, they were just alike, as administration would soon discover.

Meanwhile, Mr. Conley was working on next year's budget. It would be different from any other budget the hospital had ever had, he thought, because, with the next year's move to the new facility, it would have to fund both new and old hospitals at the same time. He was wrong about the move, but right about the budget. It would be different from any other budget the hospital had ever had because, for the first time, the budget would be cut.

Now a budget crisis came every year and had a pattern. It would begin with terrifying predictions of immense deficits, which would increase as the unions negotiated their contracts and politicians jockeyed for staff. There would be demonstrations against proposed cuts, and a deeper projected deficit would be announced, followed by pleading and compromise. Then, along about May, there would be the stunning discovery of millions of dollars of revenue that the controller had somehow overlooked, with reconciliation, smiles, and a budget bigger than the year before.

But this year the budget crisis was different. Times were, in fact, bad. People would, in fact, be laid off, and public health services would, in fact, be cut. The only question was: Which ones?

The medical department was in a particularly bad position. Dr. Stein did not like us and would not save us from any cuts. Dr. Dan had already laid off the night and weekend doctors, and we had no administrative staff whose positions he could merge and rename. Plus, in preparation for the move, the number of our patients was going to be decreased by 20 percent. So it was hard for Dr. Dan to get around the fact that he would have to cut his doctors by that same amount.

Except that the doctors did generate revenue when we saw patients, and Dr. Dan reasoned that if he could show Mr. Conley that the medical department paid for itself, at least partially, it would decrease the number of doctors he would have to lay off. So Dr. Dan began collecting data on each physician's services. Since this was not on any computer, it meant that he had to go around to every ward and look at every chart, and keep an account of what each of his doctors produced. Soon his "Productivity Reports" began to appear in our wooden mailboxes, proving how much we earned every month for the city, in theory. Although not in practice, because the billing department had no idea how much it billed for our services or any other services, nor how much it received. However, according to his accounting, the medical department earned one-half of its budget, and Dr. Dan hoped for a happy result to his efforts.

Which made me conclude that Dr. Dan was a closet idealist. Because his figures did not matter to Mr. Conley, and Dr. Dan still had to cut five physicians from his budget.

Whom would he cut? What criteria would he use? Dr. Dan spent a weekend reflecting. He would use seniority, he decided, but not mainly; he wanted young blood as well as old, energy as well as experience. He would look at board certification, comfort in doing procedures, willingness to work full-time, and other unspecified characteristics. He sketched out a form, printed it out, and called a meeting of the medical staff.

It was a short meeting. Dr. Dan explained the budget problem and handed out his forms. We looked at them. Were they mandatory?

No, they were voluntary. Although it would be easier for him to make his decision if everyone filled out a form. If someone didn't fill out a form—well, he would just have to fill it out himself.

After the meeting, a big sign appeared in Jerrie's office reminding us to fill in the forms, and there was a folder below the sign that stayed almost empty.

Then Dr. Dan called another meeting.

The budget had taken a turn for the worse, he announced, and Dr. Stein was demanding that in addition to the five doctors to be laid off in the next budget, four additional doctors had to be laid off this year. He would let us know who they would be the next week. And now Mr. Conley had a few things to tell us.

Then Mr. Conley came into the room. He looked tired. His red hair was thinner and grayer and so was his beard; his eyes were weary, and his voice was hoarse. He wanted to let us know that marketing had presented its branding campaign, and we now had a tagline and a value statement. Our new tagline was: "Laguna Honda—A Community of Care," which, he was sure we would agree, was a good description of the place. Our new value statement was: "Our Residents Come First." Marketing was still working on our new logo, our new mission, and our new name.

At this, the medical staff came to life. Heads came up from charts, journals, and tabletops. Mr. Conley was taken aback by the sudden attention.

Yes, a new name. Laguna Honda had to be repositioned and rebranded; it would not do for the new facility to be seen as an old-fashioned almshouse for the poor. The new Laguna Honda was going to be a Center of Excellence, focusing on health, wellness, and rehabilitation; and marketing had decided, therefore, that "Hospital" should be taken out of our name.

Mr. Conley looked around. Everyone was staring at him. No one spoke. And then everyone spoke at once.

If Laguna Honda was not a hospital, we asked, then who were those sick, demented, frail, one- or no-legged, coughing, yellow people we took care of every day? In their wheelchairs, gurneys, and beds? With their IVs, feeding tubes, catheters, casts, oxygen, and tracheotomies? What were they doing here? Where would they be in the new, no-hospital Laguna Honda? Would they be elsewhere?

Mr. Conley didn't hang his head exactly, but he did stop and stare into space for a moment. A vision went past his tired blue eyes. Those

patients. The ones whose beds he sat on, whose hands he, even he, Mr.
Conley, BS, MPH, executive administrator, held.

"Hospital" stayed in our name.

I t was the day before Thanksgiving.

Phoebe, our new secretary, told me when I came in that Dr. Dan
was going to notify the losers of the layoff lottery that day. He would
page them into his office, one by one. She knew who they were, of
course, and after I'd looked into her eyes—and considered the case of
Janice Gilroy—I felt pretty safe. I was paged all day long but never by
Dr. Dan, and in the late afternoon I went back to Phoebe's office to
find out who the laid-off doctors were.

Dr. Dan's choices were puzzling. He'd laid off Dr. Lydia, our oldest and longest-serving physician who'd been so helpful with Radka,
and Dr. Rajif, our youngest and last-hired physician. I could see Dr.
Lydia, who no longer needed the job financially, and Dr. Rajif, the last
hired. But he'd also laid off Dr. Stacks, tall and thin and African-
American. Had personnel told him to play it safe and choose one of
each—tall and short, white and black, young and old? His fourth
choice, though, was Dr. Talley, and I was nonplussed. Dr. Talley fulfilled every one of Dr. Dan's stated criteria: She was board-certified,
procedure-doing, and full-time. Plus, she was intelligent and cheerful, competent and beautiful. If Dr. Dan could fire Dr. Talley, he
could fire anyone.

Everyone wanted to know: What had been his criteria?

Dr. Dan wouldn't say. He didn't have to. The doctors served at
the pleasure of the medical director; he was assistant medical director, and Dr. Sonnen, upstairs, had agreed with his selection.

Over lunch, in our offices, and in the hallways, we looked at one another with a certain look. A rebellion began, like one of those fires that start with a frayed wire, a spark, and then a flame spreading under the floor and into the walls. One by one and unknown to one another, the doctors went to talk to Mr. Conley and then to Dr. Stein. It wasn't organized. But it was fierce and resolute.

On the first working day of the new year I walked into Phoebe's office to sign in. Dr. Dan was standing in the doorway, white as a ghost. Dr. Jeffers, looking solemn, was walking out. Something had happened.

I looked at Dr. Jeffers and we exchanged the glances of people who've known each other for years. Something had happened—yes. He couldn't talk about it; it was not quite as serious as his solemnity implied; I should talk to Larissa. So I found Larissa and, sure enough, although no more than forty-five minutes had elapsed since whatever had happened, had happened, she knew all about it.

"Dr. Dan and Dr. Sonnen have been fired," she told me, with a gleam in her disenchanted eyes. "First thing this morning. Mr. Conley called Dr. Sonnen into his office and told him he had to retire and Dr. Dan's job had been eliminated. And by the way, the layoffs of the four doctors were rescinded, since the elimination of his and Dr. Sonnen's positions satisfied Dr. Stein's budgetary requirements."

Now, Larissa liked Dr. Dan, but she also liked Dr. Talley. And administrative reversals of fortune warmed her Russian soul. So she was saddened, amused, and relieved all at once. Also alert. In her experience, such reversals meant other changes—abrupt promotions and demotions, capitulations, even executions—and she was usually on the wrong side. So she didn't want to talk too long. In these situations, you never knew who might be listening.

The news went around the hospital as quickly as only word of mouth can. Many nurses asked me why Dr. Dan was fired.

I could only guess. Dr. Talley was a friend of Dr. Stein's, but I didn't think that was the reason. It had more to do with Dr. Dan's pushing back against the changes coming down. He'd come to understand the uncoordinated but relentless pressure squeezing the hospital's Old Medicine into the New Health Care, and he had resisted, with flushed face and with eloquence. True, he inclined more toward the Way of Nursing than the Way of Medicine, but it was to Miss Lester's Way of Nursing, which was, in one respect at least, the same as the Way of Medicine: Both were personal, and health care was not. Dr. Dan was in the Way, and he was in the way.

Dr. Dan didn't leave immediately. He finished all the tasks he'd taken on, found a new position, and packed up his office. He sent around a thank-you note to all the staff. He signed off his patients to other doctors. Then he walked to every ward and took his leave of every nurse, and left Laguna Honda for the second time.

Then Mr. Conley himself called a meeting of the medical staff. His red beard was almost white, and there was a new bulge around his middle and bulges under his eyes, which were slightly out of focus. He no longer looked like the young Henry VIII at the time of his wedding to Anne Boleyn; he looked like Henry VIII after Anne's head was cut off.

What he wanted to tell us was that the decision to dismiss Dr. Dan and Dr. Sonnen was entirely his. Dr. Stein had no part in it. As he said this, he looked at us in a vague way and we did not believe him. He could not have dismissed the medical director and the assistant medical director without the involvement of Dr. Stein. Besides, it wasn't in him.

Also, he'd hired a search firm to find a medical director for the new Laguna Honda, someone experienced and efficient, and board-certified in medical directing. In the meantime, Dr. Jeffers would be acting medical director. Everyone looked over at Dr. Jeffers, who shrugged and smiled. That was fine with us. We liked Dr. Jeffers. He would do whatever was necessary and nothing more.

Six weeks later Mr. Conley did not show up for his morning carpool.

This had never happened before and so his carpool called the paramedics, who went over to his apartment. When he did not answer their knocks, they broke down the door. They found Mr. Conley sitting on the sofa in his work clothes, tie off, collar loosened, and dead. That afternoon the coroner did an autopsy and determined that Mr. Conley had died at seven-thirty the night before, of a heart attack due to the sudden blockage of a large coronary artery by a blood clot on top of an existing cholesterol plaque.

But we knew that Mr. Conley had died of Laguna Honda. It had just been too much. The budget cuts; the patients and the name change; the firings of Dr. Dan and Dr. Sonnen.

His memorial service took place in the recreation hall, and it was filled with staff and patients. A photo of him from his first days at the hospital, when his beard was still red and his eyes still bright, hung on an easel in the front. There was a color guard and bagpipes, and Dr. Stein bicycled over to give the encomium. Dr. Stein even cried. He felt responsible for Mr. Conley's death, he told us. Mr. Conley had been a friend of his and took on the job of transforming the old alms-house into a modern health-care facility to help him out, and he felt responsible for the death.

The next day, Dr. Stein announced Mr. Conley's replacement. It was Mirene Larose, RN, MS, CNS, also a friend of Dr. Stein's and our current co-director of nursing.

Mirene was small and wore tiny but expensive skirt-suits, with stockings and pumps; and she was warm and enthusiastic, confident and decisive. She had a wide smile and an open face, and was easy to like, especially at first. The day after her appointment, she moved into Mr. Conley's office, and the day after that she fired her only competition, the other co-director of nursing. The next week she sent around a revised organization chart that showed the previously medical departments of laboratory, radiology, and social work transferred from medicine to herself.

And that was just the beginning.

Mirene's main ally in her new job was Adrian Serf, director of marketing. He was a petite, dapper man, with well-cut brown hair, curious brown eyes, and a birdlike tilt to his head. When he arrived at Laguna Honda, he put his new marketing department in the priest's flat in the turret, redecorating its old-fashioned bathroom and kitchen in creams and taupes. The turret had its own entrance, and so he could come and go without the distraction of entering the hospital. Adrian was just about the only man left standing and he stepped up to the plate. He began attending the meetings that Dr. Dan once went to, and whenever there was a problem in the hospital—even a medical problem—there he was. He filled the niche left by Dr. Dan, although, as a lawyer, he was more concerned that nothing went wrong than that something went right.

Mirene and Adrian began making the key decisions at the hospital, in consultation with Dr. Stein and the mayor, of course. And although their decisions were not bruited about, there was a lot going on, a kind of strange, out-of-balance tension; you could feel it. Every day there were new forms, committees, directives. Nurses

THE SPIRIT OF GOD'S HOTEL

were promoted, demoted, or transferred; doctors disappeared; wards were closed. And week after week there were retirement parties and the consequent reshuffling of staff.

The final straw was the Ja Report.

Davis Ja, PhD, had been hired by Mirene and Adrian simply to document the psychiatric care in the old hospital, but he used his report in addition to lay out a kind of blueprint for the new facility. It was going to be a radically different place, his report made clear; and for the first time we, the doctors, finally understood the plans. After the move, Laguna Honda Hospital would no longer be an independent hospital but part of the County Hospital, and the director of public health would henceforth be in charge of the medical staff and patient admissions. Almost half of the new facility would be reserved for the psychiatric homeless, and the focus for the rest of the patients would be on rehabilitation and a speedy discharge. Even the model of care would be different we learned. In the new Laguna Honda, the old-fashioned "medical model" of physicians would be replaced by a "social model"—whatever that was—and "health-care workers," nurses, social workers, and psychologists not physicians, would take care of "clients."

It was a pretty stunning blueprint, although we'd had plenty of hints about where the hospital was headed. Still, we'd all been in denial. I, for one, had always thought that whatever happened, the spirit of what I privately, in my own my mind, called "God's Hotel" would somehow triumph. But after the Ja Report, I wasn't so sure and I began to wonder whether my twenty-year escape from health care was coming to an end.

Many of the doctors felt the same way and Drs. Kay and Romero, according to their temperament, wrote a brilliant rebuttal proving the Ja Report ill-conceived, poorly thought out, and illegal. Articles began appearing in the neighborhood association's newspaper about the Ja Report, letting it be known that the new Laguna Honda was slated to become a psychiatric facility for the homeless.

Next, Drs. Kay and Romero demanded an audit of the two-million-dollar Patient Gift Fund. Now, there was no policy connection between the Ja Report and the Patient Gift Fund. But there was a strategic connection because Drs. Kay and Romero had discovered that hundreds of thousands of dollars were missing from the fund, and they knew that Mirene, as head of the hospital, would be drawn into any scandal resulting from that. She would bring Adrian, as her chief advisor, along with her; also Dr. Stein, as her supervisor, and even, perhaps, the mayor. An investigation of the Patient Gift Fund might put an end to one or all of them, and, therefore, to the radical transformation of the hospital. So when Dr. Kay and Dr. Romero finished their rebuttal to the Ja Report, they requested the records of the Patient Gift Fund, going back to before Mr. Conley's arrival.

Also they submitted an ethics complaint about the financial dealings of Dr. Stein and Mr. Davis Ja.

Mirene, Adrian, Dr. Stein, and the mayor were not happy about these requests and complaints, and Drs. Kay and Romero were stonewalled for months. They received nothing, and the Ja Report was accepted as written.

But immediately after, the medical staff received momentous news. Mirene had finally hired a new medical director. It was Dr. Talley, one of our own doctors, who'd been laid off by Dr. Dan exactly one year before, and whose layoff had precipitated a rebellion. It was a typical Laguna Honda turnaround, in the premodern era known as a Turn of the Wheel of Fortune. Each of us is attached to that wheel, which is Time, and sooner or later we will go down, and sooner or later we will come up.

The medical staff was delighted with Mirene's choice. Dr. Talley was a good doctor; she knew the hospital well; she liked it the way it was and would, we felt sure, try to keep it that way. So she was a hopeful pick, a gauge, we thought, that everything would turn out all right.

Then Dr. Talley called her first meeting of the medical staff. She had several announcements, and all of them were disheartening.

First, Dr. Jeffers was retiring after twenty-eight years. We would miss him, Dr. Talley said, knowing, however, that no one was more deserving of rest and relaxation than Dr. Jeffers. Second, she had decided to move the medical director's office from its old place at the back of the hospital into the administration wing. It was time for medicine to say yes instead of no to change, she told us; to ally itself with administration and nursing—to be part of the solution, not part of the problem.

That got me a little worried.

It was true that medicine and nursing and administration had always been at odds, and with Mirene Larose, RN, MS, CNS, as executive administrator, administration and nursing had effectively been merged. So perhaps medicine should join up, too. But then I remembered what Florence Nightingale had written about the struggle between medicine and nursing and administration. That struggle was irresolvable and should not be resolved, she said, because it was in the patients' best interest. If medicine ever won control of the hospital, too much would be practiced on the patient; if administration, too little; if nursing, medical progress would be curtailed in the interest of the spiritual and emotional care of the patient.

So I worried about Dr. Talley's decision to move medicine in with administration and nursing. What did it mean about the future of medicine at the new Laguna Honda?

Her third announcement was that, due to budget cuts and with deep regret, she was laying off Dr. Kay. Her selection was in no way punitive, she said; it simply reflected the need for the medical department to meet its budgetary challenges and reorganize clinically. It was entirely her decision. Mirene and Dr. Stein had nothing to do with it.

A sigh went through the room. The last person who uttered the phrase "entirely my decision" had died of it. No one wanted Dr. Talley to die or get sick or gray or get bulges under her eyes. We wanted to support her. And Dr. Kay was an interesting choice to lay off. He was principled, and one of his principles was that he would only take care of his own patients. He almost never took call, or helped out, or covered other wards. So no rebellion broke out, and no one spoke up with passion.

Except for Sister Margaret. When Sister Margaret heard about Dr. Kay's layoff, she stormed into Mirene Larose's office, blue-and-white veil streaming behind her. Or so I heard.

"Are you a Catholic!" she shouted. "Tell me, are you a Catholic? How can you fire Dr. Kay? He's the best doctor for the hospice! . . . How can you lie? It's a sin to lie! And what did you do with the money sent by my diocese for the patients? Where is it, eh? A liar! You are a liar, and it's a sin to lie!"

Mirene knew when not to say anything. Besides, she knew that she was right to fire Dr. Kay. Because he would fight the coming changes on the beaches, in the fields, and on the streets; he was, after all, English. And though she admired the English, Dr. Kay had to go.

So Dr. Kay was laid off. Then Dr. Romero resigned. Subsequently, Dr. Kay filed a whistle-blower suit alleging that his investigation of the drained Patient Gift Fund was the reason he was laid off.

Things were changing irreversibly. The admitting ward was closed: Medicine had moved into administration; almost all the doctors I'd ever worked with were gone; and we were on some kind of Journey I didn't want to be taking, from Institution to Community. Or vice versa.

Then just a few days later, as I was driving in to the hospital in the early morning, I saw that the wraps had finally come off the new hospital—those great white wraps that had covered the rising buildings for years.

There it was.

The new Laguna Honda.

It seemed to melt in a strange way into the old Laguna Honda. It, too, had towers, although they were modern and spare, without roof tiles, decorative cornices, or copper pipes. Stuccoed in peach, taupe, and umber, the new towers were painted in the colors of the old; set into them were flat, modern windows outlined in teal.

It was time to see what the new place was like.

It was time to take the tour.

I called up Dave Jonas.

Dave was the project manager for the new facility, and he would be a congenial guide, I knew. He'd been stationed in the old hospital for such a long time that he had come to appreciate its wide-open spaces, its serendipitous meetings, and its patients. We could meet that very day, he told me, for the tour; I could come over to his office, and he would take me around.

Late that afternoon I did meet him in his office, and we left the old building, walking out of it and directly into the gardens of gray river rock, flowering lavender, and olive trees that landscaped the new buildings. You would never have known, unless you'd been there, that there had once been a wooded valley in that place, with a spring and whiskey bottles.

Dave told me we would start by looking at a neighborhood in the South Tower. "Neighborhood" was the new word for "ward." I would only have to see one neighborhood to get an idea of the patient spaces, because all the neighborhoods were pretty much identical.

Then we stopped in front of glass double doors, which opened for us, and we walked into the great room of a neighborhood. It was just as spacious and well lighted as it had been virtually. Its floors were blond wood with matching cabinets, and in the back was the nursing station, which was a simple counter with a computer. It had no doors, closets, or cabinets. It was hard to imagine having enough quiet at that nursing station to think or to discuss a patient.

Then we walked down the hall that came off the great room to see examples of the patients' rooms. I was amazed. Each two- or three-bedded "room" was actually a suite, with its own little hallway. Each suite had a bathroom, tiled in teal, cream, and taupe, large enough for the widest wheelchair and the biggest patient. Each of the "beds" was a private room, with a window that opened and a door that closed. A flat-screen television was on the wall; the new bureaus had black rubber handles so patients wouldn't hurt themselves. Under each pillow was a two-way monitor so a nurse could talk to a patient, and a patient to a nurse, without the need for face-to-face contact.

Then Dave showed me the common spaces of the neighborhood. There was the carpeted Quiet Room for reading, the dining room for eating, and a small kitchen with a shiny stove and a dishwasher, because patients would now be served on china. The new dishwasher could compost on its own. I saw the hall of offices for the nurse manager, the activity therapist, the dietician, and the medical records technician. And what about the doctors? I asked Dave. Where were our offices? And the call rooms for the doctors who covered at night?

Dave looked uncomfortable. It seemed that in the new buildings the doctors had unaccountably been overlooked. He didn't know about the call rooms, but there were no doctors' offices in the new Laguna Honda. He'd heard that we'd stay in the old building, though he couldn't say for sure.

Next we would go into the Link Building, which connected the two towers for patients. Since the elevators had some kind of electronic problem, he would take me down the stairs, which were all the way at the far end of the corridor and locked.

This was a very inconvenient place to put the stairs, I told him. Code Blues required getting from one floor to another in a hurry, and that meant not waiting for an elevator or running all the way down a corridor. And why were they locked?

Dave didn't know why the architects had placed the stairs so far away from the elevators, but they were locked for security reasons, so patients couldn't elope or do whatever they used to do in the stairwells in the old hospital. We'd gotten in too much trouble for that. Of course, staff members would have electronic keys to the stairs and the other locked places on campus on the property locator badges we would wear. There were also cameras in the stairwells for additional security, and cameras in the cafeteria and throughout the grounds.

We arrived at the lobby of the Link Building. It was stunning. The wall that faced west was almost entirely of glass, and I could just make out the ocean outside. On the other side of the glass were two ancient flowering magnolia trees, thoughtfully preserved by the Tree Subcommittee. The other walls had tapestries, raku sculptures, paintings, and glass mosaics.

Then we went to the cafeteria. Even the Swiss would have been satisfied. Spacious and white, it had small tables and colorful chairs and halogen lights. There was a new grill behind curved Plexiglas, and in the back, rows of Wolf ovens and Viking refrigerators. A cement patio gave out on to the cafeteria, looking just like the virtual patio we'd been shown so long ago, except for the absence of umbrellas and those slim young patients. I saw the gym with its two infinity swimming pools, and the outpatient clinic, furnished with the newest examining tables, computers, and equipment.

On our way out to see the new barnyard, we passed a long, low building. That was for the computer servers, Dave told me, which would control everything in the new buildings—the electricity, lights, and heat; the cameras, doors, and elevators; the medications, telephones, and computers. Naturally I wanted to see it, and we went inside. It smelled of cement and was lined, floor to ceiling, with rows of shelves on which were hundreds of black boxes, connected by thousands of wires. Each wire came from a particular room into those black boxes, Dave explained, and there were separate wires for the telephone, television, ventilation, heating, and electronic toilets.

One could only hope that those wires never got disconnected.

Last we came to the new barnyard. There was no comparison with the old barnyard. Rows of vegetable beds had been built at wheelchair level so patients could garden; the new greenhouse had accessible benches and equipment. The ducks and geese had a new pond, built to code, and the activity therapists, who would run the farm, had offices right next to the rabbits. Every animal had his or her own private room, with cement floors and warming lights. Dave showed me the little doors between their individual rooms that he'd been forced to add because the animal-rights people worried the miniature pigs and goats would get lonely with so much privacy. The little doors were so they could visit one another.

Then we walked back to his office, and he asked me to wait while he looked through his book of plans.

"I think I've found it," he said, pointing to a little box labeled PHYS. "The call room for the physicians."

I looked. It was on the third floor of the North Tower, a little box without windows, labeled PHYS. I didn't think so. More likely PHYS meant "physical plant" or "physical therapist" or even, given the complexity of the computer building, "physicist," but not physician.

I thanked Dave anyway, and as I walked back to my office, I wondered where in the new hospital the patients would drink, deal their pills, talk, and dream. For they would find places, I knew—stairwells, rooftops, a dark and windowless room labeled PHYS. Or perhaps they wouldn't. Because, although privacy had been the main reason for the new hospital, what with the cameras, the property locator badges, and the two-way microphones under every pillow, patients wouldn't have much privacy in the new Laguna Honda.

I sat down at my rickety desk. I looked out my window at the hospital wing across from me—its red-tiled roof and turret reminders of the origin of our vocation in those old monasteries. I looked at my white coat—white to remind us of cleanliness and purity of motive— at my books, and at the index cards I still kept. I wondered where the doctors would be in the new hospital, or if we would be there at all.

It was too early to say. And I still had one last lesson in my schooling at the old Laguna Honda.

Because I was still taking care of patients. Somehow, despite all the changes, life at the hospital went on pretty much as it always had. The nurses made their rounds three times a day; the doctors

took care of their patients; the therapists, social workers, and dieticians followed the strict regime laid down so long ago by Miss
Lester.

So it happened that just a few weeks after I took the tour, I was
standing in a ward, finishing up with a patient, when one of my
ex-patients, Mr. David Rapman, walked in. I recognized him right
away. His voice was unmistakable—raspy and energetic, confident and
inspired. He'd come into the ward to persuade some patients to attend
the memorial service for Don Taylor, who'd been a substance-abuse
counselor at the hospital.

"Hey! Dr. S.!" he said, with a wide, white smile. "How ya' doin'?"

"I'm excellent," I told him. "What about you?"

"Oh, doin' great, Dr. S.! Nine hundred and ninety-four days of
sobriety since I left! Best thing that ever happened to me!"

I could see that just by looking. Mr. Rapman was a far cry from
what he'd been the first and second time I'd met him. Slim, brown,
and effervescent, he had a brown-and-white ski cap on his curly black
hair and was neatly dressed—buttoned, zipped, and belted. Only his
voice connected him to that other Mr. Rapman I'd known two years
before.

I met him the first time when the nurses on the admitting ward
asked me to check up on some blood tests that Dr. Rajif, who was out
sick, had ordered. They were worried because Mr. Rapman had
gained twenty-four pounds in the past two days. Would I go over his
blood tests and then check him out?

Sure.

I went over the blood tests first. They were easy to interpret. Mr.
Rapman obviously had cirrhosis of the liver, and his liver had finally
failed. Since the liver makes the proteins that hold water inside blood

vessels, most likely the twenty-four pounds Mr. Rapman had gained was water that had leaked out of his blood vessels into his skin, abdomen, and legs. Short of a liver transplant, there wouldn't be much for me to do about that.

Then I left the office to examine him for myself.

I found him in one of the semiprivate rooms in the front of the ward. It was very quiet when I came in. There was a mound of bedclothes on the bed, and the room was stuffy with a sad and stale smell. It's not death and it's not dying, but it's on the way to both—it's a kind of stoppage: the air not moving; the patient still; the body less warm than it should be. The mound of bedclothes, I discovered, was Mr. Rapman, who wasn't moving and had the covers pulled up over his head.

I introduced myself anyway and explained why I was there, but the bedclothes did not stir. Then suddenly, I felt movement, a rush of cool, fresh air, in back of me, and a tall, vigorous woman walked in— Mr. Rapman's sister. She stopped just behind me.

Mr. Rapman rolled the covers down then and let me do a quick exam. I started with his hands, which were cool and puffy. Then I took his pulse, which was rapid and weak. I looked at his eyes, which were yellow from the jaundice of his cirrhosis; I looked at his chest, which was covered with bruises from the lack of clotting proteins due to his failed liver. His belly was swollen, and his legs were edematous.

He was going to die soon, I told them after I'd finished—in a few weeks or maybe months. He would bleed to death all of a sudden, in a minute or two. Or he would get infection after infection, until the last one, by definition, killed him. Or he'd go into a coma—the hepatic sleep of a liver no longer able to cleanse his blood. The only thing that might save him, I explained to his sister as he watched me through half-closed eyes, was that the patients at Laguna Honda were pissy, and he was pissy, I could tell. That pissiness, that toughness, that scrappiness might—just might—save him. This time. It was impossible to know for sure. But I'd give him a fifty-fifty chance of surviving—better than I'd give anyone else so sick. Though not if he kept drinking.

"See, I told you, David," his sister said. "I've told him, doctor," and here Mr. Rapman shut his eyes completely and pulled the covers back over his head. "But he's gone back to drinking so many times."

I shrugged. I admit it. Then I murmured my condolences and left the room to write some new orders for him. And a few days later, sure enough, Mr. Rapman got even sicker; he was transferred to the County, and there he spent weeks in the intensive care unit, getting transfusions, lab tests, and many antibiotics.

When he returned, I admitted him. He looked about the same as when I'd seen him before, which, in a case like his, meant that he was better. Not dying had bought his liver a bit of time, and a few new liver cells had formed, making a bit more protein. So his clotting was a bit better, his swelling a bit less, his blood a bit cleaner.

As I was examining him this time, I realized how handsome he was. Even-featured, with unlined and unblemished brown skin, white and straight teeth, Mr. Rapman was another good-looking patient to add to my long list. Most of the patients at the hospital were good-looking, I thought, and not just because they were my patients. But we had mostly Bad Boys—old, young, or middle-aged; and who but the good-looking—or the bizarre—could have survived the obstacle course of elementary school counseling, high school principals, juvenile court, prison, and the streets they'd had to navigate to get here?

Not only was Mr. Rapman's liver a bit better, but Mr. Rapman himself was better. He was attentive during my exam and interested, although irritable and grouchy, which was also an improvement. Grouchiness is ego, is self come to life—angry, yes, but also energetic and alive. Once again his sister appeared, and this time he listened carefully to my prognosis. Anyone else would have died by now, I said, but he, like so many of our patients, had nine lives, and this was life number seven and a half.

A few weeks later he'd improved enough to move out to Claren- don Hall, and I didn't see him for a year. Then he came over to the admitting ward, to find me and to say good-bye. He was being dis- charged, and he wanted to thank me. He was still swollen, but less so; and he was upright, standing on both feet. And most of all: "I've been sober! Dr. S.! Two hundred and sixty-four days of sobriety!"

Now, two years later he was back, but not as a patient. As a volun- teer. He'd joined Alcoholics Anonymous, he told me, and he was back to attend the memorial service for his sponsor, Mr. Don Taylor.

"Don was a great man, Dr. S. He saved my life. I can't believe Don is dead!" he said, in his scratchy voice. His face was shiny, and he shifted his weight from one slim leg to the other. "Don was the spon- sor for a lot of the patients here—hundreds—and he came to me when . . . Well, you remember how angry, how irritable I was. I threw him out of my room. But he kept coming back, and finally I did the first step, Dr. S.! I admitted that I was powerless, that my life had become unmanageable, and I gave myself up to a Greater Power! I'm on the fourth step now—taking a searching and fearless moral inven- tory of myself—again, because you're never done with the twelve steps; you do them one by one and again and again, because it's a rich and depthless program, AA. Are you going to the memorial service, Dr. S.?"

I hadn't planned to, but Mr. Rapman had captivated me with his vitality, his evident wellness. He was no longer not ill, but well. In fact, his wellness exuded through his skin, his rocking to and fro on his feet, through his voice, hair, and eyes. And while medicine had done a good job of saving Mr. Rapman from death, it was something else that had made him well, and that something seemed to have been Don Taylor. So I decided to go to the memorial service.

The chapel was closed for renovation, and so Mr. Taylor's memorial service was being held in the library, which was also a good place for a memorial service.

The library was quiet and airy; it smelled of books and paper, and had an enormous inlaid oak table at its entrance, with legs carved into lions. Like the chapel, the library was from an earlier time than the celadon tiles of our operating room or the metal hair dryers of our beauty parlor. It was from the time when to be free meant to be free from work, free to read and to think.

When I arrived, I was surprised to see that the library, which was huge, was completely filled with people. Chairs had been arranged in many rows, and every one was taken; people were standing in the back and on the sides in front of the bookcases. Since there was no other place to sit, I sat on top of the carved table in the back and looked out across the sea of people. Next to the rows of folding chairs I saw many wheelchairs; canes and dirty denim jackets were hanging from the chair backs; and quite a few bare shoulders had tattoos. With me in the back were staff—a few doctors, nurses, dieticians, psychologists. In spite of the crowd, it was quiet, with just a little whispering here and there.

In the front, a blown-up photo of Don Taylor had been made into a poster and put on an easel, and as I looked at it, I remembered him. He wasn't very big and not particularly outgoing, and he wasn't handsome either. Low-set ears, flat nose, eyes tilted downward at the corners, it was the face that alcohol in utero sometimes produces. So he must have started out not only with genetic alcoholism but with environmental alcoholism, too.

Just on the minute, the first speaker got up from his chair and went to the front. He was clean-shaven, wearing a starched open-collared white shirt and Levi's, precisely creased. He was Don's cousin, he told us, a very distant cousin, but he knew Don well because when Don was twelve, he moved in with him and his family. Don's mother had died of alcohol when he was three, and his father died of drugs when he was eleven, and it had taken him a year to find another family.

Don was a sweet guy, as everyone here knew; a great guy, but he didn't do well in school, and in his late teens he took to drugs and alcohol and even crime. Nothing big—thefts and burglaries—and, eventually, he went to prison. Which was good for him and lucky, as he always said, because in prison he joined Alcoholics Anonymous. And he cleaned up; he became sober and more than sober. He walked every one of the twelve steps, and when he got to number eleven, he prayed and meditated and asked the Power greater than himself to show him His will, which was for him to become a sponsor in AA. Which he did.

And what a sponsor!

Don was the sponsor of all sponsors—a guide, an elder brother, a true friend. Always there when you needed him; always there when you thought you didn't need him, too. When he got his job at Laguna Honda, he was so happy! He loved his work. When he lay in the hospital, dying of the disease he got from drugs, he was more lonely than scared. All he could talk about was his patients. How were they doing? Without him?

The thing was—Don had found himself, found his path, which was to help others see what he'd seen: That we are all powerless; that there is a higher power; that what makes us truly happy is love.

The room was very quiet. The tattooed arms did not fidget; the gold-ringed ears did not turn.

Then Mr. Rapman stood up. He's a good speaker—his hoarse but energetic voice, white teeth, shiny face, snappy brown eyes. He held the microphone in one hand and, as he talked, shifted his weight from leg to leg.

"Don was my friend," he said. "And he was the friend of most everyone here. No one will ever know how many people Don saved and helped through their bad times. When I was here and I was angry, and they sent Don over, I threw him out of my room—many times. But he kept coming back. Finally I let him stay, and he came every day. He saw all his patients every day, Saturdays and Sundays, too. You could call him anytime. And I stopped drinking, and my life became manageable, and after I left the hospital, Don became my sponsor. He saved my life and many other lives."

Mr. Rapman fell silent and, microphone in hand, looked out over the crowd. The heads on the tattooed arms nodded and murmured, and suddenly I understood that there was a whole nexus of life at the hospital I'd never been aware of. I'd known, of course, that many of the addicted knew one another, and talked and gossiped in the glass bus-stop shelter where smoking was still allowed. Yet it had never occurred to me before that their chatting might not only have been gossip and old history, but the same kind of questioning that my group spent our time, in our cubicles, at our lunch tables, doing— about the death of a patient, the meaning of life, how to live, and how to die.

As I, too, looked over the quiet crowd, I wondered how many of those I called Bad Boys and Bad Girls were, in reality, spiritually thirsty and spiritually sick. Perhaps they were the most sensitive, the most easily hurt of all my patients, the most tortured by the human fate of knowing we are going to die. Perhaps the tattooed, prematurely aged, skinny, and solemn patients in front of me were the real empaths, and my patient, Mr. Rapman, had something to teach me— that my life was unmanageable, that I might think about giving it up to a higher power, and that the twelve never-ending steps were, like the pilgrimage, for me also to tread. How was I any different from these quiet, attentive people, touched, even transformed, by the life of someone now dead?

Mr. Rapman sat down, and others came up to the microphone. Each spoke of how Don had saved his life, and the memorial service went on all afternoon. Don Taylor had saved many lives. And really saved them—not just saved them from death but saved them for life, in the same way that Mr. Rapman was not only no longer ill but well.

I don't know what a saint is, except a person sanctified by the Vatican, and though Don was a Catholic, I doubt he will ever be sanctified. But if he was not a saint, he was for sure a bodhisattva, someone who came to the end of a certain path, had an overwhelming realization, and then turned around and came back. Not to a glorious martyrdom either, but to the daily egregious errors, the foolish irritability of Mr. Rapman. And sure enough, over the next few weeks I saw photos of Don Taylor appearing like those of any saint, over the beds of his quiet, invisible disciples.

As for Mr. Rapman, I've kept up with him a bit. Today is his 1,724th day of sobriety, and he has gone back to school. He wants to go into juvenile justice—to teach or act in some way so that others, especially the kids, don't have to go through what he went through.

Mr. Rapman was the last lesson in my schooling at the old Laguna

Honda, and I knew it at the time. It was the capstone; it summarized almost everything I'd learned. There was the importance of modern medicine, with its intensive care units, transfusions, and antibiotics. Without that "medical model of care," Mr. Rapman would never have survived his fatal liver disease. But modern medicine was not enough. Mr. Rapman also needed the Way of Laguna Honda, the Way of Hildegard and premodern medicine—tincture of time, the little things, Dr. Diet, Dr. Quiet, and Dr. Merryman—to heal completely. But even that had not been enough. It took Don Taylor, with his enactment of meaning and of love, to save Mr. Rapman's life for good.

After Don Taylor and Mr. Rapman, I took a sabbatical from the hospital. But when the day finally came—move-out, move-in day—I made sure to be there.

Ever since Dr. Dan realized that the move would need careful planning, administration had been organizing. Mirene and Adrian did not use Dr. Dan's cottage-industry plan, however; instead, they hired three professional consulting firms who spent two years and almost half a million dollars preparing the staff and the patients. There had been innumerable memos, focus groups, and PowerPoint presentations, monthly training sessions, and mock move days. Also many delays. The firing of Dr. Sonnen and Dr. Dan, Mr. Conley's death, Drs. Kay and Romero's complaints; the visits of the Department of Justice. Most delaying of all had been the problems with the new buildings themselves.

Because a few of those wires in the computer building did get disconnected and then reconnected not quite correctly, so that when the toilet flushed on the fourth floor of the South Building, the heat turned off on the third floor of the North Building. There was the flooding of the fifth floor of the North Building whenever it rained. There were the rats who were eating the wires. There were the state inspectors who mutually disagreed on what was required for permits. There were problems with the electronics of the elevators, the stair-wells, the hidden cameras, and the automatic locks. And those were just the problems we heard about.

But ten million dollars and thirty-six months delayed, the move days were set: December 7 and December 8—Pearl Harbor Day for the first half of the patients to move, and Buddha's Enlightenment Day for the second half. Which seemed to me to be ironic and propi-tious both, and I volunteered to come in and help out.

On the first move day, I parked my car in its usual spot and, as instructed, went over to the recreation hall, which was filled with chairs and tables and staff. I signed all the required forms: I promised not to abuse any of the patients and affirmed that if I was abused, I knew whom to call. I was given my assignment, which was to monitor the elevators in the new building. Only one of the elevators was work-ing, and my job, therefore, was to make sure that only patients used them and that everyone else took the stairs.

Were the stairs unlocked? I asked the staff member checking me in.

She looked puzzled, but reassured me that, yes, the stairs were . . . not locked. Then she handed me a special cell phone in case I needed to call Command Central, and gave me a purple move-day T-shirt to put over my clothes. Everyone—doctors, janitors, volunteers— was supposed to wear a move-day T-shirt, blue for staff and purple for volunteers. It would help identify me, and I could keep it as memorabilia.

It was lightly raining when I walked out of the old hospital and into the lobby of the new. I checked the stairs. Yep, they were locked, and the cell phone for communicating this to Command Central hadn't been charged. So I put the T-shirt aside, sat down in one of the new chairs in the new lobby, and waited for my friends to arrive. T-shirtless, they were all moving in—the speech therapist, the activity therapist, the doctors, the psychologists, and as they came in, we chatted and got caught up. Then Dr. Jeffers, who was also volunteering, showed up, and together we wandered the new hospital. Eventually we came to the cafeteria and were greeted by the old MHRF nurses whom Mirene had moved over from the County. Their job that day was to sit outside the new cafeteria and monitor the patients as they came over from Old to New.

What had happened was that the official corridor between the Old and the New had not been finished in time. Actually it had been finished but hadn't yet passed inspection, so the state agreed to let it be used if it was lined with white plastic, lighted by construction lights, and only one patient at a time came through. So staff members were positioned at either end, and when a ward was emptied, its patients were brought down in the old elevators to wait their turn in front of the corridor. When all was clear, a signal would be given, and the next patient would leave the old hospital, enter the corridor, and then come through. Since it was the first time any patient had been inside the new hospital, each one, as he or she came out of that tunnel, would crane his head around, blinking in the bright light and trying to see this new world, precisely like an infant popping out of the birth canal. Then each would be whisked away to his or her new room, and the next patient would start on his journey from Old to New.

It was a great place, the right place, to be for the move, and Dr. Jeffers and I sat down to watch.

By the end of the day, half of the patients had been moved. The next day the rest of the patients would be moved and the old hospital closed.

On my way home, I reflected on how meticulously the move had been prepared and how well it had gone. Only one thing was missing: No one had planned a ritual to mark the end of the old hospital, and that was too bad. Some kind of final Miss Lester parade, with the priest and his incense, and doctors and nurses walking the wards, laying the ghosts to rest, acknowledging the suffering and devotion those old wards had seen.

I needn't have worried. Because a kind of ritual did occur, spontaneously, in the old organic way, and a more beautiful one than anyone could have planned. It was the next day, with Dr. Grace.

Dr. Grace was the Buddhist of Laguna Honda. I say that although there were many Buddhists at Laguna Honda, by birth or predilection, but Dr. Grace was the Buddhist of the Buddhists. She lived at Zen Center, and she was the person whom everyone went to when there was something awful to think through or grieve through. She never judged; she always listened; she didn't say much; yet afterward, whatever it was would feel different—peaceful, still painful perhaps, but with a sweetness. She'd started at the hospital eighteen years before in order to practice medicine in the AIDS ward. It was in the middle of the epidemic, and the treatments were not very effective. She told me once that she and Dr. Tommy, her partner on the AIDS ward, had signed over 1,500 death certificates.

Then one day, two and a half years before, Dr. Grace came in to attend a meeting on her day off, and on her way home, a car swerved and hit her head-on. Her car was crushed, and she was helicoptered to the ICU. She sustained twenty-eight fractures and severe abdominal trauma, and was in a coma for months. She woke up on the Fourth of July. Her mind was clear but her arms and legs took years to heal, and she was still in a wheelchair.

She hadn't been back to Laguna Honda since the accident. But she wanted to come for the move, and so she and I arranged to meet up on the second day of the move in her old AIDS ward.

I found her in the middle of the empty ward. Its patients were already in the new hospital, and its walls already stripped of their corkboards, pictures, and paintings. Sitting in her wheelchair, Dr. Grace was very still, as she had come to seem since the accident, but also full of life and even more beautiful than before.

"I didn't think it would be so intense," she said, as soon as she saw me. "To be back. To remember all those patients. All those deaths."

Next to her was Dr. Tommy. He, too, hadn't been back for years, and he, too, had come back for the move. He'd always been ironic, and this day he was wearing an overcoat, felt hat, and heavy black-plastic 1950s glasses.

"I went to a Leonard Cohen concert last night," he explained, "and decided to dress as Leonard Cohen for the move."

Then we all took off together for the new hospital.

I pushed.

Dr. Grace was much loved, and every ten feet or so, someone—a patient, a staff member, a volunteer—recognized her, called out, came over, and gave her a hug.

"Are you coming back?" each one asked. Even the demented patients.

It took us quite a while, but eventually we did make it through the central hall and down the elevator to the mouth of the corridor that led from Old to New. We waited in line, and then it was our turn to walk through the white tunnel with the light at its end. And as dramatic as it had been the day before, it was even more dramatic pushing Dr. Grace with Dr. Tommy dressed as Leonard Cohen at my side. Because from that side, going from Old to New, I couldn't tell whether it was the tunnel of birth or of death. It was white and clean and bright, and the light at the end got bigger and bigger.

Then we popped out, and Dr. Grace saw for the first time the cream and taupe walls of the new Laguna Honda, the halogen lighting, the huge windows, and the art glass.

"How beautiful!" she exclaimed.

We walked all around. We looked at the aviary, now a topiary, alas, the birds not having survived their renovation. We saw the cafeteria, the beauty salon, the great rooms with their coffeemakers and soda dispensers, balconies, and views, and Dr. Grace was thrilled. She'd been in a lot of hospitals and patients' rooms herself during the last few years and knew what was important. The flat-screen televisions! The windows that opened! The under-the-pillow speaker and monitors! The teal-and-cream tiled bathrooms!

In the late afternoon we made our way back to the old hospital, sneaking in a very illegal way back in a wrong-way mode through the tunnel, from New to Old. Which could only mean that it was the tunnel of death, and we were revenants, I suppose, if you want to keep that metaphor.

We ended up just at the intersection of Old and New, in the lobby of the Old with its 1930s WPA frescoes and telephone-switchboard office. This was where everyone ended up. The last of the patients coming out of the elevator and going through the tunnel; staff walking back from the New to stand in a crowd around Dr. Grace: Dr. Benicia, Dr. Jeffers, Mirene, Adrian, Dr. Talley, talking, laughing, telling stories of the day. Whenever someone left, the heavy glass-and-bronze doors would open to give a view of the Florence Nightingale statue, outside looking in.

Finally we put Dr. Grace in her van, and I went back to the new hospital. The evening was coming on, and I walked around the neighborhoods. The nurses were putting their old books and policy-and-procedure manuals on the counters, and taping up on the walls their curling paper schedules. The patient chart racks had been moved, and there they were. Behind, in the dining room, the medical records people had taken up their usual positions, sitting at the new dining tables, randomly thinning charts. The patients were in front in the great room, drinking their coffee and talking together.

Last I walked back to the old hospital.

It was empty. Not a single person was left, by accident or by design. Not one Bad Boy or Bad Girl; not a single little old lady or little old man; no sleeping Chinese janitor, having dozed off during his break in one of the chairs upstairs. There was no one in the stairwells or the elevators. Heavy chains now locked the doors of the wards. I looked through a window: Inside the ward, it was dark, an old calendar still on the wall, a doomed plant on the floor.

The hospital, the old hospital, was empty.

And it felt empty.

I'd wondered for years what the move would be like. I'd always assumed that the spirit of the place was created by its architecture—its arches, towers, turrets; its open wards with the solaria at the end, reminders of medieval hospitality. But now that it was empty, I could see that the spirit of God's Hotel was not in the old building, and yet it wasn't in the new, either. That spirit, I realized at that moment, was neither just the building nor just the people in it. It was some kind of amalgam, made up of the way the hospital looked and felt, what went on inside it, and the people inside it, too. Perhaps that spirit could not be transported. And when the iron praying mantis came to tear the old building down—afterward, nothing would remain.

Or perhaps, after the shock had settled, after the spirit of God's Hotel had spent the requisite forty-nine days that a spirit has to wander in the Bardo, or however long for the spirit of a building, it would reincarnate in the New, stunned a little by its fresh young body, confused, a little surprised.

I stood there in the old building for a long time. I couldn't decide, one way or the other, whether the spirit of God's Hotel would live or die.

I thought about the new facility. It was beautiful but it wasn't warm. If the old hospital was a decrepit, sprawling farmhouse, then the new facility was a five-star hotel, shiny, sterile, impersonal.

I imagined what it would be like to work there. It would not be like the old place, where the open wards had been so inviting to wander. It would take mental effort for me to visit my patients in the new neighborhoods, negotiating locked doors and locked stairwells, and entering each patient room, one by one. When the electronic records came online, the paper charts would go, and with them, the freedom of flipping through pages, recognizing the handwriting of my friends, and writing the real story of a patient. I would spend my time at a computer instead, providing health-care data so that administration could prove that Laguna Honda provided cost-efficient, culturally competent care in a nonabusive setting, with a focus on short-term rehabilitation and discharge. When would I see my patients, sit on their beds, and listen to their stories?

Maybe it would turn out all right, though. Maybe after everything settled down, and the patients figured out where they could go to read and spit, think and dream. After the hidden cameras broke and the wires in the computer building permanently crossed, the locked doors sprang open and substitute linen closets emerged. Clutches of patients would once again gather in special places of their own—the smokers in a new Harmony Park, the Chinese mahjong players, the Hispanics, the Bad Boys and Bad Girls—and the spirit of God's Hotel would reappear, in a new body, yes, but alive and still recognizable.

I thought about everything that had happened to me in that old place, and how important it had been. Being in that old hospital changed my life. It had allowed me to explore Hildegard and understand her Way, which was slow—fussing and fiddling, removing obstructions, nourishing *viriditas,* and calling in Dr. Diet, Dr. Quiet, and Dr. Merryman for every patient. It had allowed me to go on pilgrimage and realize how it was possible to be happy and cold and wet all at once, and to know the quiet that underlies activity.

Perhaps I could have had those experiences . . . someplace else.

But no place else could I have discovered the hospitality, community, and charity that were in the walls and the air, because you had to be there for a long time to feel them and the kindness that was their source. And no place else could I have discovered the "being myself" with my patients, or the "just sitting," or the *anima* at the back of the eyes.

I learned commitment there—throwing myself into the mix, regardless. Before, I'd stood back from my patients—not a lot, but a little; I was wary of the transference and the countertransference. I threw myself in, but not completely, only for that fifteen-minute visit, that two-hour workup, that two-month or even six-month period. But gradually I learned from Dr. Curtis, from Christina and Lacy, from Dr. Dan, Don Taylor, and so many others that that wasn't being the best doctor. The best doctor walks with you to the pharmacy and stands with you until you drink your medicine. They taught me that the real name for the transference and the countertransference was love, and that the doctor-patient relationship was, above all, a relationship. So in the end, if it was the end, and whatever happened in the future, I had to agree with what Dr. Curtis told me on my very first week—God's Hotel was a gift.

Acknowledgments

First and foremost, I thank the patients, staff, and doctors of Laguna Honda Hospital, past, present, and, I think, future. I've used pseudonyms to protect privacy, but you know who you are.

Nevertheless, here in the acknowledgments, in no particular order, I'd like to mention especially certain staff, patients, doctors, and mentors: Elizabeth Cutler, Paul Hendrickson, Monica Banchero, September Williams, Hosea Thomas, Ann Fricker, Larry Funk, Eric Jamison, George Brown, Guenter Risse, Jack and Wendy Pressman, Joan Cadden, Mary Anne Johnson, Craig Wilson, Grace Dammann, Theresa Berta, Johnnie Brooks, Phoebe Lim, Paul Brizendine, Chris Winkler, Brian Dolan, Julie Bresciani, Patrick Monette-Shaw, and Ellen Ficklen. Each one taught me some thing, and often many things, that changed me for the better.

Next I thank my first readers. Rebecca Moore, who freely gave her time and energy to this project, despite her own intense and demanding work. No one has been more passionate and concerned that this book be the absolute best it could be. Patricia Wick, whose critical reading and antipathy to adverbs, adjectives, and any hint of cant forced me to sculpt my prose; and Eleanor Sweet, whose laugh, and whose tears, are worth so much to me.

Others to thank include Oliver Sacks, who was just wonderful. Hearing from me, an unknown writer, he was immediately enthusiastic, generous, and emphatic that I must write this book, as was his assistant, Kate Edgar.

Many thanks to my agent, Mary Evans, who is at once warm and demanding, insightful and romantic, and has such very good ideas and instincts. Her input was crucial in the evolution of my book proposal into a real book.

Rebecca Saletan has been everything I could ask for in an editor: enthusiastic, supportive, wise with her critique, protective, and a lot of fun. Her assistant, Elaine Trevorrow, always came through. Publicity and marketing—Marilyn Ducksworth, Mih-ho Cha, Kate Stark, and their teams—have been great. Special thanks to Riverhead's publisher, Geoff Kloske, for his belief in the book.

Others without whom *God's Hotel* might not have come into being, and certainly not in the way it did, include Jennifer and Robert Leathers, who set the example of true hospitality for us all. I'd like especially to thank their sons, Jeff and Ed, and also Allison and Katie Wick for their excitement, curiosity, and fresh perspectives.

Who else? Glen Worthey and the other librarians at Stanford University Library. Meg Newman for being a wonderful physician. Dan Wick for his bravery under fire. Art Sweet for giving me his energy, his love of life, and some, at least, of his intrepidness.

And last, Jenny, for being a warm and loving partner, and for creating a stable, warm, and loving home with me for many years.

Notes

INTRODUCTION: HOW I CAME TO GOD'S HOTEL

Page 6. *Hildegard of Bingen's Medicine* was not a great book: It really wasn't. It was too presentist; it did not contextualize Hildegard's medicine; it was more a book of medicine than a book of history; and yet, it was still worth reading. See Wighard Strehlow and Gottfried Hertzka, *Hildegard of Bingen's Medicine*, trans. Karin Anderson Strehlow (Santa Fe, NM: Bear & Company, 1988).

Page 8. Laguna Honda, Dr. Major said, was probably the last almshouse in America: It's hard to know for sure. Originally, Laguna Honda was the San Francisco Almshouse; and, according to the Centers for Medicare and Medicaid Services, it was the last hospital in the country with open wards, so perhaps that entitles it to be called the last almshouse in America. On the almshouse in America, see Charles Rosenberg, "Almshouse or Hospital: Reforming the Public Hospital," in *The Care of Strangers: The Rise of America's Hospital System* (Baltimore, MD: Johns Hopkins University Press, 1995); and David Wagner, *The Poorhouse: America's Forgotten Institution* (Lanham, MD: Rowman & Littlefield Publishers, 2005).

CHAPTER ONE: FIRST YEARS

Page 14. The changes in medical financing of health maintenance organizations: In the 1970s a fundamental shift took place in medicine, engineered not by doctors but by economists. Taking the idea from the newly publicized medical payment system of the People's Republic of China, where doctors got paid only when their patients stayed well, economists proposed that the best way to manage the ever-rising cost of medical care would be if doctors were paid preemptively, to maintain their patients' health. Instead of getting paid for what they did when a patient got sick, doctors would get paid a fixed amount per patient per month, regardless of how sick or well a patient was during that month. It would be up to the doctors to manage their own budget, and, economists thought, doctors would

simply have to learn to be efficient. They did learn, too. Since doctors have no
control over the three determinants of health—people's behaviors, luck, and
genetics—they learned that the only way to manage their budgets was not to
accept patients who were sick, unlucky, or genetically challenged. Some did this
by placing their practice in an old Victorian house, on the third floor, with no
elevator, neatly excluding the sick or disabled; others by advertising yoga and
meditation, which would be of interest only to the healthy. Doctors also realized
that the longer it took them to order a test or do a procedure, the more efficient it
was for their budget. For a clear explanation of how economists understand
medicine and health care, see Sherman Folland, Allen C. Goodman, and Miron
Stano, *The Economics of Health and Health Care*, 6th ed. (Upper Saddle River, NJ:
Prentice Hall, 2009).

Page 14. (DRGs): The DRG—diagnosis-related group—was based on the same concept as health-management organizations, but applied to hospitals. In this
scheme, hospitals would be paid a fixed amount per diagnosis, per patient, per
hospitalization, regardless of how much or how little care a particular patient
received. Hospitals' incentives would then become, economists were sure, efficiency, and they were right. Cadres of middle managers were hired to make sure
that doctors put the most remunerative diagnosis first on their list of discharge
diagnoses (instead of the most important diagnosis), and that doctors discharged
patients as soon as possible—and usually sooner. One unintended consequence:
Patients were discharged when they were still sick, and often had to be readmitted for another hospitalization soon after. This was not efficient, and medical
costs continued to increase. In the health-care act of 2010, this same model of
paying a lump sum based on diagnosis was extended to home care and long-term
care.

Page 17. There was a waiting list of more than two hundred patients: From Laguna
Honda Hospital's Annual Report, 1993.

Page 18. She showed me a sample of her previous day's admission: A handwritten
note sometimes takes longer than the cutting and pasting of electronic health
records, but it has much more information. With our handwritten notes, I knew
at a glance who it was who wrote the notes and just how much credence, therefore,
to put into its conclusions.

Page 19. A microscope, with boxes of slides: The microscope, centrifuge, and slides
would be the first things to go, when Laguna Honda was discovered by modern
health-care efficiency. A new law required all "laboratories" to be certified, with
annual inspections and policy-and-procedure manuals, and Dr. Major determined that, what with all the extra bureaucracy, it was more cost-effective to send
our slides across the city to a laboratory. The microscope, centrifuge, and slides
were taken away, and we were no longer able to examine our patients' blood, urine,
or sputum ourselves.

Page 28. It was never easy to track down a discharging doctor: It still isn't. This
should be one of the great advantages of the electronic health record: a clearly
written discharge note by the actual discharging physician, with a readable name
and accurate cell phone and beeper numbers. But the discharge note is often cut

and pasted by a medical student with no knowledge of the patient, and the discharging doctor often randomly chosen by computer. For some reason, the cell phone and beeper numbers are never up to date.

CHAPTER TWO: THE LOVE OF HER LIFE

Page 42. "We'll never have it this good": It was no illusion of Dr. Jeffers's that we would never have it so good. Laguna Honda at the time was a well-run place, as the typed two-page Annual Report of 1992 made clear. The hospital easily passed its annual inspection. No services were cut, despite it being a recession year. The hospital had no influenza cases, a two-hundred-patient waiting list, and a new laundry system.

Page 47. Dr. Weitz explained its theory to us: For a thorough history of the "System of the Fours," see Elizabeth Sears, *The Ages of Man: Medieval Interpretations of the Life Cycle* (Princeton, NJ: Princeton University Press, 1986). See also the diagram of the System of the Fours by Peter S. Baker in "Byrhtferth of Ramsey, De Concordia Mensium Atque Elementorum," Victoria Sweet, *Rooted in the Earth, Rooted in the Sky: Hildegard of Bingen and Premodern Medicine* (London: Routledge, 2006), 162.

CHAPTER THREE: THE VISIT OF DEE AND TEE, HEALTH-CARE EFFICIENCY EXPERTS

Page 62. The consulting firm of Dee and Tee: You can't blame the city. The state had recently passed a law requiring that county health departments compete with private health-care providers, and the city, therefore, had to come up with an "enterprise solution." Later, I learned that our city's system was by no means Dee and Tee's only opportunity to reengineer a hospital. At about the same time as our Laguna Honda experience, Dee and Tee was brought in to help the finances of Beth Israel-Deaconess Medical Center in Boston. For the results, which paralleled our experience at Laguna Honda, see Dana Beth Weinberg, *Code Green: Money-Driven Hospitals and the Dismantling of Nursing* (Ithaca, NY: Cornell University Press, 2003). She writes, "For the most part, frontline employees' input was unsolicited; they did not participate in the task forces or meetings [40]. . . . Overlooking the therapeutic value of nurses' relationships with patients, administrators insisted that the hospital could not afford to indulge nurses with the luxury of getting to know their patients [179]. . . . The very restructuring strategies that [the hospital], following trends in the hospital industry, adopted to solve its problems were themselves a problem [183]. . . . In fact, there is some evidence that trying to wring greater productivity out of employees increased the hospital costs [186]."

Page 63. Looking at the payroll, especially at the laundry: Laundry was one of our oldest departments. It was down in the basement, spread out across the length of a long ward, and every floor above it had a large metal basket affixed to the wall and leading to a chute in the basement. A hundred years ago the laundry had been staffed by patients to help pay for their own care. It was still a pleasant place, its wooden shelves filled with stacks of clean-smelling, starched sheets, gowns, and white coats. Laundry did all the hospital's laundry, and actually made a profit for the city because it also did the laundry for many other hospitals. All day long, vans pulled up to deliver dirty laundry and take away the newly cleaned. It was a busy place, but not cost-effective, and Dee and Tee calculated that it would make more sense to contract out the laundry services. The city agreed, and Dee and Tee was awarded their 10 percent of savings for the first two years. But it did not share in the increased costs of their plan, which ended up being considerable because the laundry workers continued to work for the city; the city no longer received reimbursement for doing the laundry of other hospitals; and it still had to pay for its own laundry, including the additional expense of transporting it to outside contractors.

Page 65. The closing of the state mental hospitals: For a history, see "Politics of Deinstitutionalization" in Steve M. Gillon, *That's Not What We Meant to Do: Reform and Its Unintended Consequences in Twentieth-Century America* (New York: W. W. Norton & Company, 2000). According to Gillon, it was the Community Mental Health Act of 1963 that crippled state mental hospitals. Crafted by Robert Felix, MD, it was a reaction to the conditions of state mental hospitals, revealed in a *Life* magazine article, "Bedlam," in 1946, and the 1948 film *The Snake Pit*, in conjunction with the development of thorazine in 1952. President Kennedy submitted a reform package, and Dr. Felix promised community mental-health centers in lieu of state hospitals. In addition, in order to encourage discharges from mental hospitals, Medicaid decided it would no longer reimburse states for treating patients in mental hospitals, but would reimburse them for treating patients in a facility "not designed solely for the treatment of mental illness." What happened? Only 768 of the 2,000 promised community centers ever materialized, but mental patients were discharged from the state hospitals anyway. The population of mental patients fell from 504,600 in 1963 to 138,000 in 1980, and many went to the streets or to nursing homes. By 1977, 87 percent of the 1.3 million patients in nursing homes had a diagnosis of chronic mental illness (Gillon, 103). At Laguna Honda, about one-third of my patients had a serious mental illness. Later, Dr. Felix admitted that closing the state mental hospitals was the worst mistake he ever made.

Page 67. He thought he was a vending machine: Jimmy's psychosis is not uncommon. For instance, see Dr. Swait Pawa and others, "Zinc Toxicity from Massive and Prolonged Coin Ingestion in an Adult," *American Journal of the Medical Sciences* 336(5) (November 2008): 430–33, which describes a thirty-eight-year-old schizophrenic who ate coins. See also Dr. Daniel R. Bennett and others, "Zinc Toxicity Following Massive Coin Ingestion," *American Journal of Forensic Medicine and Pathology* 18(2) (June 1997): 148–53.

Page 69. He had the right to refuse psychiatric medications: For what happened to the mentally ill after the Mental Health Bar became concerned with their rights, see Rael Jean Isaac and Virginia C. Armat, *Madness in the Streets: How Psychiatry and the Law Abandoned the Mentally Ill* (New York: The Free Press, 1992), especially chapter seven: "From the Right to Treatment to the Right to Refuse Treatment" (142–60).

Page 71. When the first effective treatment for mental illness was discovered: For a history of lobotomy, see Jack D. Pressman, *Last Resort: Psychosurgery and the Limits of Medicine* (Cambridge, UK: Cambridge University Press, 1998). On thorazine, see Isaac and Armat, *Madness in the Streets,* "Psychoactive Drugs, The Last Domino" (221–46). Many of our ideas about the coercive effects of treating mental illness come from the psychiatrist Thomas Szasz, cofounder and chairman of the American Association for the Abolition of Involuntary Mental Hospitalization. For instance, see Thomas Szasz, *The Myth of Mental Illness: Foundations of a Theory of Personal Conduct* (New York: HarperCollins Publishers, 1974). Dr. Szasz did not believe that there was such a thing as mental illness. Instead, he wrote, "[P]sychiatric diagnoses are stigmatizing labels. . . . Those whose behavior makes others suffer and about whom others complain are usually classified as 'psychotic.' . . . If there is no mental illness there can be no hospitalization, treatment, or cure for it. . . . There is no ethical, moral, or legal justification for involuntary psychiatric intervention. They are crimes against humanity" (267–68).

Page 75. Based on research by a PhD graduate student: This was Erving Goffman, who wrote the influential *Asylums: Essays on the Social Situation of Mental Patients and Other Inmates* (Chicago: Aldine Publishing Company, 1961). His ideas came out of his one year of fieldwork where he posed as a student of recreation and community life at a large mental hospital. As he admitted, he "came to the hospital with no great respect for the discipline of psychiatry" (x), and his year in one did not change his mind.

Page 77. The traditional requirements for a nun: The three requirements were: stability, obedience, and chastity. Nurses were originally nuns and monks; as the French for nurse—*infirmier* from *infirmarian*—shows. To this day, nurses are called "sisters" in England.

Page 79. Florence Nightingale wrote her *Notes on Hospitals*: What a woman she was! For a good biography, see Mark Bostridge, *Florence Nightingale: The Making of an Icon* (New York: Farrar, Straus & Giroux, 2008). Born in 1820, she lived until 1910, and her life, therefore, spanned the Victorian era. Never married and educated at home, at twenty-seven Nightingale experienced a call from God, and would have entered a monastery, probably, had she been Catholic. But she was Protestant, so she decided, instead, "to devote herself to works of charity in hospitals and elsewhere, as Catholic sisters do" (85). Eventually, she trained as a nurse in Germany and bought its strict system back to England, instituting the ideals and practices of nursing we take for granted today. Her *Notes on Nursing* is still a worthwhile read; see Florence Nightingale, *Notes on Nursing: What it is, and What it is not* (New York: D. Appleton and Company, 1860). During the Crimean War, she worked in army hospitals, and realized that the most important attributes of a hospital were cleanliness, fresh air, and quiet. She toured hospitals throughout Europe and then wrote up her ideal hospital in *Notes on Hospitals*, also fascinating reading. See Florence Nightingale, *Notes on Hospitals*, third ed. (London:

Longman, Roberts, and Green, 1863). She begins the book with the unfortunately still pertinent line: "It may seem a strange principle to enunciate as the very first requirement in a Hospital that it should do the sick no harm. It is quite necessary, nevertheless, to lay down such a principle." In view of Dee and Tee's recommendations about the head nurses and their consequences, her observation is astute: "Practically a nurse can really supervise only as many persons as she can see from one point" (114). Laguna Honda, with its open wards, solariums, wide corridors, and floor-to-ceiling windows, was built on this Nightingale plan.

Page 80. Dee and Tee's report: I was able to find the executive summary of the report, but not the full report, even from the librarian of the Dee and Tee library. For a copy of the executive report and a summary of the full report, see http://cityofsf.net/site/courts_page.asp?id=3972. It is contained in the Civil Grand Jury Reports, 1995–1996, IX; the Dee and Tee executive report is Appendix G.

CHAPTER FOUR: THE MIRACULOUS HEALING OF TERRY BECKER

Page 91. He reminded me of an aphorism I loved: The classic article of Dr. Peabody's is still worth reading; see Francis W. Peabody, MD, "The Care of the Patient," *Journal of the American Medical Association* 88 (1927): 877–82. "Look out for all the little incidental things that you can do for his comfort. These, too, are part of the 'care of the patient.' . . . The good physician knows his patients through and through, and his knowledge is bought dearly. Time, sympathy, and understanding must be lavishly dispensed, but the reward is to be found in that personal bond which forms the greatest satisfaction of the practice of medicine. One of the essential qualities of the clinician is interest in humanity, for the secret in the care of the patient is in caring for the patient" (882).

Page 92. The good, the better, and the best doctor: From Swami Nikhilananda, *The Gospel of Sri Ramakrishna* (New York: Ramakrishna-Vivekananda Center, 1977). Ramakrishna compares the three types of gurus to three classes of doctors: "There are three classes of physicians. The physicians of one class feel the patient's pulse and go away, merely prescribing medicine. As they leave the room they simply ask the patient to take the medicine. They are the poorest class of physicians. . . . There are physicians of another class, who prescribe medicine and ask the patient to take it. If the patient is unwilling to follow their directions, they reason with him. They are the mediocre physicians. . . . Lastly, there are physicians of the highest class. If the patient does not respond to their gentle persuasion, they even exert force upon him. If necessary, they press their knees on the patient's chest and force the medicine down his throat" (469). I interpret "forcing the medicine down his throat" for the modern physician as walking to the pharmacy with the patient, waiting for the medication to be dispensed, and watching the patient swallow down his pills.

Page 93. The police department would deliver 2,356 wrapped presents: Christmas was a special time at the hospital, with a decorated tree and a special meal, although the impetus for the celebration did wax and wane over the decades. According to Miss Lester, it had waned almost completely by the late 1950s: "It was Christmas, and Mr. Moran, the administrator at the time, called me up. Let's go sing Christmas carols to the patients, he said. So we did, just the two of us. We walked around all the wards and sang Christmas carols. Later the volunteers got involved, fund-raising for those presents, and then wrapping all of them, with the police department coming over to deliver them" (oral interview, December 12, 2007).

Page 96. My master's thesis into an article for publication: For the article, see Victoria Sweet, "Hildegard of Bingen and the Greening of Medieval Medicine," *Bulletin of the History of Medicine* 73 (1999): 381–403.

Page 103. The twenty-eighth time: I'm sorry to have to report that this is not hyperbole. When I reviewed Terry's records, I counted twenty-eight emergency-room visits for the care of her open wound.

Page 106. My first job, therefore, as gardener-doctor: In the premodern era, the connections between gardening and doctoring were many, profound, and went both ways. Sometimes the doctor was thought of as a gardener, and sometimes the gardener was thought of as a doctor, whose medicine was *laetamen* (fertilizer)—the different types of fertilizers being analyzed just like medications as to their proportions of humors and of qualities. For a modern-day parallel, where the gardener is enjoined to be a good doctor of the soil, see Masanobu Fukuoka, *The One-Straw Revolution: An Introduction to Natural Farming* (Mapusa Goa, India: Other India Press, 1992).

Page 111. *Physis:* For a history of Nature, and mechanism and vitalism, see Max Neuburger, "A Historical Survey of the Concept of Nature," *Isis* 154 (1944): 16–29, and Max Neuburger, *The Doctrine of the Healing Power of Nature Throughout the Course of Time (from Hippocrates to the Middle of the Nineteenth Century)*, Linn J. Boyd, trans. (New York: 1932).

CHAPTER FIVE: SLOW MEDICINE

Page 115. Dr. Kay, our hospice director: I was impressed by Dr. Kay the first day I met him. It wasn't just his clipped English accent, though I liked that, or his well-tailored suits, or his Harvard degree, or even that he was an oncologist, that most serious of medical specialties. I was impressed by his name tag. He came into our doctors' office, sat down to use the computer, and introduced himself formally as he put out his hand.

"I'm Dr. Kay," he said. "MD, CNA."

I shook his hand. "CNA? Certified nursing assistant?"

"Yes," he replied, leaning forward and showing his badge to me. "David Kay, MD, CNA. I just finished my training as a nursing assistant. It took me twenty years to realize how little I knew about nursing, and how important it was, especially in oncology, and especially here."

"What do you mean?"

"You learn how to brush a patient's teeth, which isn't easy, especially if there are mouth sores or yeast. You learn how to turn a patient, how to make a bed, how to feed a patient, and how to give sips of water. It's a lot of work, a skill, and an art. Doctors need to learn it."

Page 115. Miss Lester: I interviewed Miss Lester in December of 2007. I also interviewed some of Miss Lester's staff, who were still working in her now ten-years-vacant office. Did they remember her? Of course! What did they remember? "Everything got done. She did it herself. Give her something in the morning, and it was done by three-thirty. She ran this place tight but—have a family problem, she just melted. She could come back tomorrow and run this place." Silence. Then, "There would be a lot of people who wouldn't be here anymore, if she did" (oral interview with staff, October 9, 2009).

Page 119. The Latin *curare* split into cure and care: Actually, the derivation is a little ambiguous. *The Oxford Latin Dictionary* defines *curare* to mean both *care* and *cure*, but *The Oxford English Dictionary* derives the English *care* from the Germanic *cur*, and the English *cure* from Latin *cura*. On the other hand, Carl Darling Buck, using Julius Pokorny's etymology, seems to disagree, since he defines the Middle English *cure* as meaning *care for* and *care* as well as *cure* (307). See Carl Darling Buck, *A Dictionary of Selected Synonyms in the Principal Indo-European Languages: A Contribution to the History of Ideas* (Chicago: University of Chicago Press, 1965), 307.

Page 119. For more than a thousand years the nuns ran the Hôtel-Dieu: For this story, see Louis S. Greenbaum, "Nurses and Doctors in Conflict: Piety and Medicine in the Paris Hôtel-Dieu on the Eve of the French Revolution," *Clio Medical* 13: 247–67. "For the first time, the full range of medical interventions: admitting, examining, diagnosing, feeding, treating and discharge . . . were vested in the hands of physicians under whose direction the nurses of the Hôtel-Dieu were to serve [247]. . . . On May 6, 1789, all appeals exhausted, the prioress notified the administration that her nuns would physically prevent the entry of workmen into the St. Paul ward" (254).

Page 121. The Department of Justice arrived, and in its wake, still a second investigative agency, the Health Care Financing Administration: To summarize the gist of it: The DOJ arrived at the hospital in February 1997 to investigate violations of CRIPA (Civil Rights of Institutionalized Persons Act). Their findings were submitted May 6, 1998; a second findings letter was submitted April 1, 2003, and in May 2008 there was a settlement letter. As for HCFA, it investigated the hospital at the same time, and its letter came on June 8, 1998. Laguna Honda's plan of correction, its letter said, was unacceptable. The hospital must decrease patients by 140 beds and add social dining by September 9, 1998, or face the withdrawal of Medicaid and Medicare reimbursement.

Page 121. Miss Lester quit—in protest, she told the newspapers: See David Tuller, "Director of Nursing Quits Laguna Honda / Abrupt Departure as Staff Dwindles," *San Francisco Chronicle*, August 29, 1997. For Dr. Stein's rebuttal, see the same article.

Page 122. Study done at the hospital: See J. S. Kayser-Jones, "Open-Ward Accommodations in a Long-Term Care Facility: The Elderly's Point of View," *Gerontologist* 26(1) (1986): 63–69. Its abstract explains: "A field study of residents' satisfaction with open ward accommodations revealed that 88% of the respondents preferred the open ward to any other type of room accommodation."

Page 123. The eighteen-page DOJ letter ended: For the letter, see www.justice.gov/crt/about/spl/documents/laguna_honda_98_finding.pdf. I've summarized only the most important issues here. The letter was a tough one, and it must have been difficult for Dr. Stein and the mayor not to have felt attacked by it. We, the doctors, certainly felt attacked, and this even though the medical staff was off the hook—the DOJ acknowledged that the medical care at the hospital was excellent. I did recognize the hospital I knew in their letter, though. Patients did wander off; alcoholic patients did drink; unsafe smokers did sometimes smoke without supervision; drug abusers did occasionally succeed in using illicit drugs on campus. It was regrettably true that the violent, demented patients we admitted from the County continued to be demented and sometimes violent with us, and that the demented hoarders continued to hoard. It was all especially true after the dismissal of the head nurses, who had been that extra pair of hands and eyes that noted the patient about to wander off, that smelled the liquor, kept the peace, and filled in when an extra pair of hands was needed. The DOJ provided a long list of remedies, most of which were ultimately applied though they never did cure the patient.

Page 128. Vision Three of her first book, *Scivias*: For excellent colored reproductions of many of Hildegard's illuminations, see Matthew Fox, *Illuminations of Hildegard of Bingen* (Santa Fe, NM: Bear & Company, 2002).

Page 141. How expensive economists thought doctors were: For instance, economists often suggest replacing MDs with mid-level providers as a cost-saving measure. Yet the math doesn't work out, at least in our city, where mid-level providers often earn as much as physicians, while carrying half the caseload.

Page 142. Where Laguna Honda's Way of Slow Medicine could be tested for efficiency: It is in the measuring of the "efficiency" of hospitals and doctors where the devil is really in the details. For instance, in acute hospitals economists often use mortality rates or readmission rates as a measure of efficiency, which is not the same thing at all as measuring success at diagnosis and treatment. In Britain, the National Institute for Health and Clinical Excellence (acronym, NICE) measures efficiency using the QALY (cost per Quality-Adjusted Life Year), where 1 is perfect health, and 0 is death. NICE defines treatments as cost-effective if their incremental cost-effectiveness ratio is £20,000 or less per QALY. "The Quality Adjusted Life Year (QALY) has been created to combine the quantity and quality of life. The basic idea of a QALY is straightforward. It takes one year of perfect health-life expectancy to be worth 1, but regards one year of less than perfect life expectancy as less than 1. Thus an intervention which results in a patient living for an additional four years rather than dying within one year, but where quality of life fell from 1 to 0.6 on the continuum will generate: 4 years extra life @ 0.6 quality of life values 2.4 less 1 year @ reduced quality (1−0.6) 0.4; QALYs generated by the

intervention 2.0." See the article, "QALY," at http://www.medicine.ox.ac.uk/
bandolier/booth/glossary/QALY.html. (I have condensed, slightly, the explanation of the calculations.)

Page 143. The ecomedicine unit: We did three studies at Laguna Honda to see if
some of the medications that patients arrived with could be discontinued. We
found that they could be discontinued 90 percent of the time. Several years later
a formal study was published that looked at a similar issue; it found that 50 percent of medications could be discontinued without adverse effects and with
improvement in health and well-being. See Doron Garfinkel and Derelie Mangin,
"Feasibility Study of a Systematic Approach for Discontinuation of Multiple
Medications in Older Adults: Addressing Polypharmacy," *Archive of Internal Medicine* 170(18) (2010): 1648–54. The figure for the money spent on patients' meals
comes from an oral interview I had with Steve Konefklatt, director of food services, on November 23, 2009. In addition to seven dollars for the food itself, he
had eighteen dollars per patient, per day, to spend on its preparation and service,
he told me.

CHAPTER SIX: DR. DIET, DR. QUIET, AND DR. MERRYMAN

Page 145. An important conference about Hildegard: This was the "Hildegard von
Bingen in ihrem historischen Umfeld: Internationaler wissenschaftlicher Kon-
gress zum 900 jährigen Jubiläum, 13–19. September 1998, Bingen am Rhein."
Many of the conference papers were later published in Alfred Haverkamp and
Alexander Reverchon, eds., *Hildegard Von Bingen in ihrem historischen Umfeld:
Internationaler Wissenschaftlicher Kongress zum 900 Jährigen Jubiläum, 13–19 Septem-
ber 1998, Bingen Am Rhein* (Mainz, Germany: Philipp von Zabern, 2000).

Page 146. She even wrote a kind of autobiography: What Hildegard wrote was an
autobiographical letter to an inquiring admirer, and this letter, and information
in other letters were pulled together into a *Life of Hildegard* (the *Vita Hildegardis*)—
by her monk secretaries, Godfrey and Theodorich, probably with her help. However, since the *Life* was written with a particular viewpoint—namely getting
Hildegard declared a saint—it highlights the religious, spiritual, and miraculous
aspects of her life. But there are many other sources for her biography, including
the hundreds of letters she wrote, and even an eyewitness report made by a Papal
Inquisition sent to Rupertsberg in 1232 to interview her nuns. Much work has
been done on Hildegard, and today there are many biographies; see chapter one in
my book *Rooted in the Earth, Rooted in the Sky: Hildegard of Bingen and Premodern
Medicine* (New York: Routledge, 2006), or see Sabina Flanagan, *Hildegard of Bingen: A Visionary Life,* 2nd ed. (New York: Routledge, 1998).

Page 147. She wrote two additional books of visions: These are the *Book of the
Rewards of Life (Liber Vitae Meritorum)* and the *Book of Divine Works (Liber Divinorum Operum)*. Several illuminated copies of the *Liber Divinorum Operum* still exist,
although none from Hildegard's own scriptorium. The costumes she designed for
her nuns to wear in her play were white robes, gold rings, and long, white, silk veils
topped by golden crowns, with angels and a lamb worked into them. Rumor had it

that her nuns also wore these costumes on holidays, which Hildegard did not deny: "It is true that a woman who is married should not show her hair, nor decorate herself with crowns of gold . . . but this isn't the case for virgins, who are not ordered to cover their hair, just as it is quite proper for them to dress in white" (Epistola CXVI, *Patrologia Latina*, vol. 197: 1116, cols. 336 C and D). For a fascinating interpretation of the play in the context of Hildegard's own life, see Gunilla Iversen, "'O Virginitas, in Regali Thalamo Stas'; New Light on the Ordo Virtutum: Hildegard, Richardis, and the Order of the Virtues," in *The Dramatic Tradition of the Middle Ages*, Clifford Davidson, ed. (Brooklyn: AMS Press, 2005), 63–78.

Page 149. The Hildegard Haus: When I was there, the Hildegard Haus was growing many of the medicinal herbs recommended by Hildegard, including, in addition to those I've listed: hyssop, bertram, wormwood, thistle, fennel, parsley, mauve, lily, lettuce, achillea, arnica, hop, salvia, and fig.

Page 153. *Unknown Language* was the most mysterious: The Wiesbaden library has a copy of the *Riesencodex*—the collection of Hildegard's works made in her own scriptorium—on its website; see http://www.hlb-wiesbaden.de/index.php?p=202. It includes *Unknown Language*. See also, Sarah L. Higley, *Hildegard of Bingen's Unknown Language: An Edition, Translation, and Discussion* (New York: Palgrave MacMillan, 2007).

Page 156. Slowly I began to understand Hildegard's *methodus medendi*: Hildegard does not provide a how-to manual of her method; I have inferred it from her description of disease states. For instance, the fact that she uses the color of the face, the tone of the skin, or the brightness of the eyes to describe a condition suggests that she observed the face and eyes, and touched the skin. For what she would have done in taking a pulse, I have combined her descriptions of different pulses with what we know about the premodern method of taking a pulse. For example, see Faith Wallis, "Signs and Senses: Diagnosis and Prognosis in Early Medieval Pulse and Urine Texts," in *The Year 1000: Medical Practice at the End of the First Millennium*, Peregrine Horden, ed. (Oxford, UK: Society for the Social History of Medicine, 2000), 265–78. Of course, the Chinese use the pulse in diagnosis as well; for a comparison of the traditions, see Shigehisa Kuriyama, "Varieties of Haptic Experience: A Comparative Study of Greek and Chinese Pulse Diagnosis" (PhD diss., Harvard University, 1986).

Page 159. Dr. Diet, Dr. Quiet, and Dr. Merryman: The Latin is *Si tibi deficient medici, medici tibi fiant. Hæc tria: mens laeta, requies, moderata diæta. Mens laeta* was rendered as "Dr. Merryman," although I'm not sure that is quite right. A *merryman* was a jester, a buffoon, a clown who performed at horse shows and circuses—a Patch Adams, perhaps. *Mens laeta* was more of a joyous spirit, a cheerful heart, a light mind, so it might be better understood as Dr. Lightheartedness, Dr. What-Me-Worry?, Dr. I'm-Rooted-in-Life-and-It's-Just-Flowing-Through-Me-Unimpeded-by-Worry-Irritability-or-Sadness.

Page 165. First, every Swiss citizen had to buy basic health insurance: For more on the Swiss system, see Uwe E. Reinhardt, PhD, "The Swiss Health System: Regulated Competition Without Managed Care," *The Journal of the American Medical Association* 292(10) (2004): 1227–31. Reinhardt argues that the Swiss system is "superior, more cost-effective, and more equitable" (1227), but economists cannot agree on exactly why. Some think it is because the Swiss system is more price-transparent, with more consumer control; Reinhardt suggests that it is due to "pervasive government regulation" of insurers, drug prices, and markets. What was interesting to me about the system was the absence of lawyers—in terms of malpractice, of regulation, and of oversight—and that the power of medical decision making seemed to be still in the hands of physicians and patients. Most important, though, was the medieval regime of the Swiss. They ate and drank moderately, walked a lot, and had real vacations: They had not forgotten Dr. Diet, Dr. Quiet, and Dr. Merryman.

Page 167. Loiasis: I remembered what Dr. Em told me with the help of *The Oxford Textbook of Medicine* (5.426–5.427).

Page 169. The Hospital of Saint Bruno: I have called the hospital the "Hospital of Saint Bruno," but that is as much a pseudonym as "Dr. Hoefer," though for a different reason. I don't remember the name of the hospital where the rehabilitation unit took me. There *is* a hospital in the French pre-Alps called the Hospital of Saint Bruno, with the same history, look, and function, but I've been unable to verify that it was indeed the hospital with the doctors' dining room and that wonderful cognac.

CHAPTER SEVEN: DANCING TO THE TUNE OF GLENN MILLER

Page 179. My new ward, E6, was one of the dementia wards: When I organized my index cards, I found that the thirty-four patients of E6 fell neatly into three categories. There were the very old, whose average age was eighty-nine (ages eighty-two to ninety-six); a middle group, whose average age was sixty-six (ages sixty-three to seventy-one); and a youngish group, whose average age was fifty (ages forty-four to sixty). Their age corresponded to why they were on E6: the elderly with an absent, frail, feeble kind of demented state; the middle group with hypertension, diabetes, and consequent strokes; and the young group with head trauma, psychiatric, and drug-abuse issues, and also, usually, some rare disease.

Page 179. Although it was a dementia ward, it was not an Alzheimer's ward: One problem with trying to understand the history of dementia is that what we call dementia wasn't always called dementia; and what was called dementia wasn't necessarily our dementia. For instance, Galen, writing in Greek, called the forgetfulness of old age *morosis*, and early Latin writers such as Isidore of Seville called it *amentia*. For a history, see Axel Karenberg and Hans Förstel, "Dementia in the Greco-Roman World," *Journal of Neurological Science* 244 (1–2) (2006), 1-2: 5–9; Frances Boller, "History of Dementia and Dementia in History," *Journal of Neurological Science* 158(2) (1998): 125–33; and N. C. Berchtold and C .W. Cothman, "Evolution of the Conceptualization of Dementia and Alzheimer's: Greco-Roman Period to the 1960s," *Neurobiology of Aging* 19(3) (1998): 173–89. Hildegard used both *amentia* and *dementia*, and her prescriptions suggest that she accepted Galen's ideas that they resulted from a cooling and drying of the brain. For instance: "The herb, balsam, is more hot than cold. And if someone becomes demented, let him drink often a potion made from balsam and fennel. As for his regime, he should not use oil but butter [*pace* the Cholesterolationists!] and should not drink wine or even water, but simply beer [*pace* the Prohibitionists! And the Puritans!]. He should avoid foods that are drying. He should eat aged and delicate foods instead, which will bring good juices to his blood." (From "De Balsamita [9] Lit, 45" CAP. CXCV, column 1202-D–1203-A; "Liber Simplicis Medicinae [Physica]" in *S. Hildegardis Abbatissae Opera Omnia*, ed. Jacques-Paul Migne, vol. 197). [my translation]. These recommendations must have been in order to warm and humidify a cool, dry brain.

Page 180. Dr. Pinel became fascinated by a group of patients: The quote is from Henry Maudsley in his *Responsibility in Mental Disease* (New York: D. Appleton and Co., 1876), 73. For Esquirol's list of causes of dementia, see Jean-Étienne Dominique Esquirol, *Mental Maladies: A Treatise on Insanity,* E. K. Hunt, trans. (Philadelphia: Lea and Blanchard, 1845), 423–24.

Page 180. In it, he defined dementia: "Dementia is a cerebral affection, usually chronic and unattended by fever, and characterized by a weakening of the sensibility, understanding and will. . . . Incoherence of ideas, and a want of intellectual and moral spontaneity are the signs of this affection" (Esquirol, *Mental Maladies,* 417).

Page 181. Dr. Alois Alzheimer published his case: For an account of Dr. Alzheimer's discovery, see David H. Small and Roberto Cappai, "Alois Alzheimer and Alzheimer's Disease: A Centennial Perspective," *Journal of Neurochemistry* 99 (2006): 708–10. In the photo of Auguste D., however, she looks more like a patient with a pituitary tumor than one with simple dementia. One wonders.

Page 181. So in the 1980s a crucial redefinition was made: The story of how Alzheimer's was redefined from a rare presenile dementia to the common dementia of old age is well told by Peter J. Whitehouse and Daniel George, *The Myth of Alzheimer's: What You Aren't Being Told About Today's Most Dreaded Diagnosis* (New York: St. Martin's Press, 2008). For a contrary view that accepts the notion that the plaques are, in fact, the disease, see Small and Cappai, "Alois Alzheimer." At autopsy, up to 45 percent of the brains of demented patients show Alzheimer's plaques and tangles, but, confusingly, so do up to 30 percent of brains without clinical dementia. Whitehouse and George suggest that the plaques and tangles may not be the cause of dementia but the brain's reparative response to some other process, and that medications to dissolve or prevent the tangles and plaques may be harmful.

Page 191. Dr. Pinel had also observed that work was therapeutic for the demented: Pinel wrote eloquently that "Nothing is more worthy of remark than the calm and tranquility which formerly reigned among the patients of the Bicêtre when the merchants of Paris furnished a great number with manual labor, which fixed their attention, and proved agreeable by a slight attendant recompense. I have been always prevented by circumstances from procuring land, and have been limited to subsidiary means, choosing the attendants from among the convalescent patients. In the hospitals of Holland much expense is saved by giving the duties of attendants to convalescents. The object of labor would be fulfilled in its whole extent by adjoining to a hospital a vast enclosure, or, rather, to convert it into a sort of farm, of which the laborers should be under the care of convalescents, and the products from the culture of which should go to their use" (Pinel, *Treatment of the Insane*, trans. Galt, 41). It was mainly the "peonage" suits of the 1970s, based on the Thirteenth Amendment outlawing slavery, that put a stop to the practice of letting patients work (Isaac and Armat, *Madness in the Streets*, 139).

Page 193. Saint Isidore wrote that dementia: *"Animus* is the same thing as *anima,* but it is *anima* of life, and *animus* of judgment. Whence philosophers say life remains without *animus* and *anima* endures without mind." Translated by Priscilla Throop in *Isidore of Seville's Etymologies* (Charlotte, VT: Medieval MS, 2005), vol. 2, book 11, verse 11. The Latin is: *Item animum idem esse quod animam; sed anima vitae est, animus consilii. Unde dicunt philosophi etiam sine animo vitam manere et sine mente animam durate; unde et amentes (Isidori Hispalensis Episcopi, Etymologiarum sive Originum,* libri xx, edited by W. M. Lindsay, London, Oxford University Press, 1911). I interpret *animus* as signifying spirit, and *anima* as soul.

Page 195. Matthew in the New Testament: "Then shall the King say unto them on his right hand, Come, ye blessed of my Father, inherit the kingdom prepared for you from the foundation of the world: For I was an hungred, and ye gave me meat: I was thirsty, and ye gave me drink: I was a stranger, and ye took me in. . . . Inasmuch as ye have done it unto one of the least of these my brethren, ye have done it unto me" (Matthew 25:34–40). These lines were the explicit foundation of monastic hospitality. "Christ's association with the outsider was central to the monastic understanding of hospitality." From Julie Kerr, *Monastic Hospitality: The Benedictines in England, c. 1070–c. 1250* (Rochester, NY: Boydell & Brewer, 2007), 26.

Page 198. He presented his recommendation to the board of supervisors: The only possibility that Dr. Stein didn't examine closely was the one I'd seen at the Hospital of Saint Bruno—that is, renovating Laguna Honda. He did observe that a renovation would be costly and result in one-third fewer beds, and, in view of the coming wave of disabled Boomers, thought it would be a foolish choice. Ironically, one-third fewer beds would be the exact number of beds we would be left with in the new hospital. And renovation of the old place would be done anyway, though not for patients but for the city's administrators. For the full text, see Mitchell H. Katz, "Options for Laguna Honda Hospital. White Paper." San Francisco Department of Public Health (1998); twenty-eight pages at www.victoriasweet .com/documents.

Page 198. The bond for a new Laguna Honda did go on the ballot: The arguments for and against Proposition A take up twenty-two pages, and though I have been fair to the gist of them, I have left out the passion and occasional vituperance in their arguments. For instance, the disability-rights advocate called the hospital a "warehouse" and the bond a "boondoggle for special interests," while Sister Miriam wrote that no other place she'd ever been was as inspiring as Laguna Honda. The supervisors voted 9 to 2 in favor of putting the bond on the ballot—one of the two no votes being the new mayor, who, nonetheless, made sure to arrive for the groundbreaking and, eventually, for the ribbon-cutting ceremony.

Page 201. It is best understood with a diagram: For more on this see the conclusion in *Rooted in the Earth, Rooted in the Sky*. See also *Byrhtferth's Enchiridion*, Peter S. Baker and Michael Lapidge, eds. (Oxford, UK: Oxford University Press, 1995), 14–15. Hildegard, too, had a picture of how it all worked; it was the illumination I'd marveled at when I began my research. For an essay on the implications of the premodern geocentric cosmos, see Giorgio de Santillana and Hertha von Dechen, *Hamlet's Mill: An Essay Investigating the Origins of Human Knowledge and Its Transmission Through Myth* (Boston: David R. Godine, 1992).

Page 205. With bated breath: The evaluation of archaeological resources makes these concerns apparent; see David Chavez and Jan M. Human, "Archaeological Resources Evaluations for the Laguna Honda Hospital's Institutional Master Plan." San Francisco, California, 1994.

CHAPTER EIGHT: WEDDING AT CANA

Page 219. *Community* comes from the Latin *communio*: This etymology comes from *The Oxford Latin Dictionary*. Laguna Honda was, in actual fact, surrounded by a wall of neatly piled, round rocks. The story I heard was that it had been built by patients out of the cobblestones no longer used for city streets. That wall did define the community—inside it was Laguna Honda; outside it, wasn't.

Page 222. Its second letter arrived: This is the letter titled "Re Investigation of Laguna Honda Hospital and Rehabilitation Center," and signed by Ralph F. Boyd, Jr., dated April 1, 2003, and from the Department of Justice. It is thirty pages long, and I summarize here only its most important demands. It did make some good points. We did have patients who could have been discharged if we'd had places to send them. But there were few apartments renting for what our patients could afford to pay; there was not a single locked facility in the city to discharge our demented patients who wandered; and no board-and-care facilities in the city accepted patients in wheelchairs. Besides, there was an unspoken agenda, or so it seemed by the choice of works the letter favored: Laguna Honda "violated" the ADA; it "failed," "refused," "delayed," "isolated" its patients. It "discriminated" against them; it was not "proactive" in discharging patients; it merely "perceived" that there was no place to send its patients. For the letter, see Laguna-Honda-findings2.pdf at victoriasweet.com/documents.

Page 223. Administration installed the minimum data set: The MDS coordinator did have to be smart and full-time, though; the form was twenty pages long, and the manual for filling it out was 538 pages.

Page 224. The team did find eight patients to discharge: Statistics about discharges were never easy to come by, but Laguna Honda's Quality Management did give me an accounting of two of the hospital's patient assessments. The first (1999) assessment in response to the first DOJ letter asserting that 80 percent of Laguna Honda patients could be discharged, found eleven patients to have discharge potential within thirty days (most likely patients on the Rehabilitation Ward); and thirty-five additional patients within ninety days (most likely patients on the longer-term rehabilitation wards). The other 1,036 patients—that is, 90 percent—had no discharge potential. In the second assessment (2003) demanded by the second DOJ letter, 990 patients out of the then 1,040 patients—again 90 percent—had no discharge potential [personal communication].

Page 224. Lawyers who, in the 1970s and 1980s, constituted the "Mental Health Bar": For an excellent account of how the state mental institutions were closed by an idealistic group of lawyers coming out of the radical 1960s, see Isaac and Armat's *Madness in the Streets.* They trace the antipsychiatry movement from R. D. Laing and Thomas Szasz in the 1960s to the creation of the federally funded Protection and Advocacy, Inc., in the 1970s to the alliance of the Left and Right in the 1980s and the consequent deinstitutionalization and abandonment of the mentally ill to the streets. By 1989, they write, much of the homeless problem could be accounted for by the displaced mentally ill: 42 percent of homeless men and 48 percent of homeless women had major mental illness (*Madness in the Streets*, 5). "Unsurprisingly, the civil libertarian lawyers who have spoken up on behalf of the 'homeless' are far from eager to advertise their own immense role in today's tragedy. More than any other single group, they have been responsible for changing our laws governing civil commitment, making it impossible to hospitalize and to treat many of the most severely ill patients" (*Madness in the Streets*, 13).

Page 224. *Davis* had many demands: For the *Davis* settlement, see www.pai-ca.org. For *Olmstead*, see *Olmstead, Commissioner, Georgia Department of Human Resources Et Al. V. L.C., by Zimring, Guardian Ad Litem and Next Friend, Et Al.-*527 U.S. 581 (1999) at www.supreme.justia.com. For a sense of how the lawyers of PAI viewed the settlement, see: http://www.dredf.org/press/laguna_settles.html.

Page 225. But it did fund TCM: TCM's initial budget was 1.5 million dollars. During its first year, TCM screened all of Laguna Honda's patients and found seventeen patients it thought dischargeable. Of these, five died during the assessment period, implying that a discharge would have been out of the question. Nine were so sick that they had to be admitted to the County; only two were discharged (Minutes of the Joint Conference Committee for Laguna Honda Hospital and Rehabilitation Center, January 2005). After three years of operation, TCM had discharged 139 patients, so about four per month. It was not clear, however, how many of those patients would have been discharged anyway (from the TCM Monthly Report, May 2007), Aggregate Data Report. Similarly for TCM Monthly Report, December 2008. There is a section labeled TCM Program Outcomes, but by that is meant only how many total patients ("consumers") were discharged from Laguna Honda. The report found at www.sfdph/tcm/rtz/december 2008 shows an average of 5.2 discharges per month over the preceding forty-eight months. Nevertheless, lawyers for Protection and Advocacy, Inc., continued to assert, "The TCM assessment shows that 80% of residents could be cared for in the community" (www.bazelon.org). Of interest, 49 percent of families and friends of those screened did not support a discharge. What happened to its patients after the TCM discharges was not public information as far as I could tell. When I asked, the TCM staff did not know or would not say. In any case, "nobody has ever actually proved that community-based care was either more humane, more therapeutic, or less expensive than state hospital care" (*Madness in the Streets*, 287).

Page 226. The city's Mental Health Rehabilitation Facility: The MHRF was funded in 1987 by Proposition C, a twenty-six-million-dollar bond to build a skilled nursing facility for the psychiatrically disabled of San Francisco. It took ten years to build, but by 1996 was up and running with 156 beds. According to a psychiatrist who worked there, its program was quite successful; most of its patients did not return to the streets. Discharging patients was always the MHRF's biggest problem, and eventually it was just about filled with treated psychiatric patients who were homeless and had nowhere to go. Which was why Dr. Stein decided to turn it into a psychiatric board-and-care facility and why he was trying to discharge its patients—legally or not—to Laguna Honda. See SF4 LagunaHonda.org/media.html.

Page 229. It was crowded and televised: For a transcript, see San Francisco Board of Supervisors, City Services Committee, *Transcript of Laguna Honda Admissions Policy Hearing Audiotape*, June 24, 2004. Dr. Stein seemed a little disingenuous when he portrayed Mr. Charles to the supervisors as "a psychiatric patient Laguna Honda didn't feel comfortable with" (7). Dr. Stein's quote was: "The money [to place Mr. Charles] would come from Laguna Honda's budget" (24).

Page 234. Happy from *hap*, as in what happens: *Hap* is "chance" or "fortune" and *happy* is "a feeling of great pleasure or contentment of mind, arising from satisfaction with one's circumstances or condition" (*The Oxford English Dictionary*). As an example, it quotes Palladius: "It is simply the *hap* of a seed to turn into a tree." ("Hit is bot happe of plante a tree to gete.")

Page 234. I would be pilgriming: A *peregrinatio* is a traveling away from home; a *peregrinus* is a foreigner, an alien (*The Oxford Latin Dictionary*). A pilgrim is a person who travels to a holy place, a traveler, wanderer, beggar (*Middle English Dictionary*).

Page 237. A patient set the fire: Dr. Romero was "pressured to admit the arsonist who went AWOL from SFGH" (*Transcript of Audiotape*, 16). The next year a nurse explained to the state surveyors that there was no individuality to the patients' spaces because the fire marshals wouldn't allow it (Department of Health and Human Services, Centers for Medicare and Medicaid Services, *Statement of Deficiencies and Plan of Correction for Laguna Honda Hospital and Rehabilitation Center*, completed February 21, 2006, p. 119). The quote is attributed to a nurse in a discussion from 2005, but this is probably a misprint.

CHAPTER NINE: HOW I FELL IN LOVE

Page 255. Charity came into the West: On the history of charity and how it turned into welfare, see James William Brodman, *Charity and Religion in Medieval Europe* (Washington, DC: Catholic University of America Press, 2009); see also Gertrude Himmelfarb, *The Idea of Poverty: England in the Early Industrial Age* (New York:

Knopf, 1984); and *With Us Always: A History of Private Charity and Public Welfare*, Donald T. Critchlow and Charles H. Parker, eds. (Lanham, MD: Rowman & Littlefield, 1998). *The Oxford English Dictionary* defines *charity* as Christ's love; God's love for man; man's love of God and his neighbor.

Page 256. The Greeks called that emotion *eleos*: *Eleos* is "the feeling of pain caused by the sight of some evil, destructive or painful, which befalls one who doesn't deserve it and which might be expected to befall ourselves . . . and soon" (Aristotle, *Rhetoric*, 2:8, 1386a from the online version at http://rhetoric.eserver.org/aristotle/rhet2-8.html. Translated by W. Rhys Roberts).

Page 262. The conflict between Dr. Stein and us was escalating: For a passionate account, see the "Letter to the Laguna Honda CEO" by Dr. Romero and Dr. Kay at victoriasweet.com. For a summary of the Flow Project and the MHRF, see George Wooding, "LHH Policy Questions—Parts 1 and 2," January and February 2010, http://www.miralomapark.org/miralomalife/miraloma-life-online-january-2010/andhttp://www.miralomapark.org/miralomalife/miraloma-life-online-february-2010.

Page 263. This was the best place to send those patients at the MHRF: For what happened at the MHRF, see Janice Cohen, MD, "Doctors support Proposition D" at www.beyondchron.org/news/index.php?itemid-3229. The Omnibus Budget Reconciliation Act of 1987 (OBRA) contained the Nursing Home Reform Act, which stipulated that a psychiatric patient could be in a skilled nursing facility only if he had a physical as well as a mental condition.

Page 265. Using the BioPsychoSocialSpirtual model: For copies of Mirene's proposal, the response, and Mirene's response, see the documents at www.stoplhhdownsize.com, and also at the SocialRehabGrant_Application.pdf at victoriasweet.com.

Page 265. Its report was brilliant: See Health Management Associates, "The San Francisco Department of Public Health: Its Effectiveness as an Integrated Health Care Delivery System and Provider of a Continuum of Long Term Care Services." For a copy, see www.victoriasweet.com. I have summarized only its most significant points in the fifty-seven-page report.

Page 266. Citizens for Laguna Honda: For information and documents on Proposition D, see www.sf4LagunaHonda.org. The best source in general, though, for documents and the politics of Laguna Honda is the website run by Patrick Monette-Shaw: www.stoplhhdownsize.com.

Page 267. Laguna Honda failed its recertification as a hospital: See LHH06report .pdf at victoriasweet.com. I have obviously summarized the most important issues in the 274-page report. It isn't quite as long as it seems, however, because three of its horror stories are repeated three times in three different places for three different kinds of infractions. Quite a few of the citations are so picayune that it's hard to believe that there was not a hidden agenda behind the report. For instance, an F250 citation was given for "weight loss" in an obese patient who was dieting. An

F248 citation was given because it took two weeks to fix a patient's television. There was an F252 citation for a wheelchair with cracked upholstery; an F371 citation because a paper-towel receptacle required touching of the receptacle; another because of a soiled oven mitt; and a third for scratched cutting boards. My two favorites are the F253 citation because the solarium was filled with wheelchairs and the F457 citation for our open wards. Regarding the citations for violent patients, all occurred because of patients admitted during the months of the Flow Project, when Dr. Romero's decision about not admitting certain patients was overruled.

Page 277. "Mr. Zed wrote a poem for Paul": Mr. Zed was part of the poetry group at Laguna Honda. There were some very good poets in it, and once a year a booklet is published of their best poetry. With Mr. Zed, the difficulty of having to follow privacy laws for patients comes into focus. The real Mr. Zed naturally wants his work to have his real name attached to it, and so do I. But as his physician, I am not supposed to reveal identifiable patient information. A compromise is that I will put anyone wishing to contact Mr. Zed in touch with him, with his permission. Since I also particularly love his "Letter Needing No Stamp," I quote it here:

To His Supreme Holiness, the Lord:
I sometimes wonder how you can bear
The dreadful burden of knowing everyone's thoughts.
The anguish, the heartbreak, the agony.
How can you even relax?
Maybe you try not to get too involved.
Or maybe you spend all night, weeping.

Why did you create such a sad world?
Why don't sandwiches grow on trees?
Why do infants die?
Why do honest people get cheated?
Why do the poor get crushed to the wall?
Personally I would turn down your job in a second.
You can't buy a pie or go to the movies.

And there are always people denouncing you and cursing you.
Some say you had a crazy son who said
I am the Way and the Life.

We must all pray that you never resign or become bitter.
As sad as things seem to be here
Without you they'd be infinitely worse.
Thank God for God
Stay in there buddy
Have a martini once in a while
Create a new universe.

CHAPTER TEN: IT'S A WONDERFUL COUNTRY

Page 287. And there was a rare form that did affect adults: I thought Steve must have the rare Becker muscular dystrophy, and not the more common Duchenne muscular dystrophy.

Page 292. The Committee to Save Laguna Honda: See "Proposition D for San Francisco, 2006: Zoning Changes to Limit Services at Laguna Honda Hospital and Other Residential Health Care Facilities" at www.sf4LagunaHonda.org. There were two organizations: San Franciscans for Laguna Honda, which sponsored Proposition D, and the Committee to Save Laguna Honda. Sister Miriam and Miss Lester, despite her retirement, were members of both; Drs. Kay and Romero, although they supported Proposition D, were members of neither.

Page 293. *Chambers* **class-action lawsuit against the city:** See *Mark Chambers et al. v. City and County of San Francisco, Co6-06346 WHA First Amended Complaint for Declaratory and Injunctive Relief,* filed October 12, 2006. It had many subsidiary demands, in addition to those I focus on here, including that the lawyers bringing the suit would monitor compliance and receive up to $200,000 per quarter to do so (27). For a summary of the politics around *Chambers,* see George Wooding, "Hi Sean," 2009, and George Wooding, "Laguna Honda Hospital Policy Questions—Parts 1 and 2," www.miralomapark.org, January and February 2010. For the lawyers' view, see www.bazelon.org. Bazelon is proud of being the same group that closed the state mental hospitals and is now intent on closing the states' long-term-care institutions. Some thought that Dr. Stein and the mayor may have helped organize *Chambers* so that they could save money by downsizing the hospital and using its beds for the homeless. The chronology is suggestive, according to Wooding. A meeting was held at the Office for Disability first with its director, Susan Mizner, the *Chambers* lawyers, and the Independent Living Resource Center, which would become the organizational plaintiff on *Chambers.* Right after the meeting, Mizner wrote Appendix A of the Controller's Report, where she calculated that it would be cheaper to discharge patients than keep them at Laguna Honda. Although she noted that 40 percent of the hospital's patients had mental-health and substance-abuse needs, she did not include those costs in her analysis and estimated their medical costs as 0. See Susan Mizner, "Estimates for Housing, Medical and Supportive Care Costs for People Discharged from Laguna Honda Hospital," in Appendix A of Ed Harrington, Controller, "Laguna Honda Replacement Program: Where Do We Go from Here?" San Francisco, May 19, 2005, pp. 7–10, at www.disabilityrightsca.org/advocacy/lhh/HarringtonReplacement.pdf.

Page 294. Although the mayor and Dr. Stein seemed sanguine about its demands: On the *Chambers* settlement: "It's a win for the client and a savings for the city; so it's a win-win," Dr. Stein explained to the newspapers. Quoted by Elizabeth Fernandez, "S.F. to Subsidize 500 Housing Units for People Leaving Laguna Honda," *San Francisco Chronicle,* November 28, 2007. The seventh plaintiff on *Chambers* was the Independent Living Resource Center, whose head also sat on the mayor's Long-Term Care Coordinating Council.

Page 299. Mrs. Han fell to her death: Mr. Conley's comments are quotes from the interview with Dan Noyes: "Feds Investigate Laguna Honda Hospital" (http://abclocal.go.com/kgo/story?section=news/iteam&id=5133815), [March 19 2007]. The doctor's comments are from follow-up reporting also by Dan Noyes. "Did Budget Cuts Lead to Patient's Death? Doctor Offers Insight" (http://abclocal.go.com/kgo/story?section=news/iteam&id=5135013), KGO, 2007 [cited March 20, 2007]. It also describes Noyes's attempt to interview the mayor.

Page 300. *The Wall Street Journal* contacted Mr. Conley: For the resulting article, see Lucette Lagnado, "Battle on Home Front," *The Wall Street Journal*, May 7, 2007. Since Ms. Lagnado interviewed two of my patients, I tried to contact her in case she might want to understand their medical issues. She did not return my calls, and she did not get their stories right.

Page 301. One hundred thousand dollars turned up in his budget: Mr. Conley revealed the new money for a public relations firm and a media position to the Health Commission on April 16, 2007. The firm, Wide Angle Communications, would "support the hospital's journey from institution to community," Mr. Conley said. His announcement of the new Director of Community Relations, Adrian Serf, was on October 29, 2007. Adrian had been the spokesman for the mayor's transition team and his job would be to "handle negative publicity and improve the hospital's community and media relations." For the minutes of these Health Commission meetings, see www.sfdph.org/dph/files/hc/jcc/lhh/minutes.

CHAPTER ELEVEN: RECALLED TO LIFE

Page 322. She was of the rare breed of Bad Girl: Bad Girls were just like Bad Boys, only fewer and badder. They used drugs; had been in prison; had acquired numerous drug-and prison-related diseases; been in car accidents; muggings, both given and received; been stabbed and attacked; had undergone many surgeries; and had bad luck. Unlike most of the Bad Boys, the Bad Girls were often prostitutes with all those medical complications, too. However, that was not what made them "bad" in my eyes. What made them "bad" was that they had spunk. They were tough; they continued to live life the way they wanted regardless of the consequences. So, they were Bad in the sense of good, just like "cool" means "hot."

Page 322: Now, a stroke on the right side of the brain: This is so for all right-handers and many left-handers, though not true for 15 percent of the left-handed, who are wired in the opposite fashion, so that a left-sided stroke is devastating in the way I recount here. At least that is the dogma. In my experience, though, left-handers do not have quite the same experience, but a more fluid, less rigid dichotomization of their skills and disabilities.

Page 325. Dr. Dan had not added any new medications to her regime: To be specific: Dr. Dan first increased her Haldol and oxycodone, then added Lexapro, then increased her Haldol, started Depakote, then Ativan, increased the Depakote, and increased the Haldol. For a similar story about the development of serotonin syndrome, see Ladan Zand, Scott J. Hoffman, and Mark A. Nyman,

"74-Year-Old Woman with New-Onset Myoclonus," *Mayo Clinic Proceedings* 85(10) (2010): 955–58.

Page 329. Dr. Stein had already given Mr. Conley an additional ten million dollars: I was given a hard copy of the plans for the "LHH Transition Budget: Consolidated Five Week Move—April 2010," by someone who wishes to remain anonymous. The paper is not signed, but it is dated August 2008, and it documents the additional money.

Page 330. The medical staff's budget of 2.5 million dollars and the hospital's budget of 170 million dollars: The various budgets were not easy to discover, and the actual costs of, say, the medical staff, or the hospital, were even harder to find. The best source I found is: www.sfdph.org/dph/files/lagunahondadocs. The minutes of the Health Commission are sometimes useful; they are at www .sfdph.org/dph/files/hc/hcmins. The minutes of the Laguna Honda Hospital Joint Conference Committee are also informative: see www.sfdph.org/dph/files/hc/ jcc/lhh/minutes. By July 2008 the hospital was down to 903 patients and 16 full-time equivalent physicians. By May 14, 2008, Clarendon Hall was empty of patients.

Page 330. The Department of Justice had accepted the *Chambers* settlement.... It still had two additional demands, however: Actually the settlement was confusing. There were, it seems, two separate documents. The first was a Side Letter from the US Department of Justice, dated May 23, 2008, that I saw only in hard copy. Somewhat later there was the "Settlement Agreement between the United States Department of Justice and the City and County of San Francisco regarding the Laguna Honda Hospital and Rehabilitation Center," which was easy to find at the DOJ website. It demanded that there be fundamental changes to the hospital, in terms of its structure, function, and mission. For instance, the new Laguna Honda would "emphasize a continuum of care model" (1) by expanding its rehabilitation service, and it would "introduce as much flexibility as possible into existing and ongoing construction efforts at Laguna Honda so as to maximize the adaptability of use from SNF services *to other integrated services going forward*" (4). This sentence was interpreted by many to mean the eventual transformation of Laguna Honda from hospital to rehabilitation facility. Other demands were that "Every individual will be team evaluated, based upon his need and ability, not on the availability of services nor on the disability of the patient" (4); that efforts at discharge "shall continue even after an individual expresses initial opposition to certain specific placement proposals . . . regardless of the . . . family" (6); "Homeless patients with nursing needs will be kept out of Laguna Honda" (11); and "The city shall implement the Health Management Associates report" (13). For the document, see www.justice.gov/crt/about/spl/documents/ laguna.honda_hosp_setagree_6_13_08.pdf.

Page 345. It would be so easy to just shock that ventricular tachycardia back to life: Easy in a manner of speaking. About 20 percent of people survive pulseless ventricular tachycardia, though many fewer actually survive to discharge from the hospital. For some statistics, see Mickey S. Eisenberg, MD, PhD, and Bruce M. Psaty, MD, PhD, "Cardiopulmonary Resuscitation: Celebration and Challenges," *JAMA* 304(1) (July 7, 2010): 87.

Page 346. Hildegard's lines about dying came into my mind: "For this color in the knees lying on top of the skin is the fiery breath of the life of the *anima,* because the *anima* in man is showing that his vitality is outside his body and weakness is inside and stands as if uncertain; like a person who stands at a doorway uncertain whether to stay or leave." *"Rubeus enim color iste in genis super cutem iacens igneum spiramen uite anime est, quoniam anima in homine illo uim suam extra corpus suum demonstrat et se in corpore debilem et incertam ostendit, uelut homo, qui interdum ad ianuam domus sue procedit, cum de ea egressurus est."* Laurence Moulinier, *Beate Hildegardis Cause et Cure* (Berlin: Rarissima mediaevalia, 2003), p. 270: lines 7–11. For those readers of Classical Latin: In the Middle Ages, there was no *j* or *v*; *i* and *u* were used instead. Also, the *ae* ending dropped out, and *e* was used instead.

Page 347. I had a different interpretation of DNR: The story of cardiopulmonary resuscitation and its mirror twin, Do Not Resuscitate, is complicated; for some background and clinical correlation, see Victoria Sweet, "Thy Will Be Done," *Health Affairs* 26 (2007): 825–30, and Victoria Sweet, "Code Pearl," *Health Affairs* 27 (2008): 216–20. In response to the poor outcome of resuscitation and the futile use of resuscitive measures in the terminally ill and the very old, a four-page form known as the POLST is now mandated in many states and medical trainees are now required to get advance life directives on everyone they admit. This is tedious, and the pendulum, therefore, has begun to shift the other way, with less being done than is, perhaps, indicated. For a provocative essay on this, see Boris Veysman, "Shock Me, Tube Me, Line Me," *Health Affairs* 29(2) (February 2010): 324–326.

CHAPTER TWELVE: THE SPIRIT OF GOD'S HOTEL

Page 353. Two weeks later, Sister Miriam resigned: For her resignation letter, see www.westsideobserver.com/pdfs/nov08obsview.pdf. For her thoughts on Clarendon Hall, see Sister Miriam Walsh, "Farewell to Laguna Honda's Clarendon Hall," *West of Twin Peaks Observer*, April 2008, at www.stoplhhdownsize.com/Media08-04_Observer1.html. For a short biography, see "Laguna Honda's Torchbearer, Sister Miriam Walsh," by Patrick Monette-Shaw, www.westsideobserver.com/pdfs/feb10e-mail(5).pdf. I have a lot of stories about Sister Miriam. I particularly liked that she kept a little box outside her office with scraps of paper on which were Xeroxed a list of people you might want her to pray for. You could check "mother, father, son, daughter, or the souls in Purgatory who have no one to pray for them."

Page 356. Marketing had presented its branding campaign: Much was disconcerting about these new marketing efforts. For instance, on the Laguna Honda website, many of the photos of "patients" were not actual Laguna Honda patients but photos of other patients walking in other gardens of other hospitals.

Page 361. The next week she sent around a revised organization chart: The organization chart can be found online; although mislabeled 2005, it is dated April 2, 2009; see www.docstoc.com/docs/9216131/lhh-Org-Chart-2005. For a biography of Mr. Conley and a description of his memorial service, as well as the announcement of Dr. Stein's appointment of Mirene, see *The Laguna Honda Grapevine*, issue 22, March 23, 2009.

Page 361. Mirene's main ally in her new job was Adrian Serf: Dr. Romero reported an instance when Mr. Serf went to a bedside to convince a patient not to go back to the County Hospital, in spite of Dr. Romero's orders to do so. From her "Statement of Concern—Patient Rights and Physician Responsibilities," November 17, 2009 (personal communication).

Page 362. The final straw was the Ja Report: For the Ja Report, see "Evaluation and Assessment of Laguna Honda Hospital Behavioral Care and Service Access: A Final Report," www.victoriasweet.com/docs. It simply put into its recommendations the unpublished document "Building a National Center of Excellence in Long-Term Care and Rehabilitation," LH Organizational Development Initiative Document (February 25, 2009) (personal copy). For Dr. Kay and Dr. Romero's report, see "The Ja Report, A Job Half Done: A Critical Analysis" at www .stoplhhdownsize.com/A_Critical_Analysis_of_the_Ja_and_Associates_ Report_on_LHH_Services.pdf. Another critique was written by the city's long-term care ombudsman, Benson Nadell, "Thoughts on Davis Ja Report: The Move Away from a Medical Model of Care," October 6, 2009, www.stoplhhdown size.com/Thoughts_on_Davis_Ja_Report.pdf.

Page 362. The old-fashioned "medical model" of physicians would be replaced by a "social model": Of everything in the Ja Report, perhaps the most eye-opening was the idea that the "medical model" should be replaced by the "social care" model. It took me a while to understand this. Apparently the "medical model of care" did not mean the modern disease/cause/treatment/scientific method of modern medicine. Rather, in the long-term-care world the "medical model" meant a specific architectural model of the hospital where patients were categorized by their disease, management was top-down, and physicians had a privileged place. The new idea was that for patients who needed nursing homes, there should be something less like a hospital and more like a home. For more on this, see www.pioneernetwork.net. But the Ja Report used "medical model" in a still different way to mean "favoring physical health over mental health and substance abuse" (21). And it connected the "imposition of the medical model" to the "professional dominance of MDs" (20). When all was said and done, though, the social model of care was in fact a code for taking care of the mentally ill substance abusers, those patients at the MHRF whom Dr. Stein had been trying to get into the hospital for almost ten years.

Page 363. Last, they demanded an audit of the two-million-dollar Patient Gift Fund: Laguna Honda's Patient Gift Fund was a pretty great thing. I first learned about it from Dr. Major. Nearly two million dollars had been given to the hospital over the years by grateful patients, families, and philanthropists, specifically for the unmet needs of patients—for the little daily things. It was this Patient Gift Fund that paid for Terry Becker's flight back to her family in Arkansas; for storing Paul's things; and for Radka's telephone calls to her son in Bulgaria. Dr. Major and Miss Lester had husbanded it carefully, spending only the interest on the account, and Dr. Romero knew it well from her days as medical director. When she was told that the two-million-dollar fund had been depleted, she and Dr. Kay set to work. They went through more than 1,300 documents and discovered that much of the money had been spent not on patients but on staff parties, nurse training, and administrative trips—my favorite expense being the $5,015 spent for museum-quality frames for pictures placed in the administrative suites; $745,000 could not be accounted for at all. See "Cost Shifting at Laguna Honda Hospital," at www.stoplhhdownsize.com/Part%201%20-%20LHH%20 Gift%20Fund%20Cost%20Shifting.pdf. For Dr. Kay's retaliation suit, see "Case No: 380-10-505443: Complaint for Damage and Demand for Jury Trial, Superior Court. www.stoplhhdownsize.com/Dekerr_Endorsed_Complaint.pdf. KGO-TV covered the story on May 20, 2010.

Page 364. Then Dr. Talley called her first meeting of the medical staff: Here I've used three meetings and three different memos from January 4, 2010, March 5, 2010, and May 3, 2010, to summarize what had happened.

Page 364. But then I remembered what Florence Nightingale had written about the struggle between medicine and nursing and administration: "A patient is much better cared for in an institution where there is the perpetual rub between doctors and nurses or nuns; between students, matrons, governors, treasurers, and casual visitors, between secular and spiritual authorities . . . than in a hospital under the best governed order in existence" (Nightingale, *Notes on Hospitals,* 184).

Page 366. It was time to take the tour: For a virtual tour of the new hospital, see www.lagunahonda.org.

Page 374. He'd joined Alcoholics Anonymous, he told me: The inspiration for Alcoholics Anonymous came, amazingly enough it seemed to me, from Carl Jung. The story is that he told his patient Rowland Hazard, who had come to him for treatment of his alcoholism, that his case was hopeless without a spiritual conversion. "All you can do is place yourself in a religious atmosphere of your own choosing and admit your personal powerlessness to go on living." Jung recommended the Oxford Group in England, which was where Hazard eventually did have his spiritual conversion, and then incorporated its principles into his Twelve Steps. Bill W. wrote to Jung reminding him of this story, and Jung wrote back, "The craving for alcohol is the equivalent on a low level of the spiritual thirst of our being for wholeness. Expressed in medieval language, the union with God. . . . Alcohol in Latin is *spiritus* . . . and the formula is *spiritus contra spiritum"* (Bill W.'s letter to Dr. Jung, January 23, 1961). There was something remarkable to me that the lesson that ended my apprenticeship at God's Hotel was a lesson from the man who had inspired it at the beginning.

Page 374. He was back to attend the memorial service for his sponsor, Mr. Don Taylor: Don Taylor's real name is Tom Lawlor, and since he was never my patient, I suppose it's ethical and legal to give his real name, which I'd like to do because he deserves it. His obituary reads: "R. Thomas Lawlor. Tom will be missed by the Doyle family, extended family, and a vast fellowship of friends in recovery. Tom celebrated twenty years clean, along the way touching countless other lives. Tom loved his job, patients, and community at Laguna Honda Hospital" (*The San Francisco Chronicle*, March 6, 2009).

Page 374. He was no longer not ill, but well: The root of the English *health* is *hàl*, which also gives us *hale* as in hale and hearty, and, crucially, *whole*. *Healthy*, *whole*, and *well* all come from the same root that originally meant "whole, intact." See Buck, *Dictionary*, 301-2; 307.

Victoria Sweet has been a physician at San Francisco's Laguna Honda Hospital for more than twenty years. An associate clinical professor of medicine at the University of California, San Francisco, she is also a prize-winning historian with a PhD in history and social medicine.